Handbook of Infectious Diseases

Handbook of Infectious Diseases

Edited by **Daniel Enger**

FOSTER ACADEMICS

New Jersey

Published by Foster Academics,
61 Van Reypen Street,
Jersey City, NJ 07306, USA
www.fosteracademics.com

Handbook of Infectious Diseases
Edited by Daniel Enger

International Standard Book Number: 978-1-63242-207-1 (Hardback)

Printed in the United States of America.

Contents

Preface

This book provides a comprehensive analysis of the pathogenesis of infectious disease. Infectious diseases and similar problems have been one of the unavoidable outcomes of war throughout the world. Numerous valuable and well-illustrated descriptions are included in this book as it examines the evolution of such diseases to their advancement. The contents of the book are divided into two sections namely, 'Environmental Epidemics in the Course of Therapeutic Outlook' and 'Molecular Epidemiology and Mitigation Strategy'. It would serve as a useful source to the researchers and scientists working in this discipline.

After months of intensive research and writing, this book is the end result of all who devoted their time and efforts in the initiation and progress of this book. It will surely be a source of reference in enhancing the required knowledge of the new developments in the area. During the course of developing this book, certain measures such as accuracy, authenticity and research focused analytical studies were given preference in order to produce a comprehensive book in the area of study.

This book would not have been possible without the efforts of the authors and the publisher. I extend my sincere thanks to them. Secondly, I express my gratitude to my family and well-wishers. And most importantly, I thank my students for constantly expressing their willingness and curiosity in enhancing their knowledge in the field, which encourages me to take up further research projects for the advancement of the area.

Editor

Part 1

Environmental Epidemics in the Course of Therapeutic Outlook

1

Three Cases of *Mycobacterium tuberculosis* Infection Initially Recognized by Focus Changing Examination in Gram Staining

Yoshiko Atsukawa[1], Sayoko Kawakami[1], Yasuo Ono[3], Ryuichi Fujisaki[2], Yukihisa Miyazawa[1] and Hajime Nishiya[2]
[1]*Department of Central Clinical Laboratory, Teikyo University Hospital, Tokyo;*
[2]*Department of Internal Medicine, Teikyo University School of Medicine, Tokyo;*
[3]*Department of Microbiology, Teikyo University School of Medicine, Tokyo, Japan*

1. Introduction

Patients with fever and pulmonary symptoms with consolidation shadows on chest X-ray are assumed to have pneumonia, which in most cases is bacterial-induced, and their sputa are first stained with gram stain. In patients with pneumonia, aside from cases with shadows typical of tuberculosis, the first empiric therapy is usually antimicrobial agents.

On gram staining of sputum, *Mycobacterium tuberculosis* either is weakly gram-positive or appears as colorless rods or "ghosts" (Hinson et al.,1981;Trifito et al.,1990). However, there is no description of Gram staining as useful staining for *M. tuberculosis* in the textbooks.

If tubercle bacilli could be easily detected in clinical samples with gram staining, it would be possible to detect tuberculosis more promptly and easily, which may contribute to tuberculosis control. In this paper, we present three infective tuberculosis cases in which gram staining easily detected tubercle bacilli before Ziehl-Neelsen (Z-N) staining and diagnosed by polymerase chain reaction (PCR) or culture.

Case 1

A 67-year-old man with hypertension, hyperlipidemia and atrial fibrillation visited our hospital because of lumbago, fever of approximately 38°C and an increased serum CRP level. Five years earlier, he had undergone resection of a prostate tumor. Two years prior to the current admission, thymectomy was performed because of myasthenia gravis and he was administered 20 mg/day prednisolone and 150 mg/day cyclophosphamide. One month earlier, he developed swelling on the back of the right hand. Gram staining of pus from the back of the hand showed many neutrophils with no bacteria when focus was adjusted on the nucleus of neutrophil, but contained gram-positive granular rods with slightly longer focus and brightening colorless rods with slightly shorter focus, suggesting the presence of *M. tuberculosis*.

The bacilli were positive (2+) on Z-N staining(Fig.1,2,3,4). The presence of *M. tuberculosis* was confirmed by PCR.

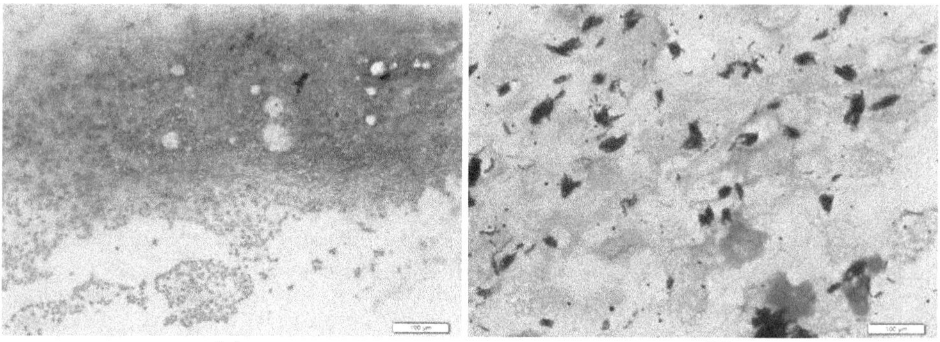

(a) (b)

Fig. 1. Gram staining and Ziehl-Neelsen staining of the pus in case 1. Gram staining of pus under a hundred-fold focus (a) and Ziehl-Neelsen staining of the pus (b). The sample contained 2+ bacilli on Ziehl-Neelsen staining(X 1000). The presence of *M. tuberculosis* was confirmed by PCR.

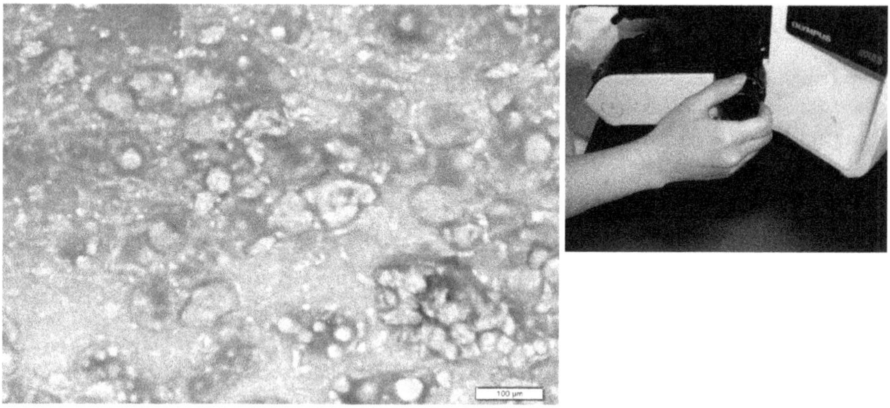

Fig. 2. Gram staining of pus under ordinary focus in case1. Gram staining of pus (X 1000) under ordinary focus in case 1. The purulent samples contained abundant of neutrophils without any causative bacteria. The small right upper figure shows left hand catching dial at ordinary style.

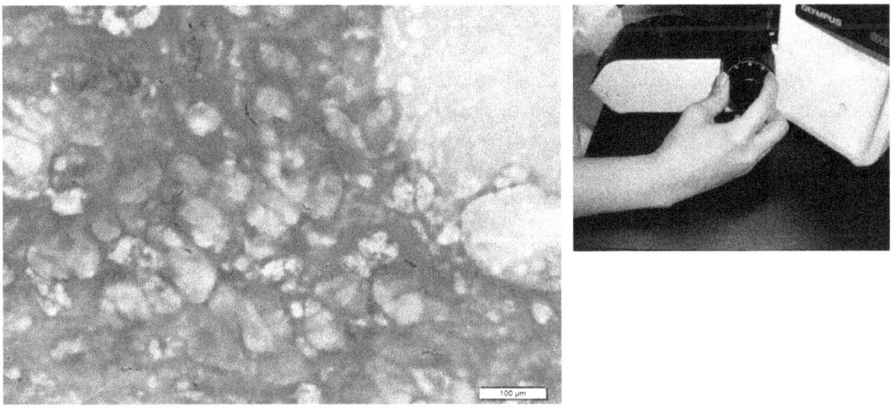

Fig. 3. Gram-positive cord-like bacilli in Gram stain in case 1. Turning the dial to adopt a slightly longer focus distance clearly showed gram-positive cord-like bacilli. The small right upper figure of hand catching dial showed position of the hand making longer focus.

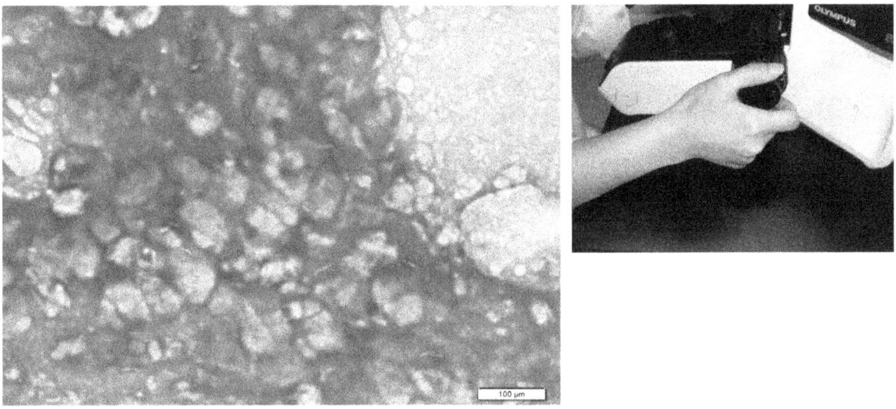

Fig. 4. Brightened rods and colorless bacilli in Gram stain in case 1. A slightly shorter focus distance revealed brightened rods and colorless bacilli in Gram stain. The small right upper figures of hand catching dial showed position of the hand making shorter focus.

Case 2

A 62-year-old man with type II diabetes mellitus presented to our hospital because of fatigue and loss of appetite. Five months earlier, he had undergone surgery for cancer at the base of the oral cavity (T4N0M0). Fifty days prior to the current admission, he noticed general malaise, loss of appetite, and fever. He was seen in our hospital, at which time the serum sodium level was 115 mEq/l. His temperature was 38.1°C. He had hypoxemia and hypoalbuminemia. Antimicrobial therapy was started. On the fourth hospital day, bilateral pleural effusion was detected, and pneumonia and congestive heart failure were suspected. On the fifth hospital day, he gradually lost consciousness. Gram staining of his sputum revealed many gram-positive cocci and gram-negative bacilli, with large numbers of neutrophils and oral epithelial cells. With small changes in focus under the microscope, some bacilli showed a change in staining pattern from gram-positive to unstained neutral. The sample contained 3+ bacilli on Z-N staining, and the presence of *M. tuberculosis* was confirmed by PCR and culture(Fig. 5,6,7). Electrocardiogram and laboratory data suggested the existence of ischemic heart disease, and he died after a decrease in blood pressure. However, the exact cause of death was unclear. Autopsy revealed the existence of miliary tuberculosis with no myocardial infarction.

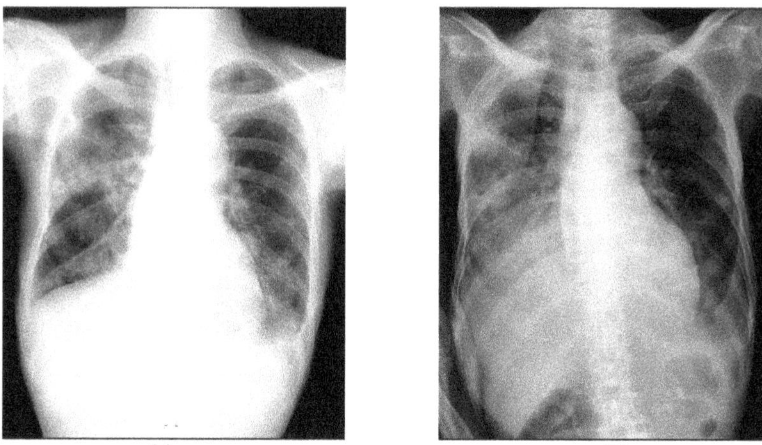

(a) (b)

Fig. 5. Chest X-rays in case 2. On admission consolidation was detected in the right lung (a). Consolidation shadows and pleural effusion were detected in the right lung on the sixth hospital days (spine position) (b).

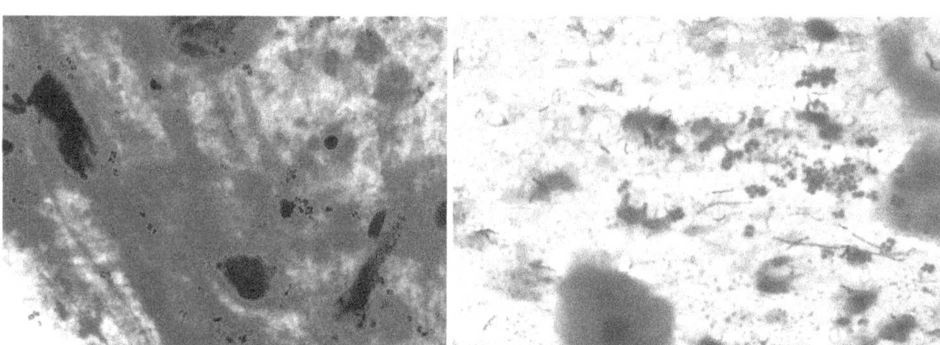

(a) (b)

Fig. 6. Gram stain and Ziehl-Neelsen staining of the sputa in case 2. Gram staining of his sputum revealed many gram-positive cocci and gram-negative bacilli, with large numbers of neutrophils and oral epithelial cells (X 1000) (a). The sample contained 3+ bacilli on Ziehl-Neelsen staining(X 1000) (b), and the presence of *M. tuberculosis* was confirmed by PCR and culture.

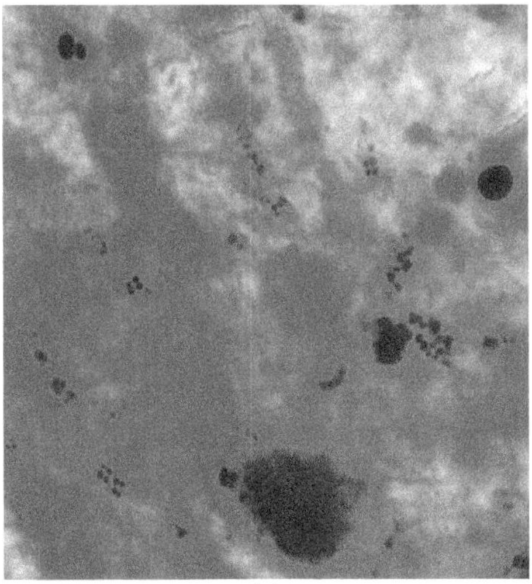

(a)

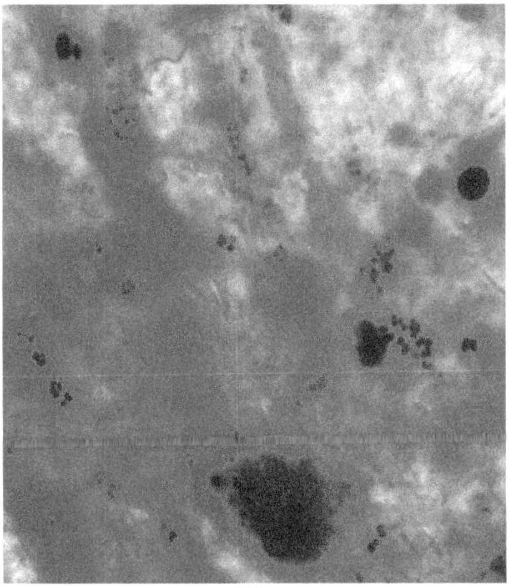

(b)

Fig. 7. Changing focus examination of sputa in case 2. Gram staining of pus in case 2 (X 1000). Turning the dial to adopt a slightly longer focus distance clearly showed gram-positive cord-like bacilli (a) and to adopt a slightly shorter focus distance revealed brightened rods and colorless bacilli (b).

Case 3

A 75-year-old man was transferred to our hospital to receive additional therapy for pneumonia that was treated unsuccessfully at another hospital. He had been treated with home oxygen therapy for chronic obstructive pulmonary disease for the past 19 years. Thirteen days earlier, he was admitted to another hospital because of pneumonia in the left lung. Several antimicrobial agents (meropenem, ciprofloxacin, imipenem/cilastatin, and vancomycin) were successively administered, but were ineffective. After being transferred to our hospital, he was administered biapenem in addition to minocycline and micafungin. Z-N staining of his sputum, done only once on admission, was negative. His inflammatory laboratory data improved slightly, but thirteen days later, the data showed abnormal levels again and hypoxemia emerged. Biapenem was changed to tazobactam/piperacillin. Gram staining of the sputum showed a large number of gram-negative rods with many neutrophils; the bacteria were confirmed to be *Burkholderia cepacia*. However, the sputum contained gram-positive granular rods, which were observed as brightened rods with a change in focus, suggesting the presence of *M. tuberculosis*. The bacilli were recognized to be positive (2+) for Z-N staining(Fig. 8,9). The presence of *M. tuberculosis* in the sputum was later confirmed by PCR.

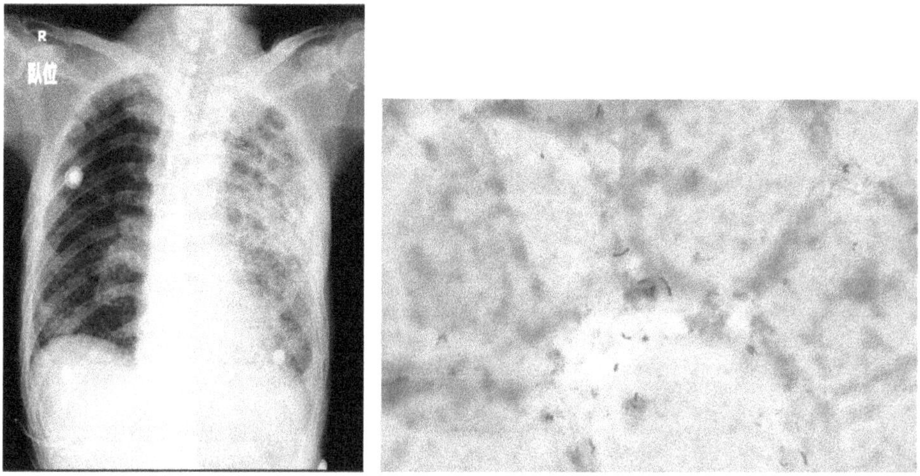

(a) (b)

Fig. 8. Chest X-rays and Ziehl-Neelsen staining of the sputa in case 3. On the seventh hospital days the part of consolidation in the upper of the left lung with emphysematous lung was persisted after successively and ineffectively administration of broad spectrum antimicrobial agents (a). Ziehl-Neelsen staining of the sputum were recognized to be positive (2+). The presence of *M. tuberculosis* was later confirmed by PCR.

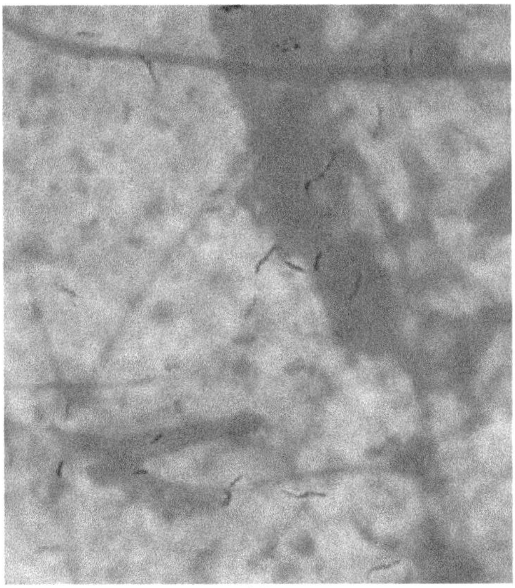

(a)

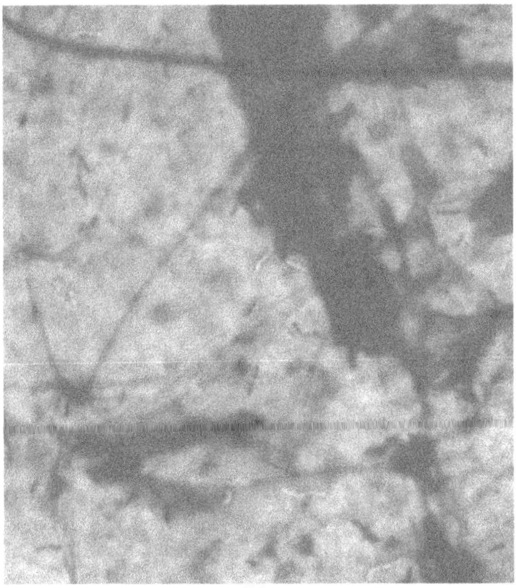

(b)

Fig. 9. Changing focus examination of sputa in case 3. Gram staining of pus in case 3 (X 1000). Turning the dial to adopt a slightly longer focus distance clearly showed gram-positive cord-like bacilli (a) and to adopt a slightly shorter focus distance revealed brightened rods and colorless bacilli (b).

2. Discussion

Gram staining is a useful technique for detecting bacteria in infectious diseases. But when infections with tuberculosis is probable, special staining, such as Ziehl-Neelsen staining is essential in detecting of *Mycobacterium tuberculosis* .

Hinson (Hinson et al., 1981) and Trifiro et al. (Trifiro et al. ,1990) observed tubercle bacilli as ghost mycobacteria in Gram staining of clinical samples.

In some textbooks one and/or two patterns of gram-stained tubercle bacilli have been described. *M. tuberculosis* often shows neutral staining (Raviglione & O'Brien,2008) , often appears as beaded gram-positive bacilli or fails to stain at all (Inderlied, 2004), or shows weak gram-positive staining and appears as colorless rods or "ghosts" (Fitzgerald,2005).

We presented a technique of Gram staining for detecting infective tuberculosis in clinical samples, the focus chaining technique (Atsukawa et al., 2011). It is a very useful procedure as an easy and rapid initial diagnostic tool to recognize highly infective tuberculosis because it can be directly applied to clinical specimens, such as sputum and pus.

Recently, we experienced a case with tuberculosis meningitis, in which Gram staining of cerebrospinal fluid with predominantly neutrocytic pleocytosis was useful as an initial adjunct to the diagnosis of tuberculous meningitis(Kawakami et al., 2012).

There are two types of samples for which the changing focus procedure on Gram staining is useful. One is purulent samples including pus without any causative bacteria. In the samples search for tubercle bacilli should be made. In an usual fixed focus, we might miss the ghost bacilli (Figure 2). The changing focus procedure is done in three steps as follows. 1) Firstly, in the ordinary focus, weakly stained gram-positive long bacilli or no conspicuous bacilli are found in samples(Fig. 2,6a), 2) with a slightly longer focus distance the gram-positive thin cord-like bacilli can be clearly observed(Fig. 3,7a,9a), and 3) with shorter focus distance the gram-positive bacilli have changed into the brightened, colorless or ghost bacilli(6)(Fig. 4,7b,9b).

The other is the samples with various amounts of gram-negative and/or gram-positive organism. Especially in purulent sputum, the existence of abundant of organisms with neutrophils usually leads a diagnosis of bacterial pneumonia. In the case2, the Gram staining showed many gram-positive cocci (Fig. 6a) and in the case3, it showed many gram-negative rods, which were confirmed to be *Burkholderia cepacia* by culture. The diagnosis of these cases by the clinicians were bacterial pneumonia and antimicrobial agents were administered.

In the ordinary procedure of Gram staining of purulent sputa, neutrophils firstly are brought into focus to check the adequacy of the safranin-staining and after once setting a focus, there is no need to change it. In the focus gram-negative and/or -positive organisms usually being also brought into focus and only we have to do is to investigate phagocytosed bacteria to catch causative organisms. However, in the focus, tubercle bacilli are weakly stained as unclear thin cord-like positive rods or sometimes inconspicuous neutral crystal-like fragments among abundant of gram-negative and/or gram-positive organism. In addition, the number of tubercle bacilli is far less than the other gram-negative and/or -positive organisms. These facts may explain why tubercle bacilli are most likely to be missed so far in Gram stained purulent sputum with various organisms and the staining have been recognized as useless one in detecting pulmonary tuberculosis. In pulmonary tuberculosis with atypical features as in case 2 and 3, sometimes the delay of Z-N staining of sputum, which is sometimes done after the first antimicrobial agent's therapy has proven unsuccessful, lead to the delay in diagnosis of pulmonary tuberculosis. The delay of Z-N staining is partly due to the complexity of the staining and the need for trained staff. However, with the repeated changing focus procedure, in a slightly longer focus distance, the weekly stained gram-positive cord-like rod had changed into clear conspicuous gram positive thin bacilli though the other organism were out of focus. And with shorter focus distance brightened and colorless bacilli, "gram-neutral" or "gram-ghost", were revealed.

Our experience has shown that, even when the sample contains various amounts of organisms, repeated changing the focus of the microscope slightly longer and shorter during the examination of the slide is indispensable in searching for tubercle bacilli. The staining characteristics of the tubercle bacilli in Gram stain , biphasic stain patterns as conspicuous thin long gram-positive bacilli changing into gram-neutral, is only noticeable by changing the focus.

The patients in case1and 2 had previous surgery for cancers. The patient in case 1 also had been administered prednisolone and cyclophosphamide and the patient in case 2 had type II diabetes mellitus. The patient in case 3 had been successively and ineffectively administered many antimicrobial agents with the broad spectrum. The patients in the case 1 and 2 dead. If their tuberculosis had been diagnosed earlier, a more rapid start of anti-tubercle therapy might save their lives.

Especially, when patients have predisposing factors to active tuberculosis, such as diabetes mellitus, liver cirrhosis, hemo-dialysis, and administration of immune-suppressive drugs, careful examination on gram staining is needed along with Z-N staining. The present study showed that gram staining is an effective initial test to check for infective tuberculosis. Considering that the clinical diagnosis of tuberculosis begins with a high index of suspicion , we should always check samples of Gram staining with the focus changing procedure.

There are certain types of images to which attention must be paid to avoid misidentification on Gram staining. Crystal-like fragments are sometimes visualized as thin, brightened neutral rods. However, when changing the focus, the brightened neutral rods never change into long gram-positive bacilli as tubercle bacilli.

The tuberculosis epidemic is far from over and is aggravated by multi-drug resistant tubercle bacilli and the even more dangerous form, extensively drug-resistant tubercle bacilli.

This study showed that gram staining represents an easy and rapid procedure for recognizing highly infective *M. tuberculosis*. The ease of the procedure and the rapidity of staining will contribute greatly to initial testing for tuberculosis, not only in developing countries but also developed countries where the number of immune-suppressed patients have increased in hospitals. Further studies are needed to clarify the usefulness of gram staining in finding infectious tuberculosis in various clinical fields or situations.

3. References

Atsukawa,Y., Kawakami,S., Asahara, M., Ishigaki, S.,Tanaka, T., Ono,Y., Hishiya, H., Fujisaki, R., Koga, I., Ota, Y.& Miyazawa, Y. (2011). The usefulness of changing focus during examination using Gram staining as initial diagnostic clue for infective tuberculosis. J Infec Chemother Vol 17: 571-574.

Fitzgerald, D. & Haas, D.(2005) Mycobacterium tuberculosis, in chapter 248 of Mandell, Bennett & Dolin (ed),*Principles and Practice of Infectious Disease 6th ed* , Elsevir Churchill Livingstone, Philadelphia, Pennsylvania, pp.2853.

Hinson, M., Bradsher,W. & Bodner, J. (1981). Gram-stain neutrality of Mycobacterium tuberculosis. Am Rev Respir Dis Vol 123: 365-366.

Inderlied, B.(2004). Mycobacteria, in chapter 233 of Cohen & Powderly (ed), *Infectious Diseases 2ed ed.* Mosby Elsevir Limitted, Edinburgh London ,pp.2297.

Kawakami, S., Kawamura, Y., Nishiyama, K., Hatanaka, H., Fujisaki, R., Ono, Y., Miyazawa, Y. & Nishiya, H. (2012). Case of *Mycobacterium tuberculosis* meningitis: Gram staining as a useful initial diagnostic clue for tuberculous meningitis. J Infec Chemother (accepted)

Raviglione MC, O`Brien RJ. Tuberculosis (chapter 158) In; Harrison`s Principal of Internal Medicine 17th ed. New York; The McGraw-Hill Companies, Inc.: 2008.p.1006

Trifiro, S., Bourgault, M. & Lebel, F. (1990). Ghost mycobacteria on Gram stain. J Clin Microb Vol 28:146-147.

2

Temperature Sensitivity of the Diphtheria Containing Vaccines

Ümit Kartoğlu
World Health Organization
Switzerland

1. Introduction

Immunization managers can improve the efficiency of immunization programmes through enhancing their knowledge of a vaccine's stability.

Vaccine management is basically all the actions related to handling of vaccines at the country level from the moment they arrive until the moment they are used. These include arrival and acceptance procedures, appropriate temperature monitoring, ensuring sufficient storage volume, maintaining standards of buildings, equipment and vehicles, effective stock management, vaccine delivery systems as well as effective use of policies such as the multi-dose vial policy (MDVP) and the use of vaccine vial monitors (VVM).

The World Health Organization (WHO) and UNICEF offer standard tools to effectively monitor management performance of vaccine stores and the vaccine management system in a country (World Health Organization, 2010).

Assessments conducted in various countries on effective vaccine management (EVM) indicate that maintaining equipment at the temperature range recommended by the WHO is not always observed (Milstien J et al., 2006). Moreover, in case of such violations, no proper follow-up actions are taken. Many countries still lack appropriate temperature monitoring tools for vaccine stores and refrigerators. Among the studies documenting temperature violations there are some that indicate that temperature violations may affect the diphtheria containing vaccines (Bishai et al., 1992; Burgess & McIntyre, 1999; Hanjeet et al., 1996; Lugosi & Battersby, 1990; Jeremijenko et al., 1996; Milhomme, 1993; Thakker & Woods, 1992; Wawryk et al., 1997; Wirkas et al., 2006). It has been observed that cold chain practices tend to rather prioritize protecting vaccine from heat damage, thus often creating the risk of exposure to freezing temperatures. As a result, inadvertent freezing of vaccines is a largely overlooked problem all over the world. In a recent systematic review, comparison of the occurrence of freezing temperatures during storage and transport were found to be a global problem occurring both in the resource-rich as well as the resource-limited settings (Matthias et al., 2007).

2. Stability of diphtheria containing vaccines

National regulatory authorities (NRA) establish the expiry dates for diphtheria toxoid vaccines through a licensing process applicable for each vaccine. In this licensing process, the manufacturer provides data to support the claimed shelf life, although vaccine may still be efficacious beyond the claimed shelf life at 2-8°C.

2.1 Analysis of vaccine stability

2.1.1 Exposure to high temperatures

The stability of diphtheria toxoid is similar to that of any simple polypeptide, that is, unaffected by rising temperatures up to the point where secondary structure is lost: generally well above 50°C (Milstien et al., 2006). In monovalent or combination vaccines diphtheria toxoid is always adsorbed onto aluminium-based adjuvants. They are stable at elevated temperatures even at long periods of storage. On the contrary, diphtheria toxoid containing vaccines may change their appearance and lose potency when frozen due to freezing destroying the gel structure of the adjuvant. The shelf-life, at the temperature usually recommended by manufacturers (2-8°C), depends on the nature of the vaccine. Monovalent toxoid and combined diphtheria and tetanus toxoid vaccines have longer shelf life (usually three years) compared to DTP and DTP combination vaccines (18-24 months). In DTP and DTP combinations, the pertussis is the least stable component compared to both diphtheria and tetanus toxoids, therefore limiting the shelf-life.

Diphtheria toxoids exposed to 60°C are destroyed in three to five hours (Sporzynska, 1965).

2.1.2 Exposure to freezing temperatures

Adsorbed diphtheria vaccines, whether monovalent or combined, alter their physical appearance after freezing changes the structure and morphology of the aluminium adjuvant. Changes in pH and storage at higher temperatures have no influence on the structure of aluminium gel, but freezing causes extensive morphological changes that are visible under the phase-contrast microscope (PCM) and scanning electron microscope (SEM) (Aleksandrowicz et al., 1990; Kartoğlu et al., 2010a). The development of heavy conglomerates, floccules or other granular matter produces an increase in sedimentation rates (Shmelyova, 1976; World Health Organization, 1980; Aleksandrowicz et al., 1990; Kartoğlu et al, 2010a). The size of the granules seems to increase on repeated freezing and thawing. The time required to freeze diphtheria containing vaccines as well as all other freeze-sensitive vaccines depend on the number of doses in the vial (the greater the volume, the longer the time) and on the temperature exposed. Studies conducted by the WHO indicate that to freeze diphtheria containing vaccines around 110-130 minutes are required at -10°C, 25 to 45 minutes at -20°C, and 9 to 11 minutes at -70°C. Because of supercooling, the temperature in diphtheria containing vaccine vials falls to well below zero (-1.6°C to -2.6°C when the outside temperature is -4.2°C to -4.6°C) before reaching an unstable threshold. At the moment of solidification the temperature in the frozen vaccine rises to the scientific freezing point, which is about -0.5°C (World Health Organization, 1990). Phase change in freezing is also affected by the vibration where the vials are resting mainly by accelerating the friction among the molecules to trigger the crystallization.

The physical changes induced by freezing can be detected by the "shake test", which is the only test that can detect freezing in all aluminium adjuvanted vaccines (World Health Organization, 1980; Kartoğlu et al., 2010a). A learning guide in Box 1 under section 3.3

explains how to do a shake test. WHO has also produced an educational video explaining how to conduct a shake test (Kartoğlu, 2010c).

The amount of antigen in a frozen non-homogeneous vaccine can vary greatly, and the administration of such a vaccine may be associated with a reduced immune response. Similarly, it may also be linked an increased incidence of local reactions due to an increased amount of aluminium adjuvant in the dose drawn for injection.

In diphtheria containing combination vaccines, reduction of the potency of different components evidently varies slightly depending on the composition of the vaccine. The tetanus toxoid component in two of five DTP vaccines stored for 12 hours at -30°C showed a decrease in potency of about 30%, while there was no such decrease in vaccines kept at -5°C to -10°C. However, the potency of the tetanus toxoid component in adsorbed DT vaccine was reduced after freezing at both -5°C and -30°C (World Health Organization, 1980). This difference is undoubtedly due to the aluminium adjuvant effect of the pertussis component in the DTP vaccines when the potency is tested by animal assay. The relevance of this observation to protective efficacy is not known. Since it would be unethical to conduct studies with known frozen vaccines, real efficacy data are difficult to get as each product has its own particular threshold for freeze damage. This also shows that there is a difference between exposure to freezing temperatures and actual freezing to destroy the potency. That is why the shake test is so important to decide whether vaccines are affected by freezing.

A study performed by Serum Institute of India Ltd. on their own DT, Td, and DTP vaccines using three freeze-thaw cycles gave the results presented in Fig 1 (Serum Institute of India, 2005).

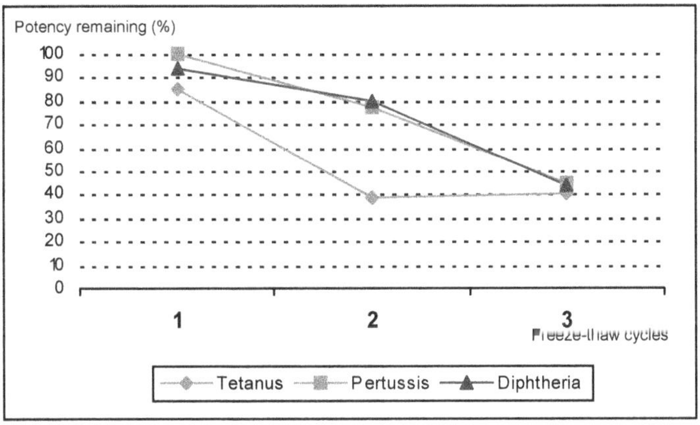

Fig. 1. Results of freeze-thaw cycles on potency of adsorbed DTP vaccine from Serum Institute of India.

3. Ensuring the optimal potency of vaccine

3.1 Temperature control requirements for diphtheria containing vaccines

To ensure the optimal potency of vaccines, careful attention is needed in vaccine handling practices at the country level. These include storage and transport of vaccines from the primary vaccine store down to the end-user at the health facility, and further down at the outreach sites. The WHO recommended conditions for storing the diphtheria containing vaccines used in immunization programmes are shown in Table 1. This Table also indicates the maximum storage periods and temperatures in each case.

	Primary vaccine store	Intermediate vaccine store		Health centre	Health post
		Province	District		
Storage temperature	+2°C to +8°C	+2°C to +8°C	+2°C to +8°C	+2°C to +8°C	+2°C to +8°C
Maximum storage period	6-12 months	3 months	1-3 month	1 month	According to session plan

Table 1. WHO recommended storage temperatures and maximum storage periods of diphtheria containing vaccines in a country cold chain system (World Health Organization, 2011).

Since the diphtheria containing vaccines are sensitive to freezing, the vaccines should be protected from being exposed to freezing temperatures both during storage and transport. Use of frozen icepacks is the major source of freezing in transport. Although for years, organizations recommended conditioning of icepacks as the best practice to prevent freezing in cold boxes, serious compliance problems have been observed and reported in the field. In principle, if used with freeze-sensitive vaccines, icepacks should be fully conditioned before being placed in the cold box with the vaccines (World Health Organization, 2002a). In order to do so, the frozen icepacks should be kept at room temperature until the icepack temperature has reached 0°C, that is, when the icepack contains a mixture of ice and water. The only way to check whether this is the case is to shake the icepack and verify whether the ice moves about slightly inside its container through listening to a slush noise. Conditioning requires both space and, more importantly, time, therefore patience. An area of approximately 1 m^2 is needed to condition 25 icepacks, a number usually required for loading one large cold box. This practice is generally found to be impractical and unrealistic because it requires more than one hour at an ambient temperature of +20°C. The practice of wrapping the freeze-sensitive vaccines to protect them from frozen icepacks and avoid freezing is found to be ineffective and no longer recommended by WHO (World Health Organization, 2004).

Although conditioning of frozen icepacks is said to be followed in the field, in a recent systematic review the occurrence of freezing temperatures during transport was found to be 16.7% in developed countries compared to 35.3% in developing countries. This difference is not statistically significant, potentially indicating that the current transport practice common to all countries - vaccines placed with frozen ice packs inside of insulated carriers - is placing vaccines at risk, regardless of the resource setting in which it is conducted (Matthias et al., 2007). In the six studies that analyzed the exposure of vaccine shipments to freezing temperatures as they travelled through both shipment and storage segments of the cold chain from either national or regional stores all the way to peripheral health centres, the findings were even more striking. In these studies, between 75% and 100% of the vaccine shipments were exposed to freezing temperatures at least once during the distribution process (Matthias et al., 2007). These comprehensive studies suggest that the risk of damaging freeze-sensitive vaccines is present in virtually every stage of the cold chain.

Between 2002 and 2004, WHO conducted a series of controlled laboratory studies and field tests (Nepal, Myanmar, Turkey and Zimbabwe) to assess the impact of using cool water packs (pre-cooled to a temperature between +2°C to +8°C) on the cold life of the vaccine transportation boxes and on the shelf life of the vaccines (Kartoğlu et al., 2009). Evaluations were conducted to verify the assumption that cool water packs can safely replace the use of icepacks for the transport of vaccines and, thus prevent the freezing of vaccines. Based on the recorded temperatures, the remaining shelf life of the vaccines were calculated through vaccine vial monitor (VVM) reactions using the Arrhenius equation[1]. Based on the results, investigators defined "cool life" (+2°C to +20°C) as a safety margin such that all vaccines except OPV can safely be transported with cool water packs even in hot climates and up to a repetition of four times (Kartoğlu et al., 2009). Fig 2 illustrates the impact of temperatures to vaccine shelf life calculated based on VVM reaction.

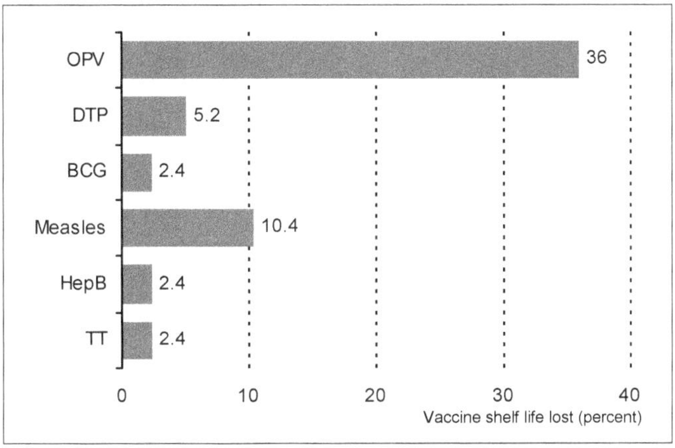

Fig. 2. Temperature impact on life loss of vaccines calculated on the basis of VVM reaction (Each transportation is assumed to be done at a continuous ambient temperature of +43°C for a period of 48 hours with a minimum temperature reading inside the vaccine transport box recorded as 11.5°C, a maximum of 25.3°C, and an average of 18.9°C throughout each journey. This scenario was repeated four times.)

Following this study, the Performance, Quality and Safety project at WHO has included the definition of "cool life" in passive cooling equipment performance specifications and now requires additional testing for cool life in prequalification of passive containers (World Health Organization, 2011a). Cool life (*with cool water-packs at +5°C)* is measured from the moment when the container is closed, until the temperature of the warmest point inside the vaccine storage compartment first reaches +20°C, at a constant ambient temperature of +43°C (World Health Organization, 2011a).

[1] The Arrhenius equation gives the quantitative basis of the relationship between the activation energy and the rate at which a reaction proceeds. Both VVM and vaccine degradation due to time and temperature exposure follow Arrhenius equation. For details on how a VVM works, please refer to section 3.2 Vaccine vial monitors and diphtheria containing vaccines.

The above results demonstrate that the use of cool water packs is a safe practice for vaccines, including diphtheria containing formulations. This clearly indicates that water packs can safely replace frozen icepacks without any damage to the vaccine potency or any major impact on vaccine shelf life. Successful implementation of this vaccine transport system has been observed in Moldova during an assessment (Babalioğlu & Kartoğlu, 2004). One drawback to the use of cool water packs could be the refrigeration volume required to store water packs to cool for use when needed. Therefore, volume requirements for introduction of cool water packs should be carefully calculated. Countries may consider conducting a temperature monitoring study in their vaccine cold chain before introducing cool water packs. Special study protocols should be used for this particular purpose (World Health Organization, 2005).

3.2 Vaccine vial monitors (VVM) and diphtheria containing vaccines

A vaccine vial monitor (VVM) is a label containing a heat-sensitive material which is placed on a vaccine vial to register cumulative heat exposure over time (World Health Organization, 2002, 2011b, 2011c). The VVM, which was introduced in 1996 for Oral Polio Vaccine (OPV), became available for all other vaccines including diphtheria containing vaccines in 1999 (World Health Organization, 2005). Today, all diphtheria containing presentations come with VVM through the United Nations (UN) procurement agencies. VVM clearly indicates to health workers whether a vaccine can be used. VVM is designed to meet the vaccine's heat stability curve, allowing a margin of safety (World Health Organization, 2011b, 2011c). Correlation between the vaccine vial monitor and vaccine potency was tested with OPV and good correlation was found (World Health Organization, 1999b).

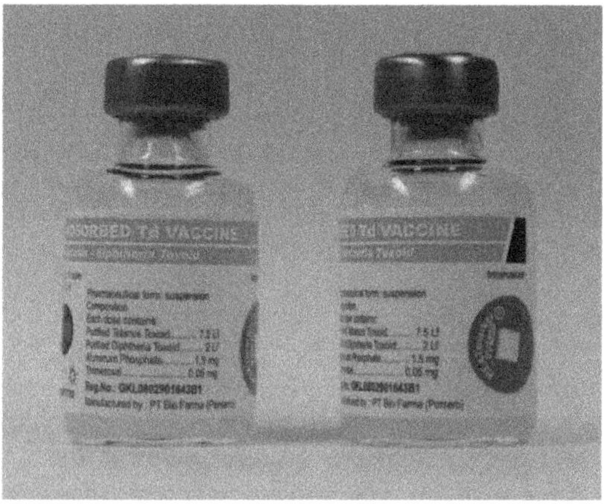

Photograph: PT Biofarma, Indonesia

Fig. 3. Vaccine vial monitor on Td vaccine (PT Biofarma, Indonesia).

The inner square of the VVM is made of heat sensitive material (monomer) that is light at the starting point and becomes darker with the combined effect of time and heat exposure. This change (polymerization) is cumulative and irreversible. Until the temperature and/or duration of heat reaches a level known to degrade the vaccine beyond acceptable limits, the inner square remains lighter than the outer circle. At the discard point, the inner square reaches the same color as the outer circle. This reflects that the vial has been exposed to an unacceptable level of heat and the vaccine degraded beyond acceptable limits. The inner square will continue to darken with heat exposure until it is much darker than the outer circle. Whenever the inner square matches or is darker than the outer circle, the vial must be discarded.

The below Fig 4 explains the interpretation of VVM.

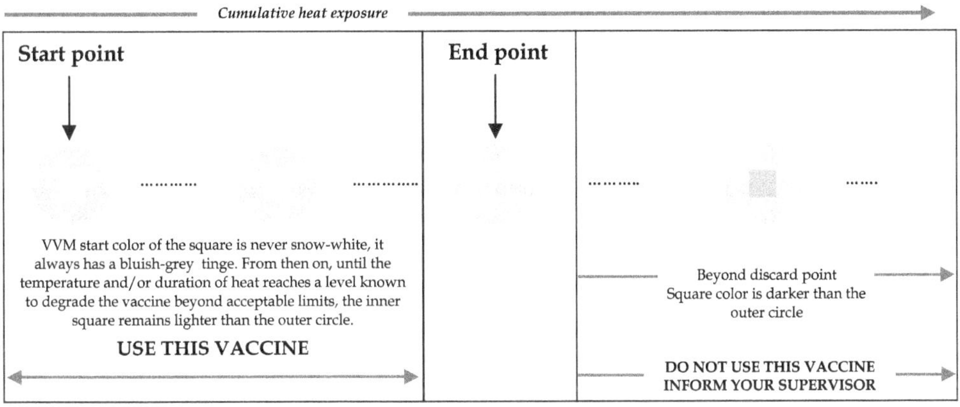

Fig. 4. VVM interpretation guidelines (Milstien et al., 2006).

A direct relationship exists between the rate of color change and temperature:

- The lower the temperature, the slower the color change.
- The higher the temperature, the faster the color change.

VVMs are located either on the label or on the top of the cap or on the neck of the ampoule depending on the following conditions. Diphtheria containing vaccines fall in the first category and VVMs in these vaccines are applied to their labels (World Health Organization, 2011b, 2011c):

- For multi-dose vials containing a vaccine that can be used in subsequent sessions: regardless of the vaccine presentation (liquid, freeze-dried or two vial combinations of liquid and freeze-dried), the VVM must be permanently attached to the label of the vaccine vial and must remain readily observable before, during, and after use, until the entire contents of the vial have been used.
- For vaccines that must be discarded at the end of the session or within 6 hours, whichever comes first: the VVM must be attached to the vaccine vial or ampoule and must remain readily observable until the vial or ampoule is opened, but not observable after opening. In order to achieve this requirement, the VVM must be located on the flip-off top of a vial or on the neck of an ampoule.

There are four different types of VVMs designed for different stability profiles (Table 2). Reaction rates are specific to four different models of VVM, relating to four groups of vaccines according to their heat stability at minimum two specific temperature points.

Category (Vaccines)	No. of days to end point at +37°C	No. of days to end point at +25°C	Time to end point at +5°C
VVM 30: High Stability	30	193	> 4 years
VVM 14: Medium Stability	14	90	> 3 years
VVM 7: Moderate Stability	7	45	> 2 years
VVM 2: Least Stable	2	N/A*	225 days

*VVM (Arrhenius) reaction rates determined at two temperature points

Table 2. VVM reaction rates by category of heat stability (World Health Organization, 2011b).

The above table does not give specific references to vaccine products, and only refer to the stability profile. Same type vaccines made by different manufacturers may have different heat stability characteristics and may therefore be assigned to different categories by WHO. In general, DT and Td combinations are either with VVM14 or VVM30 depending on their stability characteristics. DTP combination vaccines are usually with VVM14 mainly due to limiting component of pertussis.

Vaccines with VVMs including diphtheria containing ones can be taken out of the cold chain if health workers and others persons handling the vaccines have been trained to interpret VVM readings correctly and to discard any vial bearing a VVM that has reached its discard point. Although most of the out-of-cold chain studies are conducted with HepB vaccine and OPV, recent studies show that taking vaccines with VVMs out of the cold chain can successfully be implemented without compromising vaccine potency (Guthridge et al., 1996; Halm et al., 2010; Hipgrave et al., 2006; Huong et al., 2006; Lixia et al., 2007; Nelson et al., 2004; Otto et al., 2000; Zipursky et al., 2011). WHO recommends all Member States to consider adoption of policies permitting the use of vaccines beyond the cold chain where warranted for routine immunization activities or on a limited basis in certain areas or under special circumstances, such as (World Health Organization, 2007a):

- national immunization days;
- hard-to-reach geographical areas;
- immunizations provided at home - including hepatitis B vaccine birth dose;
- cool seasons;
- storage and transportation of freeze-sensitive vaccines (DTP, TT, DT, Td, hepatitis B and Hib vaccines) where the risk of freezing is greater than the risk of heat exposure.

In 2007, WHO has celebrated the 10 year anniversary of VVM introduction. Detailed information on the event as well as many other visuals and documents on VVM can be reached at http://www.who.int/immunization_standards/vaccine_quality/vvm_10years/en/index.html (World Health Organization, 2007b).

3.3 Shake test: detecting freeze-damage to diphtheria containing vaccines

Practices inadvertently exposing vaccines to sub-zero temperatures are widespread in both developed and developing countries and at all levels of health systems. (Bishai et al.,

1992; Burgess & McIntyre, 1999; Hanjeet et al., 1996; Lugosi & Battersby, 1990; Jeremijenko et al., 1996; Milhomme, 1993; Thakker & Woods, 1992; Wawryk et al., 1997; Wirkas et al., 2006). The most recent systematic literature review of vaccine freezing practices showed that inadvertent freezing occurs across all parts of the cold chain (Matthias et al., 2007). Between 14% and 35% of refrigerators or transport shipments were found to have exposed vaccines to freezing temperatures. In studies that all segments of the distribution chain were studied, between 75% and 100% of the vaccine shipments were exposed to sub-zero temperatures.

When a vaccine containing an antigen adsorbed to an aluminium adjuvant (e.g. hepatitis B, diphtheria toxoid, ..) is damaged by freezing, the loss of potency can never be restored, the damage is permanent (Dimayuga et al., 1995; World Health Organization, 1980).

Freezing affects the adsorbed vaccines by changing their physical form. Freezing does not affect non-potency parameters (such as acid content, pH; flocculating ability (Lf); ratio of free aluminium to aluminium phosphate; free formaldehyde; and thiomersal content). After freezing, the lattice (made up of bonds between the adsorbent and the antigen) in a vaccine is broken, whether monovalent or combined. Separated adsorbent tends to form larger, heavier granules that gradually settle at the bottom of the vial when this is shaken. It has been observed that ice crystals formed during freezing force aluminium particles to overcome repulsion, thereby producing strong inter-particle attraction resulting in aluminium particle coagulation/agglomeration. Thus the particles become bigger and heavier. As a simple physics rule, these heavy particles sediment faster than particles in never frozen vaccines. The size of the granules seems to increase on repeated freezing and thawing cycles.

As shown in Fig 5, diphtheria containing vaccines kept at the optimal temperature (+2°C to +8°C) show a fine-grain structure under PCM. In contrast, large conglomerates of massed precipitates with a crystalline structure are observed in vaccines affected by freezing (Kartoğlu et al., 2010a). Vaccines that are exposed to subzero temperatures without freezing show identical physical characteristics to vaccines that are kept at optimum conditions. These vaccines were also found to be in full liquid state despite being exposed to -2°C over a 24 hour period.

In this study, under PCM, particles in the non-frozen samples measured from 1 µm (DTP and DTP-HepB) to 20 µm (DT). By contrast, aggregates in the freeze-damaged samples measured up to 700 µm (DTP) and 350 µm on average (Kartoğlu et al., 2010a).

Scanning electron microscopy and X-ray analysis results in frozen and non-frozen diphtheria containing vaccines are illustrated in Fig 6, 7 and 8 (With permission from Kartoğlu, U., World Health Organization, Geneva, Switzerland and Kurzatkowski, W., Institute of Hygiene, Warsaw, Poland). Scanning electron microscopy of vaccines kept at +2°C to +8°C showed uniform flocculent structure either dense or dispersed (Fig 6A). Scanning electron microscopy of vaccines damaged by freezing (exposed to -25 °C for 24 hours) exhibited conglomerates either with rough or smooth surfaces (Fig 7A and B). Phosphate content was found to be related with formation of the precipitates, lower values are mostly resulted in rough surfaces with sharp edges while higher phosphate content affected precipitates' surfaces to be more smooth. As shown in Fig 6B and 8B, X-ray analysis

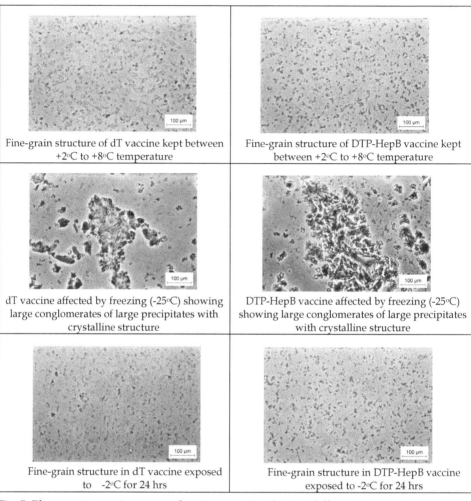

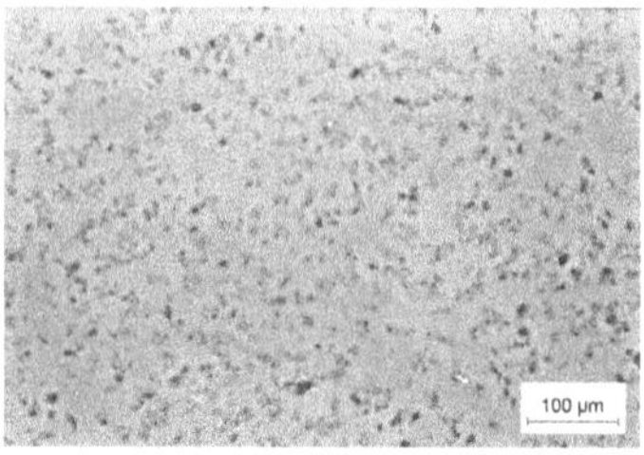 Fine-grain structure of dT vaccine kept between +2°C to +8°C temperature	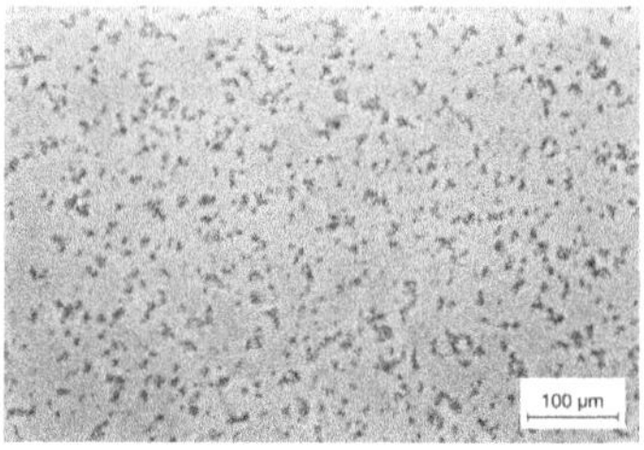 Fine-grain structure of DTP-HepB vaccine kept between +2°C to +8°C temperature
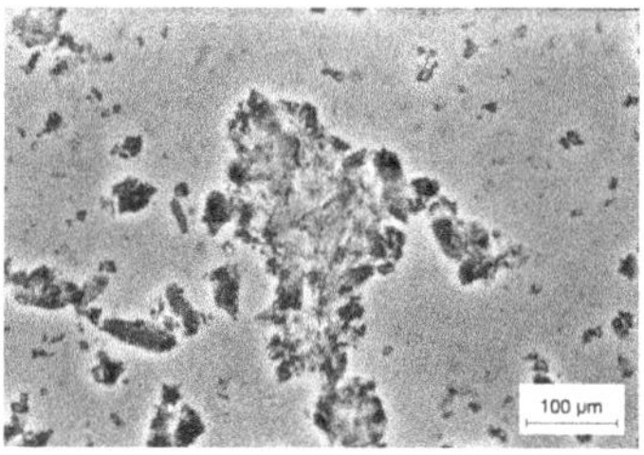 dT vaccine affected by freezing (-25°C) showing large conglomerates of large precipitates with crystalline structure	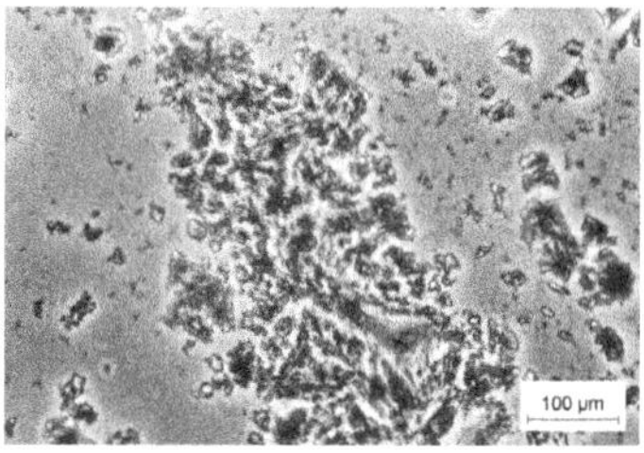 DTP-HepB vaccine affected by freezing (-25°C) showing large conglomerates of large precipitates with crystalline structure
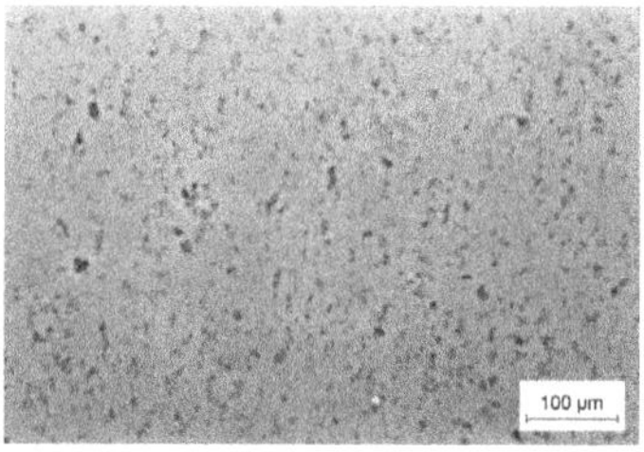 Fine-grain structure in dT vaccine exposed to -2°C for 24 hrs	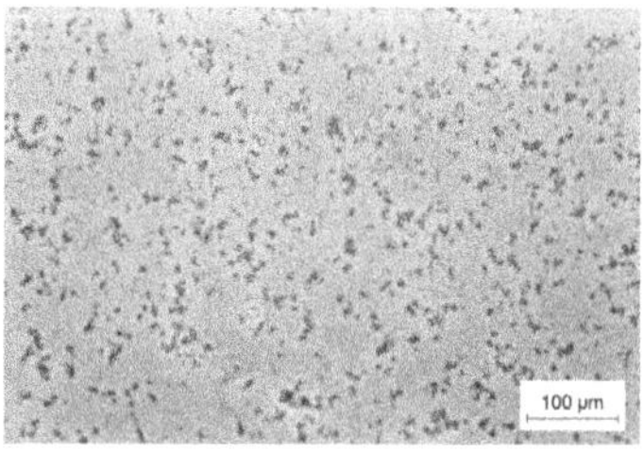 Fine-grain structure in DTP-HepB vaccine exposed to -2°C for 24 hrs

Fig. 5. Phase contrast microscopy of various vaccines kept at different temperatures (Kartoğlu et al., 2010a).

of precipitates in vaccines affected by freezing showed high aluminum content, indicating that the conglomerates are mainly aluminium clutters.

The physical changes initiated by freezing can be detected by the shake test simply by naked eyes. The shake test is designed to understand whether the vaccines are damaged by freezing based on the difference in sedimentation rates of freeze-sensitive vaccines in frozen and non-frozen vials (Fig 9). Shake test is validated by a WHO study against PCM with a 100% positive predictive value (Kartoğlu et al., 2010a, 2010b). In a typical demonstration of the shake test, two identical vials of a vaccine (i.e. from the same batch and the same manufacturer) that is suspected of having been exposed to freezing temperatures are selected; one of the two vials is purposely frozen and then thawed as the "negative control", while the second vial serves as the vial to be "tested" against this negative control. The two

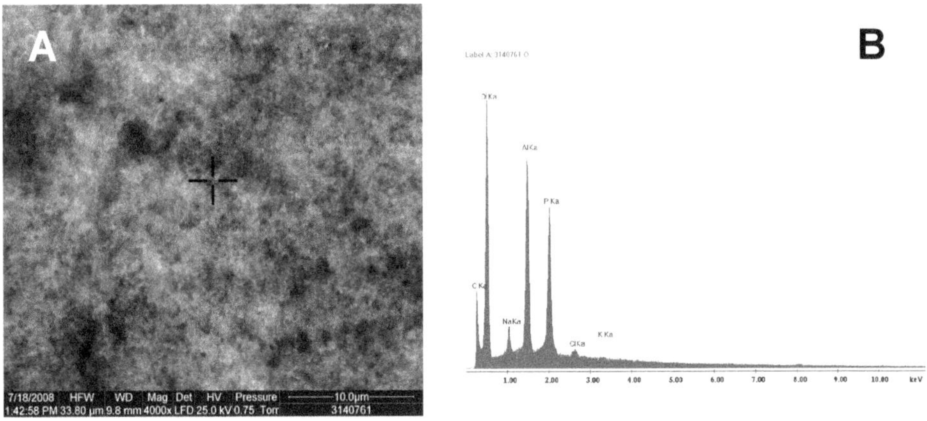

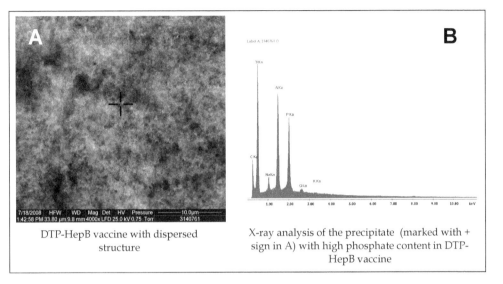

DTP-HepB vaccine with dispersed structure

X-ray analysis of the precipitate (marked with + sign in A) with high phosphate content in DTP-HepB vaccine

Fig. 6. Scanning electron micrograph (A) and X-ray analysis of the elements (B) of non-frozen DTP-HepB vaccine (kept at +2°C to +8°C at all times).

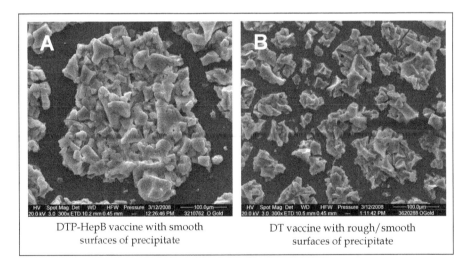

DTP-HepB vaccine with smooth surfaces of precipitate

DT vaccine with rough/smooth surfaces of precipitate

Fig. 7. Scanning electron micrographs of gold coated conglomerates of frozen DTP-HepB (A) and DT vaccines (B) exposed to -25°C for 24 hrs

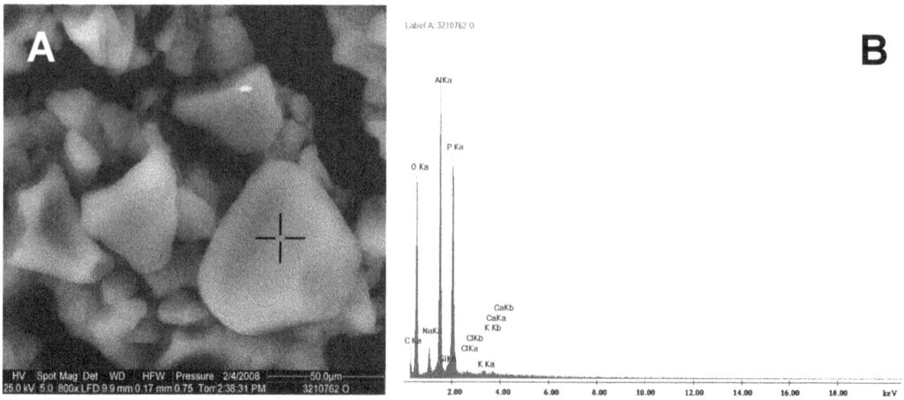

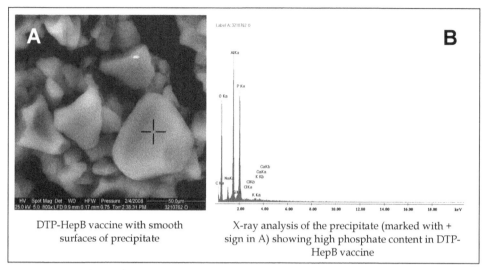

DTP-HepB vaccine with smooth surfaces of precipitate

X-ray analysis of the precipitate (marked with + sign in A) showing high phosphate content in DTP-HepB vaccine

Fig. 8. X-ray analysis of the elements of frozen DTP-HepB vaccine exposed to -25°C for 24 hrs.

vials are held together in one hand and shaken; they are then placed side by side on a flat surface. Provided the test vial has not been frozen, sedimentation is slower in the test vial than in the control vial that has been frozen and thawed. If the test vial has been frozen, the test and control vials will have similar sedimentation rates.

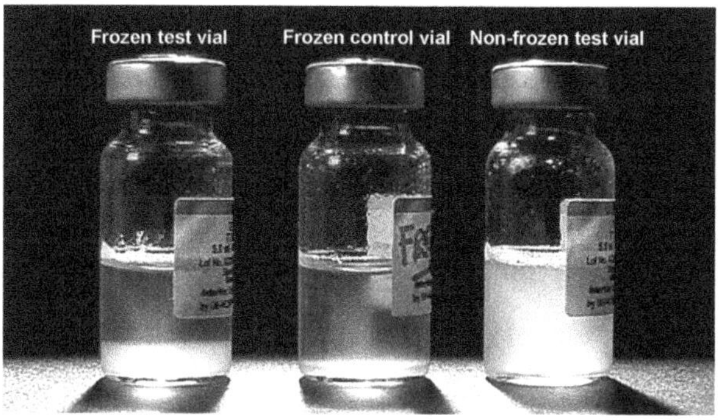

Photograph: Ü. Kıvanç (WHO)

Fig. 9. Visual difference in sedimentation rates after shake test for detecting freeze damage to adsorbed DTP vaccine (Kartoğlu et al., 2010a).

The shake test correctly identifies if a vaccine has been affected by freezing 100% of the time (95% confidence interval, CI: 0.97–1.00) and it also correctly identifies if a vaccine has not been frozen 100% of the time (95% CI: 0.99–1.00). Sensitivity and specificity of the shake test for slushy vaccines were both calculated as 100% (sensitivity 95% CI: 0.86–1.00; specificity 95% CI: 0.93–1.00). In addition to the article (Kartoğlu et al., 2010a), WHO has produced a video article illustrating all steps of the validation study. This can be viewed at http://vimeo.com/8381355 (Kartoğlu et al., 2010b).

The shake test should not be conducted under the following circumstances and vials should be discarded immediately, without the need for any confirmatory shake test (Milstien et al., 2006):

- When a solid frozen vaccine vial(s) has been found
- With a vial for which a homogeneous solution CANNOT be obtained after vigorous shaking as seen in Fig 10. In such cases, the white lump/sediment cannot be separated from the walls of the glass vial. This happens only with DTP vials that are exposed to subzero temperatures without freezing (due to P component).

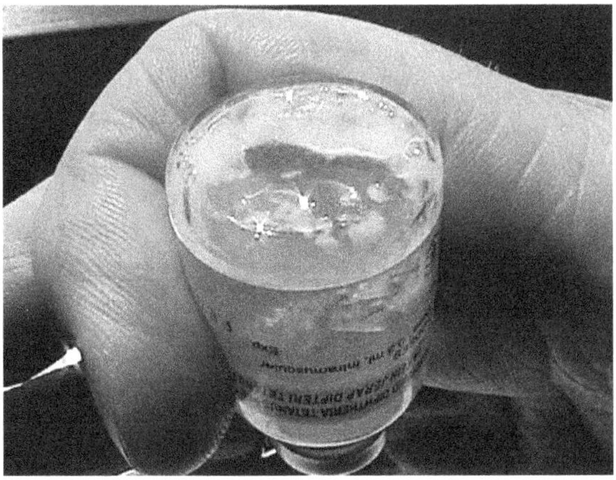

Photograph: Ü. Kartoğlu (WHO)

Fig. 10. Sub-zero temperature effect on DTP vaccine (after 10 minutes of vigorous shaking)

A learning guide to conduct the shake test is given in Box 1.

4. Summary

Diphtheria toxoids are some of the most stable vaccines in common use. They are stable at temperatures of 2 to 8°C for years, at room temperature for months, and at 37°C for weeks. At the temperature of 45°C the degradation of diphtheria toxoid is accelerated and its potency can decline during few weeks. At 53°C diphtheria toxoid lose its potency after few days, and at 60°C potency lost occurs within few hours. Freezing can reduce the potency of adsorbed diphtheria toxoid containing vaccines, however, it does not seem to affect the immunogenicity of unadsorbed products. The freezing point for adsorbed toxoids is between -5°C and -10°C. Adsorbed diphtheria toxoids containing vaccines should never be frozen.

As recommended by the WHO, all diphtheria toxoid containing vaccine products should be stored at +2°C to +8°C at all levels of any cold chain. Use of frozen icepacks at transport increases the risk of freezing the diphtheria containing vaccines. It has been observed and reported that the conditioning of icepacks for the purpose of preventing freezing during transport is not practiced in the field. Today WHO recommends to remove ice and introduce cool water packs (pre-cooled to a temperature between + 2°C to + 8°) for in-country transport of freeze-sensitive products including diphtheria containing vaccines.

<table>
<tr><td colspan="5">Name of health staff: ______________________________</td></tr>
<tr><td colspan="5">Performance assessment scale:
1. Insufficient: Health staff performs the shake test incorrectly, or not in the right order or skips it altogether.
2. Competent: Health staff performs the shake test correctly and in the right order but either misses some points or needs to be reminded and encouraged by the study coordinator.
3. Proficient: Health staff performs the shake test correctly, in the right order, and without hesitating.</td></tr>
<tr><td colspan="2" rowspan="2">NOTES:
□ This protocol must not be altered. There is only one correct way to conduct a Shake Test.
□ The test procedure described below should be repeated with all suspect batches. In the case of international arrivals, the shake test should be conducted on a random sample of vaccine. However, if there is more than one lot in the shipment, the random sample must include a vial taken from each and every lot.</td><td colspan="3">Practice no.</td></tr>
<tr><td>1</td><td>2</td><td>3</td></tr>
<tr><td colspan="2">1. Take a vial of vaccine of the same type and batch number as the vaccine you want to test, and made by the same manufacturer.</td><td></td><td></td><td></td></tr>
<tr><td colspan="2">2. Clearly mark the vial as "FROZEN".</td><td></td><td></td><td></td></tr>
<tr><td colspan="2">3. Freeze the vial in a freezer or the freezing compartment of a refrigerator until the contents are completely solid.</td><td></td><td></td><td></td></tr>
<tr><td colspan="2">4. Let it thaw. Do <u>NOT</u> heat it!</td><td></td><td></td><td></td></tr>
<tr><td colspan="2">5. Take your "TEST" vial from the batch that you suspect has been frozen.</td><td></td><td></td><td></td></tr>
<tr><td colspan="2">6. Hold the "FROZEN" vial and the "TEST" vial together in one hand.</td><td></td><td></td><td></td></tr>
<tr><td colspan="2">7. Shake both vials vigorously for 10-15 seconds.</td><td></td><td></td><td></td></tr>
<tr><td colspan="2">8. Place both vials on a flat surface side-by-side and start continuous observation of the vials until test is finished.
(NOTE: If the vials have large labels, which conceal the vial contents, turn both vials upside down and observe sedimentation in the neck of the vial.)</td><td></td><td></td><td></td></tr>
<tr><td colspan="2">9. Use an adequate source of light to compare the sedimentation rates between vials.
IF,</td><td></td><td></td><td></td></tr>
<tr><td>10. The TEST vial sediments slower than the FROZEN vial,
THEN,</td><td>10. Sedimentation is similar in both vials
OR
The TEST vial sediments faster than the FROZEN vial
THEN,</td><td></td><td></td><td></td></tr>
<tr><td>11. Use the vaccine batch.</td><td>11. <u>Vaccine damaged</u>: Notify your supervisor. Set aside all affected vaccine in a container marked "DAMAGED VACCINE FOR DISPOSAL- DO NOT USE"</td><td></td><td></td><td></td></tr>
<tr><td rowspan="2"></td><td>12. Discard all affected vaccine once you have received permission to do so.</td><td></td><td></td><td></td></tr>
<tr><td>13. Fill in the Loss/Adjustment Form.</td><td></td><td></td><td></td></tr>
</table>

Box 1. Shake test learning guide.

Heat impact on vaccines is cumulative. The VVM, which was introduced in 1996 for Oral Polio Vaccine (OPV), became available for all other vaccines in 1999. Today, all diphtheria containing products procured by the United Nations procurement agencies come with VVM. At any time in the process of distribution and at the time a vaccine is administered, the VVM indicates whether the vaccine has been exposed to a combination of excessive temperature over time and whether it is likely to have been damaged. It clearly indicates to health workers whether a vaccine can be used. With the help of VVM, vaccines can be taken beyond the cold chain under special circumstances defined by the WHO. These include national immunization days, hard-to-reach geographical areas; immunizations provided in the home - including hepatitis B vaccine birth dose; cool seasons; storage and transportation of freeze-sensitive vaccines (DTP, TT, DT, Td, hepatitis B and Hib vaccines) where the risk of freezing is greater than the risk of heat exposure.

Freezing of vaccines is a widespread problem across the world. When a vaccine containing an antigen adsorbed to an aluminium adjuvant is damaged, the loss of potency can never be restored. Freezing affects the physical form of the adsorbed vaccines through breaking the lattice structure that is made up of bonds between the adsorbent and the antigen. Separated aluminium adjuvant tends to form larger, heavier granules that gradually settle at the bottom of the vial when the latter is shaken. The shake test can demonstrate these facts and is the only test to determine whether freeze-sensitive adsorbed vaccines have been affected by freezing.

5. References

Aleksandrowicz, J.; Drozdz, M., Fieka, M. & Kurzatkowski, W. (1990). Evaluation of the physico-chemical state of aluminium hydroxide in biopreparations stored at various conditions. *Medycyna doswiadczalna i mikrobiologia,* Vol. 42, No.3-4, pp. 163-170, ISSN. 0025-8601

Babalioğlu, N. & Kartoğlu, U. (2004). *EVSM assessment: Chisinau primary vaccine store,* Republic of Moldova. 6-10 December 2004 (unpublished EVSM external assessment report)

Bishai, D.M.; Bhatt, S., Miller, L.T. & Hayden, G.F. (1992). Vaccine storage practices in pediatric offices. *Pediatrics* Vol. 89, No. 2, pp. 193–196, ISSN. 0031-4005

Burgess, M.A. & McIntyre, P.B. (1999). Vaccines and the cold chain: is it too hot... or too cold? *Med J Aust,* Vol. 171, No. 2, pp. 82, ISSN 0025-729X

Dimayuga, R.; Scheifele, D. & Bell, A. (1995). Effects of freezing on DTP and DTP-IPV vaccines, adsorbed. *Can Commun Dis Rep* Vol. 21, pp. 101–103, ISSN. 1188-4169

Guthridge, S.L. & Miller, N.C. (1996). Cold chain in a hot climate. *Australian and New Zealand Journal of Public Health.* Vol. 20, No. 6, pp. 657-660, ISSN. 1326-0200

Halm, A.; Yalcouyé, I., Kamissoko, M., Keïta, T., Modjirom, N., Zipursky, S., Kartoğlu, U. & Ronveaux, O. (2010). Using oral polio vaccine beyond the cold chain: a feasibility study conducted during the national immunization campaign in Mali. *Vaccine.* Vol. 28, No. 19, pp. 3467-3472.

Hanjeet, K.; Lye, M.S., Sinniah, M. & Schnur, A. (1996). Evaluation of cold chain monitoring in Kelantan, Malaysia. *Bull World Health Organ* Vol. 74, No. 4, pp. 391–397, ISSN. 0042-9686

Hipgrave, D.B.; Maynard, J.E. & Biggs, B.A. (2006). Improving birth dose coverage of hepatitis B vaccine. *Bulletin of the World Health Organization,* Vol. 84, No. 1, pp. 65–71, ISSN. 0042-9686

Huong, V.M.; Hipgrave, D., Hills, S., Nelson, C., Hien, D.S. & Cuong, N.V. (2006). *Out-of-Cold-Chain Delivery of the Hepatitis B Birth Dose in Four Districts of Vietnam.* PATH. October 2006 (unpublished study)

Jeremijenko, A.; Kelly, H., Sibthorpe, B. & Attewell, R. (1996). Improving vaccine storage in general practice refrigerators. *BMJ* Vol. 312, No.7047, pp. 1651–1652, ISSN. 0959-8138

Kartoğlu, U. (2007). Five senses, 14 September 2011, Available from: http://vimeo.com/8373523

Kartoğlu, U.; Ganivet, S., Guichard, S., Aiyer, V., Bollen, P., Maire, D. & Altay, B. (2009). Use of cool water packs to prevent freezing during vaccine transportation at the country level. *PDA Journal of Pharmaceutical Science and Technology.* Vol. 63, No. 1, pp. 11-26, ISSN. 1079-7440

Kartoğlu, U.; Ozguler, N.K., Wolfson, L.J. & Kurzątkowski, W. (2010). Validation of the shake test for detecting freeze damage to adsorbed vaccines. *Bull World Health Organ* Vol. 88, No. 8, pp. 624-631, ISSN. 0042-9686

Kartoğlu, U.; Ozguler, N.K. & Wolfson, L.J. (2010). Shake and tell Tell - video article. 14 September 2011, Available from: http://vimeo.com/8381355

Kartoğlu, U. (2010). Step-by-step how to conduct a shake test - educational video. 15 September 2011, Available from http://vimeo.com/8389435

Lixia, W.; Junhua, L., Haiping, C., Fangjun, L., Gregory, L.A., Carib, N., Wenyuan, Z. & Craig, N.S. (2007). Hepatitis B vaccination of newborn infants in rural China: evaluation of a village-based, out-of-cold-chain delivery strategy. *Bulletin of the World Health Organization,* Vol.85, No. 9, pp.688–694, ISSN. 0042-9686

Lugosi, L. & Battersby, A. (1990). Transport and storage of vaccines in Hungary: the first cold chain monitor study in Europe. *Bull World Health Organ* Vol. 68, No. 4, pp. 431–439, ISSN. 0042-9686

Matthias, D.M.; Robertson, J., Garrison, M.M., Newland, S. & Nelson, C. (2007). Freezing temperatures in the vaccine cold chain: a systematic literature review. *Vaccine* Vol. 25, No.20, pp. 3980–3986, ISSN. 0264-410X

Milhomme, P. (1993). Cold chain study: danger of freezing vaccines. *Can Commun Dis Rep* Vol. 19, No. 5, pp. 33–38, ISSN. 1188-4169

Milstien, J.; Kartoğlu, U. & Zaffran, M. (2006). *Temperature sensitivity of vaccines.* World Health Organization, WHO/IVB/06.10, Geneva, Switzerland

Nelson, C.M.; Wibisono, H., Purwanto, H., Manssur, I., Moniaga, V. & Widjaya, A. (2004). Hepatitis B vaccine freezing in the Indonesian cold chain: evidence and solutions. *Bulletin of the World Health Organization,* Vol. 82, No. 2, pp. 99-105, ISSN. 0042-9686

Otto, B.F.; Suarnawa, I.M., Steward, T., Nelson, C., Ruff, T.A., Widjaya, A. & Maynard, J.E. (2000). At-birth immunisation against hepatitis B using a novel pre-filled immunisation device stored outside the cold chain. *Vaccine.* Vol. 18, No. 5-6, pp. 498-502, ISSN. 0264-410X

Serum Institute of India. (2005). Personal communication.

Shmelyova, E.I. (1976). Study of stability of physical properties and biological activity of liquid and freeze dried adsorbed pertussis-diphtheria-tetanus vaccines. *Proceedings of the symposium on stability and effectiveness of measles, poliomyelitis and pertussis vaccines.* Yugoslav Academy of Sciences and Arts, pp. 159-179, Zagreb, Yugoslavia

Sporzynska, Z. (1965). Studies on the stability of toxoids. I. The effect of temperature on the immunogenic properties of diphtheria toxoid. *Experimental medicine and microbiology*, Vol. 17, pp. 130-139.

Thakker, Y. & Woods, S. (1992). Storage of vaccines in the community: weak link in the cold chain? *BMJ* Vol. 304, No. 6829, pp. 756–758, ISSN. 0959-8138

Wawryk, A.; Mavromatis, C. & Gold, M. (1997). Electronic monitoring of vaccine cold chain in a metropolitan area. *BMJ* Vol. 315, No. 7107, pp. 518, ISSN. 0959-8138

World Health Organization. (1980). The effects of freezing on the appearance, potency, and toxicity of adsorbed and unadsorbed DTP vaccines. *Wkly Epidemiol Rec* Vol. 55, No. 50, pp. 385–392, ISSN. 0049-8414

World Health Organization. (1990). Tests of the freezing point of vaccines. *Cold chain newsletter*, 90.3, pp.5

World Health Organization. (1999). *Quality of the cold chain: WHO-UNICEF policy statement on the use of vaccine vial monitors in immunization services.* WHO/V&B/99.18, World Health Organization, Geneva, Switzerland

World Health Organization. (1999). *Testing the correlation between vaccine vial monitors and vaccine potency.* World Health Organization, WHO/V&B/99.11, Geneva, Switzerland.

World Health Organization. (2002). *Guideline for establishing or improving primary and intermediate vaccine stores.* WHO/V&B/02.34, World Health Organization, Geneva, Switzerland

World Health Organization. (2022). *Getting started with Vaccine Vial Monitors.* WHO/V&B/02.35, World Health Organization, Geneva, Switzerland

World Health Organization. (2004). *Immunization in Practice.* WHO/IVB/04.06, World Health Organization, Geneva, Switzerland

World Health Organization. (2005). *Study protocol for temperature monitoring in the vaccine cold chain.* WHO/IVB/05.01, World Health Organization, Geneva, Switzerland

World Health Organization. (2007). *WHO-UNICEF policy statement on the implementation of vaccine vial monitors: The role of vaccine vial monitors in improving access to immunization.* WHO/IVB/07.04, World Health Organization, Geneva, Switzerland

World Health Organization. (2007). WHO celebrates 10 years of VVM implementation, In: Immunization standards, 14 September 2011, Available from: http://www.who.int /immunization_standards/vaccine_quality/vvm_10years_index/en/index.html

World Health Organization. (2010). Effective vaccine management (EVM) initiative, In: *EVM - setting standards for the Immunization Supply Chain*, 14 September 2011, Available from: http:// www.who.int/immunization_delivery/systems_policy/logistics/ en/index6.html

World Health Organization. (2011). *Performance Quality and Safety Devices Catalogue*, (version 2 August 2011), pp. 1-234, Geneva, Switzerland, Retrieved from http://www.who.int/entity/immunization_standards/vaccine_quality/pqs_devices_catalogue_02aug2011.pdf

World Health Organization. (2011). *PQS performance specification for vaccine vial monitor.* Retrieved from WHO/PQS/E06/IN05.2, http://www.who.int/entity/immunization_standards/vaccine_quality/who_pqs_e06_in05_rev_july2011.pdf

World Health Organization. (2011). *PQS independent type-testing protocol for vaccine vial monitors.* Retrieved from WHO/PQS/E06/IN05.VP2, http://www.who.int/ entity/ immunization_standards/vaccine_quality/who_pqs_e06_in05_vp_rev_may2011.pdf

Wirkas, T.; Toikilik, S., Miller, N., Morgan, C. & Clements, C.J. (2006). A vaccine cold chain freezing study in PNG highlights technology needs for hot climate countries. *Vaccine* Vol. 25, No. 4, pp. 691-697, ISSN. 0264-410X

Zipursky, S.; Boualam, L., Cheikh, D.O., Fournier-Caruana, J., Hamid, D., Jannsen, M., Kartoğlu, U., Waeterlos, G. & Ronveaux, O. (2011). Assessing the potency of oral polio vaccine kept outside of the cold chain during national immunization campaign in Chad. *Vaccine.* Vol. 29, No.34 , pp. 5662-5656, ISSN. 0264-410X

3

Iron and Microbial Growth

Argiris Symeonidis[1] and Markos Marangos[2]
[1]*Hematology Division and*
[2]*Division of Infectious Diseases,*
Dept of Internal Medicine, University of Patras Medical School, Patras,
Greece

1. Introduction

Iron is an essential element for the growth and development of all the scale of living organisms, and acquiring iron is crucial for the development of any pathogen. Iron participates in a large number of cellular processes, the most important of which are oxygen transport, ATP generation, cell growth and proliferation, and detoxification. It is a co-enzyme or enzyme activator of ribonucleotide reductase, a key enzyme for DNA synthesis, which catalyzes the conversion of ribonucleotides to deoxyribonucleotidides and particularly of deoxyuridine to thymidine.[1]

Iron is essential for both, the pathogen and the host, and complex mechanisms have evolved that illustrate the longstanding battle between pathogens and hosts for iron acquisition. The host has developed mechanisms to withhold iron from the microorganisms, thus preventing their growth, while the microorganisms have the capacity to adapt to the iron restricted environment by several strategies. Furthermore, iron modulates immune effector mechanisms, such as cytokine activities, nitric oxide (NO) formation or immune cell proliferation, and consequently, host immune surveillance.[2] High levels of free iron may damage or destroy the natural resistance. It catalyzes the formation of highly reactive compounds, such as hydroxyl radicals, that cause damage to the macromolecular components of the cells, including DNA and proteins.[3,4] Most environmental iron is in the Fe^{3+} state, which is almost insoluble at neutral pH. To overcome the virtual insolubility and potential toxicity of iron, ingenious transport systems and related proteins have evolved, to mediate balanced and regulated acquisition, transport, and storage of iron in a soluble, biologically useful, non-toxic form. The various proteins involved in mammalian iron transport and metabolism are presented in Table I.

2. The role of iron in normal cell growth

Iron holds an important metabolic role on the regulation of the cell cycle. It activates the cyclin/cyclin-dependent kinase complexes, favouring the progression to the S phase. Normally, all eukaryotic cells, entering the S-phase, upregulate transferrin receptor-1 expression, to obtain iron from the extracellular environment. Low levels of intracellular Fe^{3+} increase cyclin-dependent kinase inhibitor $p21^{CIP1/WAF1}$ levels, delaying or inhibiting the transition to the S-phase. As a result, Bcl-2 is down-regulated and Bax levels are increased, conditions that activate caspase-3, caspase-8, and caspase-9, and lead to apoptotic cell

Protein	Function
Duodenal Cytochrome B	Reduces Fe^{3+} to Fe^{2+} in the intestinal lumen, to facilitate iron absorbtion
Nramp1 (Natural resistance-macrophage protein-1	Divalent iron transporter expressed in phagocytes. Participates in intracellu- associated lar iron recycling.
DMT1 (Nramp2 or DCT1)	Associates and transports Fe^{2+} from intestinal lumen - Intracellular iron transporter - receives and delivers endosomal iron
HFE protein	Binds to Tf Receptor - antagonizes Tf binding
Ferroportin	Cell membrane iron transporter, both importer and exporter
Hepcidin	Allosteric inhibitor of Fp – Induces Fp internalization and degradation
Ceruloplasmin	Bivalent metal iron transporter mainly for copper and iron
Hephaestin	Facilitates iron efflux by the enterocyte
Hemojuvelin	GPI-linked membrane protein – Upregulates hepcidin gene expression
Transferrin	Main iron transporter in the systemic circulation
Transferrin Receptor-1	Main cellular receptor for iron internalization
Transferrin Receptor-2	Mainly expressed in the liver – Binds only holotransferrin
Matriptase-2	Membrane-bound serine protease - Downregulates hepcidin gene expression
Iron Regulatory Protein-1	Regulates intracellular iron homeostasis by binding to various iron regulatory elements - Cytosolic aconitase activity
Iron Regulatory Protein-2	RNA-binding protein – Regulates translation of iron protein mRNA
PCBP1	Cytosolic chaperone – Trafficks iron from endosomes to cytosolic ferritin
Lactoferrin	Tissue iron-binding protein with pleiotropic activity
Ferritin	High molecular weight protein-complex – Main iron storage protein
Mitoferrin	Inner mitochondrial membrane protein – Importer of iron to mitochondria
Frataxin	Mitochondrial iron-storage protein. Mediates iron transport to Iron-Sulfur cluster-containing proteins and iron export from the mitochondrion
ABCB7	Main mitochondrial iron exporter
Mitochondrial Ferritin	High H-Ferritin molecule with higher affinity for iron than ferritin found in the intramitochondrial space – Storage protein

Table 1. Proteins involved in iron transportation and metabolism.

death.[5] Therefore, unavailability of extracellular iron, and consequently intracellular iron deprivation, results in impaired DNA synthesis, and the cell cycle progression is arrested at the transition from G1 to S phase. Studying gene expression profile alterations in the HL-60 cell line, it has been demonstrated that, under iron-deprived conditions 11 of 43 genes are >50% inhibited. These genes are Rb, $p21^{WAF1/CIP1}$, bad, cdk2, cyclin-A, -D3, -E1, c-myc, egr-1, iNOS and FasL, all of which are essential for cell-cycle regulation and apoptosis.[6] Apoptosis of the HL-60 cells, induced by iron deprivation, was not attributed to decreased bcl-2 or c-myc expression, but to the activation of the cyclin-dependent inhibitor $p21^{WAF1/CIP1}$.[5,7] However, although this metabolic step has long ago been recognized, it appears that additional key-points of cellular growth and development, exist, still vaguely known, which are controlled by intracellular iron and iron-containing proteins, since in some cases cell cycle arrest may also occur at the transition from the G2 to M phase.[7]

Iron is highly toxic for biologic substrates, due to its high oxidative potential and its ability to generate Reactive Oxygen Species (ROS) according to the Haber-Weiss reaction: ($O_2^- + H_2O_2 \Rightarrow HO + O_2 + HO^-$).[8] The major amount of intracellular iron is stored in ferritin, and the major cellular part of active iron implementation is the mitochondria. Iron is transported in the endomitochondrial space, with the assistance of the specific transporter mitoferrin and is stored in a specific type of ferritin, the mitochondrial ferritin.[9] In the mitochondria, iron participates as coenzyme in the respiratory chains enzynes, the cytochromes, and in the formation of heme, which is incorporated in the other heme-containing proteins, hemoglobin and myoglobin. In the cytoplasm iron is usually found in the endosomes, loosely bound with transferrin, and ready to be transported to specific substrates, in various as yet poorly-defined proteins and molecules and is stored in ferritin. All the sources of non-ferritin bound iron are collectively defined by the term intracellular labile iron.[10,11,12]

Iron is a major regulator of the cell cycle, by intervening with the formation and activity of the cyclin/cyclin-dependent kinase complexes. Depletion of intracellular iron by various iron chelators leads to cell cycle arrest, particularly in the G1 and the S phase, by producing an allosteric inhibition of cyclin-A, cyclin-E, and of cdc2 and cdk2. Moreover, it decreases intracellular levels of cyclin-D and cdk4 and changes retinoblastoma protein phosphorylation.[13] In neuroepitheliomatous cells iron depletion reduces the expression particularly of the group D cyclins, and affects also negatively the expression of other cyclins.[14] Iron chelators enhance the expression of several genes, involved in the down-regulation of cell cycle progression, such as WAF1 and GADD45, in a p53-independent mechanism.[15] In addition, cdc2 (p34) protein levels, which regulate the checkpoint of the G2/M phase transition, are decreased following incubation with iron chelators.[16] A group from Sydney, Australia, specialized on iron metabolism has reported that iron depletion with deferroxamine (DFO) is associated with substantial decrease of cyclin D1 levels, through post-transcriptional modification of the protein, in a ubiquitin-independent manner, in contrast to what happens under normal conditions, in which cyclin D1 is cleared through proteasomal degradation.[17] However, the expression of other cyclins, such as cyclin-E may be induced by iron deprivation, but since this cyclin form complex with cdk2, whose expression is down-regulated, the final result is again cell cycle arrest.[16]

Excluding cyclins and cdks, many other cytoplasmic biological pathways are severely modified in relation to the concentration of intracellular iron. One of this is the retinoblastoma gene protein (pRb), which is a major regulator of the cell cycle. Under iron-deplete conditions pRp is hypophosphorylated, an effect probably mediated by lactoferrin (Lf), and cell cycle is arrested. Lf is also a cell cycle regulator. In MCF-7 cells it induces Akt phosphorylation, which is followed by phosphorylation of pRb and of two G1-checkpoint Cdk inhibitors, $p21^{Cip1/WAF1}$ and $p27^{kip1}$.[18] Hence the two inhibitors cannot cross nuclear membrane, remain in the cytoplasm and are degraded, whereas E2F transcription factor, the final inducer of the PI3K/Akt pathway, promotes the S phase entry. Lf-induced higher cytoplasmic localization of $p21^{Cip1/WAF1}$ levels are abolished when cells are treated with the PI3K inhibitor LY294002. Thus Lf behaves as an antagonist of the Cdk inhibitors.[19]

Other cell regulators, whose expression is influenced by the intracellular iron levels are p53 and Hypoxia-Inducing Factor-1α (HIF-1α). Iron is a cofactor of the enzyme HIF-1α prolyl hydroxylase, which down-regulates HIF-1α activity. Under iron-deprived conditions intracellular HIF-1α levels are increased, resulting in phosphorylation and stabilization of p53, whose levels are also increased. p53 in turn, induces transcription of the Cdk inhibitor $p21^{Cip1/WAF1}$, with the previously mentioned consequences.[20] Quercetin, a flavonoid antioxidant, strong metal chelator, increases and stabilizes HIF-1α levels in normoxia and inhibits cell proliferation, predominantly by decreasing the concentration of intracellular iron.[21] An additional cell cycle control system, influenced by the intracellular iron levels is accomplished by the cytochromes. In cells without a functional mitochondrial respiratory chain, and also in normal cells, quenching of mitochondrial ROS synthesis with MitoQ, the proliferation rate is delayed. In both cases important cell-cycle regulators such as cyclin D3, cdk6, p18^{INK4C}, p27^{KIP1} and p21$^{CIP1/WAF1}$are reduced. Therefore, functional loss of mitochondrial electron transport chain inhibits cell-cycle progression, and this may occur through the decreased concentration of ROS, leading to down-regulation of p21$^{CIP1/WAF1}$.[22]

Finally iron appears to influence also the mRNA translational process. A Japanese group investigated the interaction of the multifactorial Y-box-binding protein (YB-1), with the iron-regulatory protein-2 (IRP2) on translational regulation. Direct interaction of YB-1 and IRP2 is taking place in the presence of high iron concentration. YB-1 reduces the formation of the IRP2-mRNA complex, and both, YB-1 and IRP2 inhibit mRNA translation. However, co-administration of both proteins, abrogate the inhibitory effect of each protein alone. IRP2 binds to YB-1, in the presence of iron and a proteasome inhibitor. The interaction of these two proteins demonstrate the involvement of YB-1 and of an iron-related protein in the translational regulation.[23] The various intracellular signal pathways in which there is a known implication of iron are depicted in Table 2.

Activity	Mediator	Result
Inactivation of p21$^{CIP1/WAF1}$and p27^{kip1}	Uknown	Cell cycle progression, bcl-2 upregulation
Stabilization of cyclin D1 and -E	Uknown	Cell cycle progression, Bax downregulation
Stabilization of cdc2 (p34)	Uknown	G2 M phase progression
Activation of cyclin-A	Uknown	G1 S phase progression
P33/cdk2 complex formation	Uknown	G0 G1 phase progression
Phosphorylation of Rbp	Lactoferrin/Akt	Cell cycle progression
HIF-1α down-regulation	HIF-1$^{\alpha}$ hydroxylase	Inactivation of p53
Stabilization of mitochondrial electron transport chain	Frataxin	ROS production, cell growth
TB-1/IRP2 complex formation	Uknown	mRNA translation enhancement
Ribonucleotide Reductase	Direct action	Deoxyribonucleotide formation
PI3K/Akt phosphorylation	Uknown	Cell cycle progression, differentiation
NFκ-B nuclear maintenance/activation	Uknown	Transcriptional activation
Upregulation of IRF-1 gene expression	Uknown	Cytokines' gene expression
Upregulation of c-myc gene expression	Uknown	Cell proliferation

Table 2. Intracellular signal transduction pathways in which iron is implicated.

3. The role of iron in immune function

Since the majority of the effector functions of the immune system rely on the rapid development and fast proliferation of the immunocompetent cells, and taking into account the strong influence of cell growth, proliferation and differentiation by intracellular iron levels, it is self-evident that iron would exert significant regulatory role on the immune system. Moreover, since iron plays also a crucial role for the growth and development of many pathogens, a large variety of cellular mechanisms, dedicated to both, microbial growth and host defense, are orchestrated, upon a combat for iron acquisition or iron deprivation.[24]

The most primitive and less specific antimicrobial mechanisms of innate immunity are based on the development of proteins with high affinity to trivalent iron, such as transferrin (Tf) and Lf. These proteins are excreted by many cell types, but particularly by the neutrophils, to the extracellular space, bind iron from the circulating blood and tissues, thus creating an environment not favoring pathogens' growth. On the other hand, all pathogens elaborate specific iron-picking mechanisms from their environment, and in many instances also from the iron transporting proteins of the hosts, by synthesizing very high-affinity low molecular weight iron-chelators, the siderophores.

Lf, in addition to its iron-depriving properties, exerts various direct antimicrobial, antiviral, antifungal and antiparasitic activities. By directly interacting with the cellular surface, Lf inhibits microbial and viral adhesion, and consequently prevents the entrance to the host cells, probably by interfering to various glycosaminoglycan-type receptors and viral particles. It also acts at later phases, impairing viral DNA insertion and replication.[25] Degradation of Lf by some proteolytic enzymes, leads to the formation of lactoferricin, which shares stronger antimicrobial activity and inhibits the growth of many pathogens, included multiresistant strains of bacteria and fungi. Both, Lf and lactoferricidin can prevent bacteremia, following food contamination of milk-fed animals with strong pathogenic bacteria or fungi (*E.coli, Staph.aureus, C.albicans*) and protect the intestinal mucosa from injury.[26] Lf is also protective against the development of insult-induced *Systemic Inflammatory Response Syndrome* (SIRS) and its progression towards septic shock. This is accomplished through reduction or almost complete inhibition of the generation of intracellular and tissue oxidative stress, following LPS exposure, as measured by mitochondrial ROS expression, in a dose-dependent way. In vivo administration of Lf to experimental animals, significantly lowered LPS-induced mitochondrial dysfunction, estimated by decreased H_2O_2 release and mitochondrial DNA damage.[27]

More striking was the clarification of the ability of stress hormones and inotropes, to stimulate the growth of pathogenic bacteria. Using electron paramagnetic resonance spectroscopy and chemical iron-binding analyses it was demonstrated that catecholamines form direct complexes with Fe^{3+}, found within Tf and Lf. The formation of such complexes results in the reduction of Fe^{3+} to Fe^{2+} and the loss of protein-complexed iron. Both forms of iron, released from Tf or Lf is thereafter used as bacterial nutrient sources. Therapeutically relevant concentrations of stress hormones and inotropes in human serum could directly affect iron binding by Tf, so that the normally highly bacteriostatic tissue fluids may become significantly more supportive of the bacterial growth. The relevance of these catecholamine-Tf/Lf interactions to the infectious disease process is under ongoing research.[28]

Lf is also a very potent immunomodulator and anti-inflammatory protein.[29] It recognizes specific microbial molecules/receptors, named *Pathogen-Associated Molecular Patterns* (PAMPs), which are LPS from the gram-negative cell wall, and bacterial unmethylated CpG DNA, acting either as a competitor for these receptors, or as a partner molecule, depending on the physiological status of the organism. By interacting with proteoglycans and membrane receptors of many cells of the innate- and adaptive immune system (lymphocytes, antigen-presenting cells, endothelial cells), Lf modulates the migration, maturation and function of these cells, and thus influences both arms of immunity.[30] Bovine Lf attenuated Staphylococcal Enterotoxin B (SEB)-induced proliferation, IL-2 production and CD25 expression by transgenic mouse T-cells, an effect not induced through iron-deprivation of staphylococci, but by lactoferricin. Cytokine secretion, following SEB-stimulation by T-cell lines and by normal peripheral blood mononuclear cells, was also inhibited by Lf, suggesting a possible therapeutic applicability of this protein.[31] When given orally, Lf is easily uptaken by enterocytes, but also by the CD3+ lymphocytes of the lamina propria and the small intestinal submucosal tissue, and is mainly distributed in the cytosol. However, occasionally, it may also be distributed in the nucleus, suggesting that it might exert a direct regulatory role.[32]

Similar immunoregulatory properties have been postulated for Tf, which plays an essential role for normal T-lymphocyte growth and early differentiation. The absolute number of T-cells has been found substantially reduced in hypotransferrinemic $Trf^{hpx/hpx}$ mice, and this could not be attributed to increased apoptosis. Moreover, the differentiation of CD4-CD8-CD3-CD44-CD25+TN3 into CD4-CD8-CD3-CD44-CD25-TN4 cells was impaired, and a similar impairment of early T-cell differentiation was observed in mice with reduced levels of Tf receptor.[33]

The iron chelator DFO arrests cell cycle progression in activated T lymphocytes in the late G1 phase, before the G1/S border, by inhibiting transcription of the cdc2 gene, but has no effect on accumulation of cdk2, cdk4, or IL-2-transcripts. p34/cdc2 protein complex becomes undetectable, whereas synthesis of the p33/cdk2 protein begins and is activated as an H1 histone kinase, but this complex is insufficient to complete the G1 phase. Synthesis and early accumulation of cyclin E and cyclin E-dependent kinase are not affected by DFO, but cyclin A and cyclin A-dependent kinase are inhibited, although cyclin-A mRNA levels remain normal. Thus, DFO blocks cell cycle progression, through inhibition of cyclin A appearance, which is a major component of the p33/cdk2 complex.[34] DFO but not ferrioxamine (iron saturated DFO) inhibits growth and proliferation of the Jurkat T-cell line at the G0/G1 transition and induces apoptosis. However, iron-loaded Jurkat cells are not arrested. Silybin, a flavonoid antioxidant, free radical scavenger, acting also as iron chelator, shows a bimodal effect, inducing cell proliferation at low-, and DNA synthesis inhibition and apoptosis at high concentrations. The effect of silybin on the growth and viability of iron-loaded cells was similar to that of its iron complex, implying that the biological effects of silybin are different than those of DFO, and it probably shares pro-oxidant effect, via iron-catalyzed oxidation and generation of ROS.[35]

The high frequency of infections, reported in hemodialysis patients, when receiving intravenous (IV) iron preparations, revealed that IV iron administration is associated with time-dependent increases of the intracellular oxidative stress in many immunocompetent cell populations, resulting in dysfunctional cellular immunity. The CD4+ lymphocytes are mainly affected, with a statistically significant reduction in their survival after incubation with all doses of iron preparations. IV iron products induce also various deleterious effects on CD16+ lymphocyte populations, which may also be mediated by intracellular ROS formation.[36]

Iron tetrakis (N-methyl-4'-pyridyl-porphyrinato: FeTMPyP) is a potent antiinflammatory and scavenger of ROS. Treatment of thymocytes with FeTMPyP results in the inhibition of various mitogen-or cytokine-induced proliferation signals, and of the DNA-binding activity of NF-κB and IL-2 secretion. Inhibitors of p38-MAPK and of the ERK protein block the growth and proliferation of ConA-stimulated thymocytes, the NF-κB activation and IL-2 secretion.[37] Interferon regulatory factor-1 (IRF1) regulates the expression of genes involved in the inflammatory response and cell cycle control. IRF1 expression is transcriptionally mediated by TNF-α or IFN-γ, via iron-dependent pathways and is inhibited when cells are pretreated with iron chelators. Addition of exogenous iron reconstitutes cytokine responsiveness, indicating that iron is the target for the chelator effect.[38]

In addition to Lf, ferroportin (Fp), an iron efflux protein, strongly influences host response to infection. Murine macrophages overexpressing Fp show impaired intracellular *M.tuberculosis* killing at early stages of infection. When challenged with LPS or *M.tuberculosis* infection, control macrophages increase NO synthesis, but macrophages overexpressing Fp had significantly reduced NO and iNOS mRNA and protein production, thus limiting the bactericidal activity of these macrophages. IFN-γ reversed the inhibitory effect of Fp on NO production, findings suggesting a role for Fp in attenuating macrophage-mediated immune response.[39] Hepcidin, the allosteric inhibitor of Fp, regulates intracellular iron levels by interacting with, and promoting Fp degradation. All immunoregulatory cells express hepcidin mRNA; hepcidin mRNA expression increases after T-lymphocyte activation and in response to holotransferrin (Fe-Tf) or ferric citrate challenge. Therefore, low hepcidin expression impairs normal lymphocyte proliferation.[40]

Normal tissue macrophages are polarized, through the action of cytokines, into classically-(M1) and alternatively-activated (M2). M1 macrophages have low IRP-1 and -2 binding activity, express high levels of H-ferritin, low levels of Tf receptor-1 and internalize iron, only at high extracellular concentrations. Conversely, M2 macrophages have high IRP-binding activity, larger intracellular labile iron pool, express low levels of H-ferritin and high levels of Tf receptor-1, and effectively internalize and release iron, even at low concentrations. Iron export correlates with Fp expression, which is higher in M2 macrophages. In the absence of iron, only M1 macrophages are effectively activating antigen-specific, MHC class II-restricted T cells. Thus finally, cytokines control iron handling, by differentiating macrophages into a subset with relatively-low intracellular iron content (M1), or a relatively-high iron containing subset, endowed with the ability to recycle iron (M2).[41] Besides the classical mechanisms of antimicrobial activity (peptidic antibiotics, induction of oxidative stress, leading to respiratory burst) macrophages can deprive intracellular pathogens of necessary nutrients, and most importantly of iron. Moreover, according to the type of phagocytized pathogen, they can modulate, even the extracellular environment, impeding pathogens the access to essential nutrients. Thus various membrane transporters may remove nutrients from vacuolar compartments, degrade growth factors, and sequester other molecules, important for microbial growth, in a way similar to iron deprivation.[42]

Iron deficiency has been associated with various immune abnormalities, and particularly with impaired lymphocyte proliferation. T-cells from iron deficient mice exhibit poorer monocyte stimulatory activity following Con-A activation, as estimated by CD80 and CD86 expression on antigen presenting cells. The addition of DFO increased the expression of both markers on resting B and T cells. Lymphocyte proliferative responses to mitogens correlated positively with CD80 and CD86 expression, but negatively with the percentage of CD80+ cells. Therefore, the impaired lymphocyte proliferation of iron deficiency cannot be attributed to reduced CD80 and CD86 expression.[43]

The immunoregulatory properties of ferritin include binding to T lymphocytes, suppression of the delayed-type hypersensitivity and of antibody production by B lymphocytes, and impairment of phagocytosis by the granulocytes.

4. The role of iron in inflammatory and neoplastic diseases

Iron plays a major role in the generation and perpetuation of inflammatory processes. Many chronic inflammatory diseases are directly influenced by the intracellular and extracellular iron concentrations. Disease activity, and particularly the manifestation of serositris and various hematological disturbances in rheumatoid arthritis, systemic lupus erythematosous, Still's disease, dermatomyositis, and other collagen diseases are strongly correlated with serum and tissue ferritin levels.[44,45] Ferritin and iron homeostasis are implicated in the pathogenesis of many other disorders, including atherosclerosis, Parkinson's disease, Alzheimer disease, and restless leg syndrome. Iron contributes to the synthesis of myelin, and severely iron deficient patients exhibit impaired myelin formation. In patients with multiple sclerosis, serum and cerebrospinal fluid levels of Tf and ferritin levels have been found significantly elevated only during progressive active disease.[46] Brain tissue of patients with multiple sclerosis exhibits abnormal distribution of Tf and ferritin.[47] Ferritin binding to the inflammatory lesion and the immediate periplaque region within the white matter is practically absent, but returns to normal as the distance from the lesion increases. Therefore, the loss of ferritin binding is correlated with demyelination, accompanying multiple sclerosis.[48] Reactive Oxygen Species participate in the pathogenesis of allergic encephalomyelitis, whereas the infusion of apoferritin in experimental animals may induce a remission status.[49] Thyroid hormone upregulates ferritin genes' expression, and elevated serum ferritin levels have been reported in patients with subacute thyroiditis, which were correlated with disease activity. These levels were higher, as compared to patients with Graves' disease and Hashimoto's thyroiditis.[50]

Ferritin synthesis is regulated by the main proinflammatory cytokines (TNF-α, and IL-1α) at various levels (transcriptional, post-transcriptional, translational) during cellular development, differentiation and inflammation. Cytokine-induced cellular response to infection by various pathogens includes the upregulation of ferritin genes. Translation of ferritin is induced by IL-1β, IL-6 and TNFα, and iron is required for this regulation. Ferritin is accumulated in macrophages during various inflammatory conditions, when serum iron levels are decreased, leading to the formation of ferritin molecules with high content of iron.[51]

High heme oxygenase-1 (HO-1) expression, elevated ferritin accumulation in renal tubules and increased iron deposition in renal proximal tubules have been reported in patients with immunohemolytic anemia.[52] HO-1 degrades heme to biliverdin, carbon monoxide and free iron. HO-1 expression is induced among others, by proinflammatory cytokines and high intracellular ROS levels. This enzyme appears to have significant immunoregulatory properties, acting as inhibitor of immune reactions and participating in the pathogenesis of many inflammatory, infectious, allergic and autoimmune diseases and conditions, and has been proposed as a possible target inducing immunosuppression in allogeneic stem cell transplantation.[53]

Besides the stimulatory role on DNA synthesis, iron interferes with cell proliferation, by enhancing c-myc expression. Regulation of c-myc expression is crucial for the maintenance of cellular homeostasis. Overexpression or abnormal intracellular localization of c-myc results in the activation and deregulation of this oncogene. Surprisingly, when added to Burkitt's lymphoma cell lines, iron markedly inhibits cell proliferation, through cell cycle arrest in the G2/M transition, followed by a significant decrease in c-myc expression. A similar effect is not observed in cell lines with constitutive c-myc expression. Down-regulation of c-myc, which is independent from cell cycle blockade, leads to apoptotic cell death, implying the existence of another iron-dependent cell cycle regulatory mechanism, involving modulation of c-myc expression.[54]

Antisense oligodeoxynucleotide treatment against H- and L-ferritin chains increased the steady-state labile iron pool and the production of ROS after oxidative challenges and down-regulated Tf receptors, whereas it had no effect on the long-term growth of the cells. However, repression of ferritin synthesis facilitated renewal of the growth and proliferation of cells pre-arrested at the G1/S phase. Renewed cell growth was significantly less dependent on external iron supply, when ferritin synthesis was repressed, and its degradation was inhibited by lysosomal antiproteases.[55]

5. Iron and bacterial infections

Bacteria are confronted with a low availability of iron owing to its insolubility of the Fe^{3+} form, or its binding to host proteins. Free iron concentration in the host environment is about, or lower than 10^{-15}M and in some instances as low as 10^{-24}. Bacteria and other microorganisms need powerful and sophisticated mechanisms to acquire iron. Iron availability is a signal, alerting pathogenic bacteria, when they enter the hostile environment. When bacterial pathogens infect a host, cytotoxins damage the host cells releasing ferritin, hemolytic toxins lyse erythrocytes releasing hemoglobin, and Lf is produced by neutrophils and epithelial cells. The bacteria cope with the iron deficiency, by developing various uptaking systems: siderophores (low-molecular weight substances, with very high affinity for iron), systems for free heme and heme bound to hemoproteins (hemoglobin, hemoglobin-haptoglobin, heme-albumin, heme-hemopexin) and siderophore-based mechanisms to acquire iron from the iron-binding proteins Tf and Lf.

Pathogens encounter a period of iron starvation, upon entering their host and they sense alterations of the iron status, via the *Ferric Uptake Regulator* (FUR). The FUR protein plays a key role in the transcriptional response to iron of *Escherichia coli* and other gram-negative bacteria. The mechanism of action of FUR is repression of siderophore production and iron transport promoters. When iron is limiting, FUR protein is inactive as a repressor. This results in derepressed transcription of genes, involved in siderophore synthesis, and high-affinity iron uptake. FUR homologues are present in many bacteria.[56] In addition heme-sensing systems have been evolved by many pathogens, like *Staphylococcus aureus, Bacillus anthracis,* and *Corynebacterium diphtheriae.* For instance, *S. aureus* is able to sense heme through the heme sensing system (HssRS), two-component system that detect the presence of toxic levels of exogenous heme. Upon sensing heme, HssRS directly regulates the expression of the heme-regulated ABC transporter HrtAB, which alleviates heme toxicity.[57] In some halophilic bacteria, such as *Chromohalobacter salexigens*, iron homeostasis is coupled to the reaction to osmotic stress, through the activity of FUR. A decrease in iron and histidine requirements and a lower level of siderophore synthesis were observed at high salinity.[58]

Siderophores (named after the Greek word for iron carriers) are low molecular weight iron-binding complexes, produced and secreted by bacteria, fungi and plants. These molecules target ferric iron (Fe^{3+}), the form of iron found in well oxygenated environment in the host. Based on the metal chelating group, there are three major classes of microbial siderophores, the catecholate, the hydroxycarboxylate and the hydroxamate class. These substances exhibit extremely high affinity for iron, and hold it with three bidentate bonds. The high affinity is specific for iron, and does not extend to other bivalent cations. Siderophore production is enhanced in conditions of iron starvation, and many metabolic steps of their biosynthesis have been characterized. Siderophores have higher binding constants for iron, than do Tf and Lf, and thus are capable of detaching iron from these proteins. Their biosynthesis is confined to bacterial and fungal cells, and their expression increases the virulence of these species.[59] The most commonly encountered siderophores are described in Table 3.

Citrate
Hydroxamate class of siderophores
N,N'N''-triacetylfusarinine C
Rhodorotulic acid
Brucebactin (*Brucella abortus*)
Dihydrobenzoic acid (2,3-DHBA, *Brucella spp*)
Enterobactin (Dihydroxybenzoylserine, *E.coli*)
Enterochelin (*E.coli)*
Salmochelin (*Salmonella enteritidis, E.Coli spp, Klebsiella spp*)
Acinetobactin (*Acinetobacter baumannii*)
Pyoverdin *(Pseudomonas aeruginosa)*
Pyochelin *(Pseudomonas aeruginosa)*
Quinolobactin *(Pseudomonas aeruginosa)*
Bacillibactin (*Bacillus Anthacis, B.subtilis, other Bacillus spp)*
Petrobactin (*Bacillus Anthacis)*
Amphibactins
Agrobactin
Synechobactin
Ochrobactin
α-Hydroxycarboxylate and carboxylate class of siderophores
Aerobactin (*Vibrio spp)*
Anguibactin (*Vibrio anguillarum)*
Achromobactin *(Pseudomonas spp, marine microorganisms)*
Vibriobactin
Acinetoferrin (*Acinetobacter spp*)
Staphyloferrin (*Staph. aureus*)
Rhizoferrin
Vibrioferrin (*Marinobacter spp*)
Vanchrobactin (*Vibrio anguillarum*)
Amonabactin (*Aeromonas hydrophila)*
Mycobactin-T (*Mycobacterium Tuberculosis)*
Carboxymycobactin (*M. Tuberculosis* and other *Mycobactrerium spp)*
Yersiniabactin (*Yersinia enterocolitica)*
Rhizobactin (*Sinorhizobium meliloti)*
Desferrioxamines (A, B, C, D1, E, F, G)(*Actinomycetes spp*)
Ferric complexes of β-hydroxyaspartate
Aquachelins
Loihichelins
Marinobactins
Alterobactins
Ferrichrome class of siderophores (*Aspergillus, Ustilago, Penicillium etc*)
Ferricrocin
Ferrirubin
Ferrichrysin
Ferrirhodin
Ferredoxin
Rubredoxin
Asperchromes
Ferrichrome
Fusigen
Coprogen

Table 3. The major microbial sideropophores.

Iron loaded siderophores bind to cognate receptors, expressed at the bacterial surface. In gram negative bacteria, there is an outer membrane, external to a very thin (1-nm) peptidoglycan layer. Peptidoglycan is the structure that confers cell wall rigidity and resistance to osmotic lysis, in both, gram positive- and gram negative bacteria. In gram positive bacteria peptidoglycan is the only layered structure external to the cell membrane and is thick (20-80 nm). In gram negative bacteria the ferric-siderophores use outer membrane transporters, because they are large enough to pass through the porins (the small pores in the bacterial outer membrane that allow passive diffusion of molecules with molecular weight <600 Da).[60] The energy for the transport of these ligands across the outer membrane is delivered from the inner membrane, by a complex of three cytoplasmic membrane proteins TonB, ExbB, and ExbD.[61,62] TonB spans the periplasm, contacts outer membrane transporters by its C-terminal domain, and transduces energy from the proton motive force to the transporters. There is no need for TonB-ExbB-ExbD complex and outer membrane trasporters in gram-positive bacteria, as there is no outer membrane. Each class of siderophore is shuttled by a specific periplasmic binding protein (PBP) to the inner membrane. For example, FhuD is a siderophore binding PBP with a well-determined structure, found in gram negative and gram positive bacteria.[63] When iron-replete siderophores arrive at the microbial cytoplasmic membrane, they are taken up across the membrane by periplasmic binding protein-dependent ABC transporters in an ATP-dependent process. ABC trasporters comprise of two transmembrane domains forming a channel for the siderophore, to pass through and two nucleotide binding domains that hydrolyse ATP. The complex is internalised into the bacterium and the iron is released by proteolysis or by the action of enzymes that reduce Fe^{3+}. Fe^{2+} is incorporated into metalloenzymes or stored in bacterioferritin or in the related Dps proteins. The genes for siderophore biosynthesis and transport are usually under transcriptional control in response to the cellular pool of iron.

At the site of infection, leukocytes secrete siderocalin (also called lipocalin-2, neutrophil gelatinase-associated lipocalin). Siderocalin is also produced by epithelial cells and macrophages. Upon encountering invading bacteria, the Toll-like receptors on immune cells stimulate the transcription, translation and secretion of siderocalin. Secreted siderocalin then binds to ferric-siderophore complexes, participating in the antibacterial iron depletion strategy of the innate immune system.[64,65,66] However, pathogens produce structurally modified enterobactin-type siderophores, that are resistant to siderocalin and are known as stealth siderophores.[67] The first glucosylated siderophore described was salmochelin, a C-glucosylated enterobactin produced by *Salmonella* species, uropathogenic *Escherichia coli* strains, and some *Klebsiella* strains.[68]

Except of siderophores, gram positive and gram negative bacteria may use free heme or heme bound to host hemoproteins as iron source.[69,70] Like siderophores, this iron uptake pathway includes a TonB-dependent outer membrane receptor, while the transport across the cytoplasmic membrane requires periplasmic and inner membrane proteins comprising the ABC systems, which utilize the energy derived from ATP hydrolysis.[71] In addition, bacteria elaborate hemophores which are molecules that can remove heme from host hemoproteins. Bacterial hemophores are secreted to the extracellular medium, where they scavenge heme from various hemoproteins, due to their higher affinity for this compound, and return it to their specific outer membrane receptor.[72] An example is *Serratia marcescens,* that secretes a heme-binding protein, HasA, which functions as a hemophore that catches heme and shuttles it to a cell surface specific outer membrane receptor, HasR. The HasR receptor belongs to the TonB-dependent family of outer membrane receptors. HasAp, a gene from *Pseudomonas aeruginosa* has been isolated. HasAp is an iron-regulated extracellular heme-binding protein that shares about 50% identity with HasA and is required for *P. aeruginosa* utilization of hemoglobin iron.[73]

Pathways analogous to those described above are also utilized in gram-negative bacteria, for the uptake of iron from the iron-binding proteins Tf and Lf. Lf and Tf receptors are present in pathogenic bacteria.[74] Iron must be stripped away from Lf and ferritin prior to be transported into the bacterial cell. Two proteins, Tf-binding protein A (TbpA) and Tf-binding protein B (TbpB), function like the Tf receptor in many pathogenic bacteria, such as *Neisseria meningitides.* The expression of these genes is induced along with several other proteins under iron-restricted conditions.[70] Lf-binding protein A (LbpA) and Lf-binding protein B (LbpB) have been identified as outer membrane receptors for Lf. The extracted iron is then transfered into the periplasm. Within the periplasm, the ferric ion is complexed by ferric ion-binding protein A (FbpA). FbpA shuttles the iron to an inner membrane complex consisting of two proteins, the inner transmembrane FbpB and the cytoplasmic ATPase FbpC, finally transported into the cytoplasm.

Pseudomonas aeruginosa produces 2 siderophores under iron-limiting conditions, pyoverdine and pyochelin. Vanadium a rare metal, and probably other metallic ions, form complexes with both of these siderophores and strongly inhibit *P.aeruginosa* growth. Pyoverdin-deficient mice were more sensitive to vanadium, whereas pyochelin-negative mutants were more resistant. V-pyochelin strongly inhibits pseudomonas growth, increasing the activity of Superoxide Dismutase by about two times. Therefore, it appears that V-pyochelin catalyses a Fenton-type reaction, in which superoxide anion O^{2-} is generated, and vanadium compromises pyoverdin utilization.[75] However, in some pyoverdin deficient strains another siderophore molecule was identified, and this is quinolobactin. Its receptor is the 75-kDa iron-repressed outer membrane protein (IROMP) and the quinolobactin-mediated iron uptake system functions only in the absence of pyoverdine, and is repressed by pyoverdine.[76] Multicopper ferroxidases are enzymes that oxidize Fe^{2+} to Fe^{3+} in the microbial environment, so that iron will be transformed in a less active form, easily uptakable by microbial siderophores. *Ps. aeruginosa* possesses such an enzyme. Mutant strains are unable to grow with Fe^{2+} as iron source, because they cannot uptake iron. Thus multicopper ferroxidase represents another iron acquisition mechanism, important for virulence and pathogenicity of many bacteria.[77]

Some strains of *Vibrio anguillarum* produce a catechol-type siderophore named vanchrobactin, whose biosynthesis is under complex regulation, in an effort to adjust its production according to environmental iron concentrations.[78]

Although iron is important for all the scale of microorganisms, some types are less strictly dependent on iron than others. Moreover, growth characteristics and virulence of intracellular pathogens may vary, according to the type of infected cells. *Chlamydia pneumoniae* is an intracellular bacterium, causing chronic inflammatory disease in humans. When endothelial cells and monocytes were infected with *C.pneumoniae,* supplemented with iron and then stimulated with IFN-γ, iron had no significant effect on *Chlamydia* growth within monocytes, whereas on endothelial cells iron enhanced its proliferation and differentiation, and IFN-γ had an inhibitory effect. *C.pneumoniae* infection induced a pro-inflammatory immune response in monocytes, but not in endothelial cells and *Chlamydia* remains in a persistent-latent form within monocytes but it differentiates and proliferates within endothelial cells.[79]

Various drugs may interfere with the microbial-host battle for iron acquisition. The calcium channel blocker nifedipine enhances host resistance against intracellular pathogens, by restricting iron availability. In a murine macrophage cell line, nifedipine significantly reduced intracellular bacterial survival of *Salmonella Typhimurium* and *Chlamydophila pneumoniae*. Moreover, in mouse models of iron overload, nifedipine was capable of mobilizing tissue iron. When these mice were infected intraperitoneally with *Salmonella,* and subsequently treated with nifedipine for 3 consecutive days, bacterial counts in livers and spleens were significantly reduced and survival was prolonged, compared with placebo-treated animals. Nifedipine increased Fp expression in the spleen, whereas splenic levels of ferritin and serum iron concentrations were reduced. Therefore, nifedipine, and probably other drugs, may induce Fp expression, export iron from macrophages and thus restrict iron availability for intracellular pathogens.[80]

The *Brucella* spp are facultative intracellular pathogens. The two predominant host cell types inhabited by *Brucella* are macrophages and placental trophoblasts. These bacteria produce 2,3-dihydroxybenzoic acid (2,3-DHBA) in response to iron limitation *in vitro,* which functions as a siderophore.[81] In addition, *Brucella abortus* strain 2308 produces brucebactin, a more complex 2,3-DHBA-based siderophore.[82] It has been showed that these siderophores are not required for wild-type replication of *B. abortus* in cultured murine macrophages. Paulley et al showed that heme is an important iron source for the bacterium, during chronic infection. Heme has a key role during the stationary phase, allowing *Brucella* to maintain intracellular residence in host macrophages. Recent analysis of the known *Brucella* genome sequences revealed a homolog of the heme transporter *shuA* gene of *Shigella dysenteriae* and has been given the designation *bhuA* (Brucella heme utilization).[83,84] The gene encodes a TonB-dependent outer membrane heme transporter. In *Brucella* spp the genes involved in the transport of heme across the cytoplasmic membrane are located in an operon distant from the *bhuA* locus.[85] In other gram negative bacteria, the genes for the periplasmic binding protein-dependent ABC transporter, responsible for the transportation of heme across the cytoplasmic membrane, are located in an operon with the gene for the TonB-dependent outer membrane transporter.

6. Iron and mycobacterial infections

Mycobacterium tuberculosis (Mtb) has developed various means of attacking the host system. One such crucial strategy is the exploitation of the iron resources of the host system. When Mtb evade the mammalian immune system, it resides within macrophages in an early phagosome, whose maturation to the late phagosome and phagolysosome stages is blocked. The control of the intraphagosomal environment is crucial. Macrophages digest senescent erythrocytes and degrade heme, thus accumulating iron. Iron mainly egresses the macrophage bound to Tf, although a part of it is incorporated into ferritin in the cytosol. Other main iron sources for the macrophage are the hemoglobin-haptogobin complex, taken up via the hemoglobin scavenger receptor CD163 during hemolysis, and iron bound to Tf and Lf that enters macrophages, via the transferrin-transferrin receptor and lactoferrin receptor pathway, respectively.[71] Iron is exported from the cell via Fp-1 which is the receptor for hepcidin. In the presence of inflammation serum hepcidin is high and the binding to Fp induces conformational changes to this molecule, resulting in allosteric inhibition of its function, thus halting iron egress, and promoting internalization and degradation of Fp.[86,87]

Within its phagosome, Mtb acquires iron from the cytoplasmic sources or from the Tf/Tf-receptor complex.[88] By the time Mtb faces the low-iron environment of the phagosome, several Mtb genes, involved in the biosynthesis of siderophores, are induced. There is a dual mycobacterial siderophore system, made of mycobactins, the water-soluble carboxymycobactin, and the lipophilic mycobactin-T, which transfers iron captured by the hydrophilic carboxymycobactin, across the cell wall.[89] Mycobactin, except from participating in iron internalization, it prevents sudden influx of excess iron, when the metal becomes available. For the transportation across the cell membrane, a reductase converts Fe^{3+}-mycobactin to the Fe^{2+} form. The ferrous ion, possibly complexed with salicylic acid, is then shuttled across the membrane, either for direct incorporation into various porphyrins and apoproteins, or for storage of iron within the bacterial cytoplasm. The overall process of iron acquisition and utilization requires the activation of a number of mycobacterial genes. Mtb contains four potential iron-dependent regulators, belonging to two different families of metalloregulatory proteins. Two genes, *furA* and *furB*, encode proteins, belonging to the FUR family. The other two genes, IdeR and SirR are members of the DtxR (diphtheria toxin repressor) family. IdeR is an essential regulator with a major role in controlling iron metabolism, by repressing siderophore production, activating iron storage genes and positively regulating oxidative stress responses.[90] In Mtb-infected macrophages an upregulation of IdeR was found as part of the bacterial protective mechanism against iron-mediated oxidative stress.

Immune cell derived mediators control systemic and cellular iron homeostasis. On the other hand, iron affects the activity of transcription factors related to immune responses, and therefore, the secretion of cytokines.[91] Iron, directly inhibits the action of IFN-γ, which is crucial for the control of intracellular infections. In iron-loaded macrophages, an inhibition of IFN-γ mediated pathways is noted while intraphagosomal Mtb growth is stimulated.[92] However, IFN-γ activation of human monocytes decreases iron availability to Mtb.[93] Sow et al. examined the expression of hepcidin in macrophages, infected with Mycobacterium avium and Mtb and found that IFN-γ induced high levels of hepcidin mRNA and protein by pathways involving STAT1 activation and Toll-like receptors TLR2 and TLR4.[94,95]

Dietary iron overload, mainly in rural populations in sub-Saharan Africa, causing iron overload of macrophages and hepatocytes may increase the risk of tuberculosis. The incidence of tuberculosis has markedly increased the last decades, primarily as a result of the infection with the human immunodeficiency virus (HIV). Acquired immunodeficiency syndrome (AIDS) patients exhibit alterations in iron metabolism that lead to increased deposition of this element in the tissues. Such alterations may underlie the increased susceptibility of AIDS patients to mycobacterial infections. Many ongoing studies are aiming to investigate the Mycobacterial iron-acquisition pathways and their role in the treatment of tuberculosis e.g. synthesizing selective inhibitors of iron metabolism that may be helpful as chemotherapeutic agents. Table 4 resumes the most commonly encounterd iron uptaking mechanisms, during bacterial growth.

— Expression of receptors for iron containing proteins of the host (Transferrin, Lactoferrin, Hemoglobin)
— Adaptation of the expression of a polymorphic Tf receptor according to host's Tf structure
— Non-enzymatic reduction of Fe^{2+} to Fe^{3+} by 3-hydroxylanthranilic acid or melanin (*C.neoformans*)
— Enzymatic oxidation of the Fe^{2+} to Fe^{3+} out of bacteria in the surroundings (various ferroxidases)
— Production and release of iron-depleted siderophores and uptake of iron-saturated siderophores
— Expression of specific siderophore ligands in the outer surface of the bacterial membrane
— Production, release and uptake of heme-picking substances (ABC transporter HrtAB)
— Oxidation of heme by heme oxygenase and uptaking of the iron from the porphyrin ring
— Production and release of hemophores (removing heme from hemoproteins, for example HasA)
— Expression of specific hemophore ligands in the outer surface of the bacterial membrane (HasR)
— Elaboration of iron permease-ferroxidase complex (Ftr1-Fet3, Aft1-Aft2, CIR1, HapX/Php4)
— Production, release and uptake of specific protein iron transporters (Sit1 in C. *Glabrata*)
— Induction of iron-starving conditions in the host and upregulation of Tf receptor (Intracellular pathogens)
— Modulation of the IRPs and/or the IRE of critical genes of the host cells (Intracellular pathogens)

Table 4. Summary of the most common iron upatking mechanisms elaborated by pathogens.

7. Iron and fungal infections

The larger proportion of systemic fungal infections are opportunistic i.e. an important factor for their occurrence is a background of primary or secondary (in the majority of cases iatrogenic) immunosuppression. For all fungal pathogens iron is essential for many metabolic processes and the most intelligent and complex systems of iron acquisition from the host cells and tissues, is found among various fungal strains. Particularly for fungi, iron is a major virulence factor.[96] Many if not all, host-developed mechanisms of host defence against pathogenic fungi are orchestrated through iron deprivation. Lf, produced and released mainly by neutrophils and monocytes, represents the major fungistatic factor of human serum, milk and other fluids.[97]

Fungal pathogens require 10^{-7} to 10^{-6} M iron for their growth, and, therefore, serum and other biological fluids and tissues, containing $<10^{-15}$ and as low as 10^{-24} M of iron are normally fungistatic for all species, including Candida, Aspergillus and Zygomycetes.[98] The fungistatic properties of human serum are completely abolished by the in vitro addition of exogenous iron, and Candida albicans can grow in serum cultures with Tf saturation >90%, but not in serum with normal Tf saturation. Diseases and conditions, accompanied by a high iron burden have been associated with increased susceptibility to fungal infections. Among these are tissue hypoxia, diabetic ketoacidosis, acidosis of any other cause, tissue damage and necrosis, post-traumatic states or those induced by chemotherapy, hemochromatosis, liver disease and cancer. Patients with acute myelogenous leukemia or other hematologic malignancies have commonly an excess of iron, and particularly, non-transferrin-bound iron, which is further increased following chemotherapy,[99] either because of tissue damage or, in some cases, as a result of circulating iron complexes. Such complexes are produced by the leukemic cells and are liberated following their death, induced by chemotherapy. All the above, render leukemic neutropenic patients particularly vulnerable to fungal infections. Liver iron overload, in patients undergoing orthotopic liver transplantation, is also a predisposing factor for the development of invasive fungal infections, and such infections occur almost three times more commonly among transplanted patients with elevated levels of iron in the liver.[100]

Iron uptake by fungi is accomplished by specific transport systems, in which an initially Fe^{3+} form is reduced to Fe^{2+} iron, through the action of specific cell surface reductases (ferroxidases). Ferrous iron is then internalized by three different mechanisms. The first is achieved thank to the high affinity of the iron-containing ferroxidases for a specific type of fungal transport proteins, named permeases. The iron permease-ferroxidase complexes (Ftr1-Fet3) easily transverse the fungal wall and cell membrane, and iron is thereafter provided intracellularly. There are three types of specific transcriptional activators or repressors of the genes encoding ferroxidases and permeases, which modulate their expression under iron-deprived conditions: the Aft1 and Aft2 activators in *Saccharomyces cerevisiae* and other yeast, or the Cryptococcus iron regulator gene (CIR1) in *Cryptococcus neoformans*, the GATA-type repressors, such as Sfu-1, present in many fungal species and the HapX/Php4 in *Schizosaccharomyces pombe* and *Aspergillus* species. A second mechanism or iron acquisition involves the production of siderophores, which are excreted through the fungal wall in the deferric form, bind iron, and then are taken up by the fungi. Finally, a third mechanism is related to a fungal heme oxygenase, which takes up iron from heme.[101,102]

C. albicans possesses two high-affinity iron permease genes that are essential for its virulence. Iron permeases are encoded by iron-responsive genes, which are regulated by the specific transcriptional activator Hap43 and the repressor Sfu1. Deletion of these genes renders mutant strains non-virulent.[103] Various iron overload conditions enhance *C. albicans* growth and increase the mortality rate of infected mice. Elevated serum iron levels have been documented among patients with urogenital candidiasis. In *C. albicans* CIR1 is a gene regulating iron homeostasis, as well as calcium and cAMP signaling, cell wall integrity, and the expression of all virulence functions, including capsule and melanin formation and growth at host temperature. Hap43 protein is essential for the growth and virulence of *C.albicans* under low-iron conditions, and is accumulating in the nucleus. Hap43 is not required for iron acquisition, but it is responsible for repression of genes encoding iron-dependent proteins involved in mitochondrial respiration and iron-sulfur cluster formation. There is an association between Hap43 and the global corepressor Tup1 in response to iron deprivation.[104]

Sit1 is a combined siderophore-iron transporter, found in *C. glabrata*. For this yeast iron acquisition is necessary, not only for the growth and virulence, but also for maintaining its survival against the fungicidal activities of macrophages. Within the Sit1 transporter, a conserved extracellular *SIderophore Transporter Domain* (SITD) has been identified, that is critical for the ability of *C. glabrata* to resist macrophage killing. *C. glabrata* senses altered iron levels within the phagosomal compartment and Sit1 functions as a determinant of survival in a way that is dependent on the iron status inside the macrophage.[105]

Non-enzymatic reduction of ferric iron by 3-hydroxylanthranilic acid and melanin has been documented in *Cryptococcus neoformans*.[106] The expression of permease genes in *Aspergillus* and *zygomycetes* is upregulated during their growth and virulence.[107] The growth, survival and virulence of *Aspergillus fumigatus* and other mold species in serum is associated with the removal of iron from Tf and other iron-containing proteins.[108] This is accomplished by siderophores. HapX, a bZIP-type transcriptional regulator, is a very important gene, which sets up the adaptation mechanism to iron starvation in *A. fumigatus*. HapX represses all iron-dependent and mitochondrial-orchestrated metabolic activities, including respiration, TCA cycle, amino acid metabolism, iron-sulfur cluster formation and heme biosynthesis. Iron starvation induces significant modulation of the amino acid pool and HapX coordinates the production of siderophores and their precursor amino acid ornithine. HapX activity is restricted to iron-deplete conditions, therefore, HapX-deficiency causes significant attenuation of virulence in a murine model of aspergillosis.[109]

Fungal species are capable of synthesizing many different siderophores; however, the most important and most commonly found in *Aspergillus* and zygomycetes are N'',N', N-triacetylfusarinine C and ferricrocin. *Aspergillus* uses two iron uptake mechanisms, the reductase-permease complex and the siderophore-assisted mechanism.[110] The latter has been demonstrated in vitro, as holotransferrin, but not apotransferrin, supports the growth of *Aspergillus spp.* in iron-depleted serum culture systems. In such systems, siderophore production becomes evident following 10 h of incubation and reaches a peak at 20 h.[105] Nevertheless, not all species and strains produce siderophores. Some fungi use ferric reductases or low molecular mass iron reductants, to reduce ferric to ferrous iron, and extract it from the extracellular environment. Such mechanisms have been documented in *C. albicans*, *Histoplasma capsulatum*,[111] and in *Cryptococcus neoformans*.[112]

7.1 Iron metabolism in Zygomycetes

Zygomycosis is a difficult-to-treat systemic fungal infection, caused by the *zygomycetes*, and is associated with a high mortality rate, ranging from 50% to 100%. *Rhizopus oryzae* is the most common cause of zygomycosis. The disease is usually presented with the rhinocerebral form and is characterized by the propensity of *zygomycetes* for vascular invasion and dissemination, commonly resulting in thrombosis and tissue necrosis. The infection can rapidly extend from the paranasal sinuses to the oral cavity, to the orbit and intracranially, sometimes producing cavernous sinus thrombosis.[113] Zygomycosis almost always occurs among patients with a pre-existing immune defect, although rare cases have been reported among apparently normal individuals.[114] In the majority of cases, the course is rapidly progressive and eventually fatal, unless prompt treatment with high doses of liposomal amphotericin B (LAmB), in association with careful and may be repeated surgical debridement, can change the otherwise dismal clinical course.

Since the spectrum of diseases for which the use of immunosuppressive treatments, such as corticosteroids, cyclosporine, purine analogs (fludarabine, cladribine, nelarabin, pentostatin), rapamycin and mTOR inhibitors, various monoclonal antibodies (rituximab, bevacizumab, infliximab, basiliximab, Campath, etc) and allogeneic hematopoietic stem-cell transplantation has enlarged,[115] and since the use of systemic antifungal prophylaxis with agents that are ineffective against *zygomycetes*, mainly azole derivatives has increased, zygomycosis appears to be an emerging threat the last two decades.[116] Well-recognized predisposing factors for zygomycosis are diabetes mellitus (especially when complicated by ketoacidosis), treatment with corticosteroids, immunosuppression, prolonged leukopenia (neutropenia and lymphopenia), recent chemotherapy and tissue damage, history of allogeneic stem cell transplantation, chronic graft-versus-host-disease, and prolonged treatment with broad spectrum antibiotics and azole-type antifungal prophylaxis.

However, a common denominator of almost all of these conditions is the presence of excessive iron overload, either as high tissue iron burden, or as elevated serum Tf, and also as increased non-transferrin-bound iron.[117] In particular, it has been suggested that diabetic ketoacidosis and acidoses of any aetiology predispose to zygomycosis by facilitating the dissociation of iron from iron-carrying proteins, thus providing increased available free iron.[118] Elevated serum and tissue iron have a tremendous impact on the growth and development of *zygomycetes*.[119] There are reports of fast *Mucor* growth, with formation of intra-arterial thrombi, among immunocompromised patients with iron overload.[120,121] In a retrospective analysis of 263 allotransplanted patients, all five cases of invasive zygomycosis had significantly higher serum ferritin levels, Tf saturation, and number of previously transfused red blood cell units, as compared with matched controls. *Zygomycetes* possess a specific high-affinity iron permease gene (RFTR1), which has been characterized and cloned.[122] Analysis of the polymorphisms of this gene, has recently been proposed as a tool for the molecular identification of the different *zygomycete* species.[123] FTR1 is expressed during infection in diabetic ketoacidosis (DKA) and is required for full virulence of R.oryzae in mice. Disrupted FTR1 in multinucleated *R. oryzae* resulted in the inability of the fungus to segregate to a homokaryotic null allele. However, reduction of the relative copy number of FTR1-mRNA and inhibition of FTR1 expression by RNAi compromised the ability of *R. oryzae* to acquire iron in vitro and reduced its virulence in DKA mice. Importantly, passive immunization with anti-Ftr1p immune sera protected DKA mice from infection with *R. oryzae*.[124]

The well-documented and repeatedly reported increased susceptibility to zygomycosis of haemodialysis patients, during treatment with DFO, an iron chelator that is capable of removing tissue iron, initially appeared to be a paradox.[125,126] It became clear, however, that although DFO chelates iron, from the perspective of *zygomycetes* it is a xenosiderophore, as fungal siderophores have higher affinity for iron than DFO and therefore, are capable of easily and effectively detaching iron from it and providing it to the fungi.[101,126] This ability is particularly prominent in *zygomycetes*, and these species can remove 8-40 times greater amounts of iron from DFO than *A. fumigatus* and *C. albicans*, respectively. The rapid and effective iron uptake by *zygomycetes* results in rapid growth in serum. The growth of *Rhizopus rhizopodiformis* spores, isolated from a dialysis patient with zygomycosis while on DFO therapy, was studied in an iron-deficient medium, containing human serum at increasing concentrations, enriched with different concentrations of ferrioxamine. A serum concentration of 40% inhibited fungal growth by >50%. However, in the presence of serum, ferrioxamine produced significant growth stimulation at 24 h that persisted at 48 h (Figure 1).[127] Data from animal models emphasize the exceptional requirement of iron for *Rhizopus* pathogenicity, since administration of DFO or free iron worsens the survival of animals infected with *Rhizopus*, but not with *Candida*.[128] DFO can act as a xenosiderophore in *Rhizopus*, other members of the *Mucorales*, and probably other pathogenic fungi. It is assumed that fungal enzymes or siderophores are able to specifically bind to ferrioxamine and, because they have higher affinity for iron, strip iron from ferrioxamine and facilitate iron uptake by the fungi. A similar phenomenon does not take place with deferiprone.[129] The susceptibility of dialysis patients, treated with DFO, to zygomycosis could be attributed to the fact that uraemia results in significant retention of the iron-loaded ferrioxamine in the circulation, and that this is removed during dialysis, causing patients' serum to lose its fungistatic power and be transformed to a favourable culture medium for *zygomycetes*.[130]

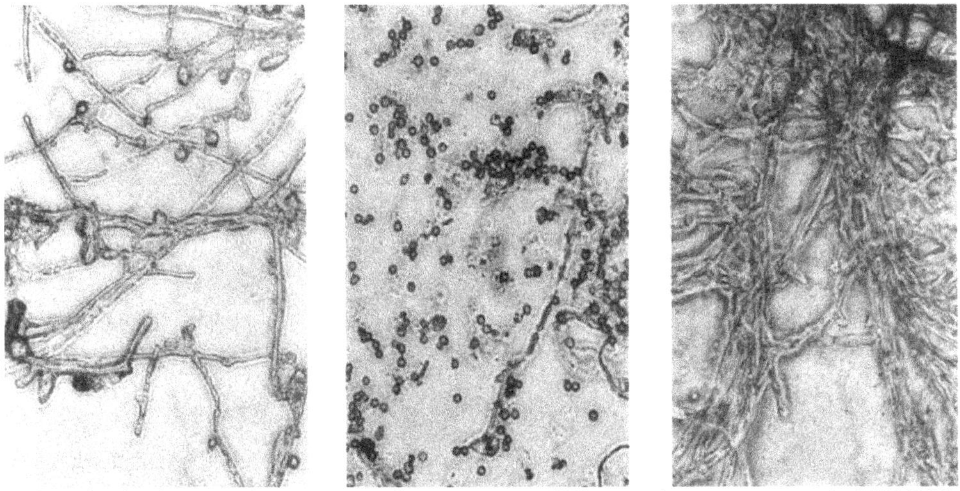

Fig. 1. Spores of Rhizopus were cultivated for 24 h at 370C in standard culture medium BDM alone (A), in BDM with 40% human serum (B) or in BDM with 40% serum + 1 MM Fe.DFO (C). Lugol stain x 500. Reprinted from Boelaert J et al. *J.Clin.Invest.* 1993; 91: 1979-1986.

7.2 The role of newer iron chelators

Since the mid-90's additional orally administered iron chelators are available. There are two newer molecules, deferiprone (DFP, Ferriprox, Apotex), which was introduced in the 1990s, and deferasirox (DFX, Exjade, Novartis), which was introduced more recently.[131] Both drugs are effective in clinical practice, but their use has not been associated with increased numbers of fungal infections and particularly, of zygomycosis. The reason for this discrepancy, as compared with DFO, may be the different chemical structure and chelating affinities of the three drugs. DFO is an exadentate chelator, has a higher molecular weight and shows a chelating relationship with the ferric iron of 1 : 1, which implies that each DFO molecule chelates one ferric ion. DFP is a bidentate chelator, and its chelating relationship is 3 : 1, meaning that each ferric iron is chelated by three molecules of DFP. DFX is a tridentate chelator, and its chelating relationship is 2 : 1, meaning that each ferric iron is chelated by two molecules of DFX.[132] The chemical structures of the three iron chelators are shown in Figure 2.

The two newer iron chelators do not act as xenosiderophores, apparently because the fungal iron uptake systems are incapable of detaching iron from them. This could be due, either to inadequate molecular access, since they are smaller molecules than DFO, or to their higher affinity for iron, which means that DFP and DFX might form more stable chemical structures with iron, that are not destabilized in the presence of fungal enzymes or siderophores. Moreover, the demonstration of clear inhibitory activity of the two newer chelators on fungal growth suggests that these molecules are probably capable of detaching iron from the fungal iron uptake molecules and holding it more strongly.[133] This has been proven in vivo, using animal models of zygomycosis, in which treatment of *Rhizopus*-

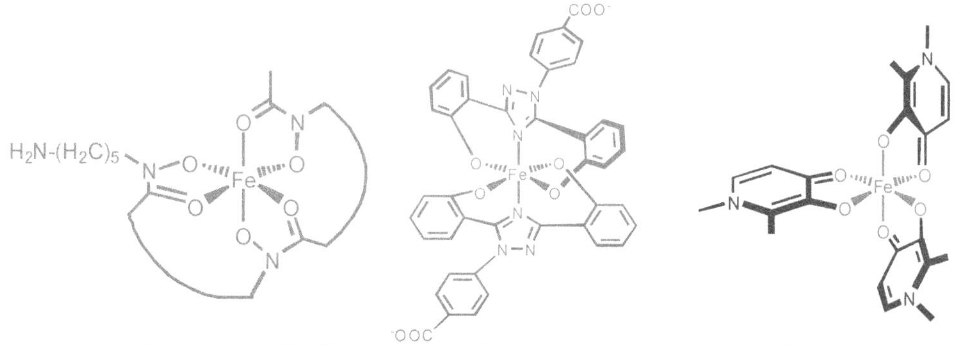

Deferroxamine (DFO) Deferasirox (DFX) Deferiprone (DFP)

Fig. 2. Stereochemical structure and mocecular chelating relationship of the three available iron chelators. Deferroxamine (DFO) has higher molecular weight (MW) and is a hexadentate, i.e. each molecule holds one ferric iron (chelating ratio 1:1). Deferasirox (DFX) has lower MW and it is a tridentate, i.e. 2 DFX molecules hold each ferric iron (chelating ratio 2:1). Deferiprone (DFP) has even lower MW and it is a bidentate, i.e. 3 DFP molecules chelate each ferric iron (chelating ratio 3:1).

infected mice or guinea pigs with DFP markedly improved survival.[133] In cultures of *Rhizopus oryzae*, DFP has fungistatic activity at 24 h, confirmed at 48 h.[129] The introduction of DFX and the recognition of the safety and efficacy profile of the drug encouraged its use in sporadic cases of systemic zygomycosis and in experimental animal studies. DFX induces an iron-starvation response in *R. oryzae* and activates RFTR1 expression. Addition of DFX to cultures of different members of the *Mucorales* produced a fungicidal effect, which was reversed by the addition of iron. The MIC90s of DFX against various *Mucor spp*. were much lower than the levels achieved by the administration of the usual daily dose of 20 mg/kg. Treatment with routine doses of DFX of diabetic ketoacidotic mice, infected with spores of *R. oryzae* led to significantly improved survival, as compared with controls, and resulted in a more than ten-fold reduction of brain and kidney fungal burden as compared with placebo-treated animals. The kidneys of DFX-treated mice had no visible hyphae and there was an effective neutrophil inflammatory reaction, whereas kidneys of placebo-treated mice had extensive filamentous fungi and manifested a poor or complete absence of a neutrophil inflammatory response.[134] In another experiment, mice infected intranasally with 10^7 spores of *R. oryzae* were treated for 7 days, starting 24 h post-infection, with either DFX 10 mg/kg twice daily or placebo. Similar to controls, infected or uninfected mice were treated with DFO 50 mg/kg. DFX was significantly more protective than placebo or DFO. As expected, DFO worsened the survival of infected mice, although it had no effect on uninfected mice. Treatment with DFX resulted in significantly increased Th1 and Th2 splenocyte subpopulations, and in significantly higher splenic and kidney levels of the proinflammatory cytokines TNF-α and IFN-γ, than those in mice treated with saturating iron or placebo.[134,135]

8. Iron, protozoan and parasitic infections

For the most intracellular protozoa, survival, growth and replication within the phagolysosomes of the macrophages is almost entirely relied on their successful iron acquisition from the host cells. These microorganisms elaborate elegant mechanisms for obtaining iron and transfer it into the iron-poor endophagosomal environment.

Legionella pneumophila requires iron for optimal extracellular and intracellular growth. Some mutants are both, sensitive to the iron chelators and resistant to streptonigrin, an antibiotic which requires high levels of intracellular iron to exert microbicidal activity. These mutants were about 100-fold more sensitive than the wild type to treatment with DFO, indicating that they have defective intracellular iron acquisition and assimilation. This strain was unable to mediate any cytopathic effect and was impaired for infectivity of an amoebal host.[136] *L.pneumophila* is engulfed into macrophages by macropinocytosis, and is not digested but proliferates intracellularly. Proliferation can be blocked by the Nramp1 protein, an iron transporter that reduces endolysosomal iron and confers resistance against invasive pathogens. However, inactivation of the PI3K pathway enhances *Legionella* infection and suppresses the protective activity of Nramp1. *L.pneumophila* abrogates phosphoinositide-dependent fusion of macropinosomes with acidic vesicles, without affecting Nramp1 recruitment. Thus *Legionella* escapes fusion with acidic vesicles and Nramp1-induced resistance to pathogens.[137]

For any protozoan pathogen iron is an absolutely necessary nutrient to effectively grow and multiply. On the other hand many antiparasistic immune effector mechanisms of innate and adaptive immunity are orchestrated through iron deprivation. Incubation of human enterocyte cell lines with IFN-γ and in vitro infection with the protozoan enteropathogen *Cryptosporidium parvum* resulted in the upregulation of IFN-γ receptors and was followed by inhibition of the parasite growth and development. IFN-γ mediated its action by inhibition of parasite invasion and by modification of intracellular Fe^{++} concentration, and this effect was partially reversed by inhibition of the JAK/STAT signaling pathway. IFN-γ directly induces enterocyte resistance against *C.parvum* infection.[138]

Toxoplasma gondii is an obligate intracellular parasite and a common opportunistic pathogen in HIV positive patients, and macrophage early nonspecific response is an important part of host defense. About 18 h following infection of mouse macrophages with a high burden of *T.gondii* tachyzoites, a strong down-regulation of the macrophage Tf receptor levels was observed. Stimulation of the mouse cells with toxoplasma lysate antigen had no effect on Tf receptor expression.[139] IFN-γ alone or in combination with IL-1, IL-6 or TNF-α significantly inhibited *T.gondii* growth in murine astrocytes. However this inhibition appear not to be mediated through induction of ROS expression, or iron deprivation, but by other, as yet unclear mechanisms.[140]

The in vitro growth of Pneumocystis Carinii can be easily suppressed by daphnetin (7,8-dihydroxycoumarin) a well-known iron chelator, through iron deprivation in a dose-dependent way. The inhibitory activity is not exerted when iron-repleted daphnetin is added to the culture system. Inhibition of *P.carinii* growth by daphnetin is associated with morphological changes, clearly determined by transmission electron microscopy.[141]

Leishmania donovani uses another mechanism to obtain iron from the labile iron pool of the macrophages. As a consequence, intracellular macrophage iron is depleted, iron sensor, through IRP-1 and -2 is activated, mRNA of the Tf receptor-1 is stabilized and is transcribed, Tf receptor expression is upregulated and Tf uptake is increased. Then Leishmania easily retrieves iron from holotransferrin.[142] *L. donovani* itself expresses a Tf receptor and their in vitro growth is inhibited by iron chelators. Moreover, in vivo administration of DFO in mice infected with Leishmania leads to a slight delay in the development of cutaneous lesions. Unexpectedly however, systemic iron delivery at early time points of infection, decreased parasite load at the site of parasite inoculation, the regional lymph node, the liver and spleen. The protective effect of iron correlated with lower IL-4 and IL-10, but higher type-1 cytokine transcripts (IFN-γ and inducible NO synthase) at the site of inoculation, as well as by increased serum levels of IgG2a.[143] An iron-dependent superoxide dismutase from *Leishmania Chagas* is expressed at low levels in the early logarithmic stage of development and increases at later stages of growth. The parasite demonstrates significant growth reduction when endogenous superoxide levels are increased, following the addition of paraquat in culture. There is a protective gene, LcFeSODB, which plays an important role in the parasite growth and survival by protecting the glycosomes from superoxide toxicity.[144]

Malnutrition alters the innate immune response against *L.donovani*. Thus, diets deficient in calories, protein, and in the metal elements zinc and iron represent a risk factor for the development of visceral leishmaniasis, and in malnourished mice, a greater parasite burden is found in the spleen and liver, which is attributed to a failure of lymph node barrier function. Lymph node cells from the malnourished group produced increased levels of PGE_2 and decreased levels of IL-10 and inducible NO synthase activity.[145] Iron deficiency may finally favor the host and impair *L.donovani* growth. When iron availability is restricted the parasite's growth may be reduced and the infection attenuated.[146]

Another *Leishmania spp*, *Leishmania amazonensis,* elaborates an inducible ferrous iron transport system through LIT1, a novel parasitic membrane protein. LIT1 is only detectable upon intracellular invasion of the parasite and its expression is accelerated under iron-deprived conditions. *L. amazonensis* lacking LIT1 protein abolishes its virulence and its replicating capacity within macrophages.[147]

Trichomonas vaginalis is the most common non viral pathogen, transmitted sexually and is highly-dependent on iron. *T. vaginalis* is adhered to vaginal epithelial cells, through specific surface proteins (AP65, AP51, AP33 and AP23) named adhesins. Free iron, heme and hemoglobin induce AP65 mRNA and protein expression on the parasistic membrane, thus favoring virulence. Heme-induced AP65 expression was about 10-fold higher in a low-iron culture medium, indicating that *T. vaginalis* can use heme as an alternative source of iron, important to its growth and regulation of expression of the adhesin genes.[148] An iron-responsive promoter and other iron regulatory elements (IRE) in the 5'-UTR of the ap65-1 gene, as well as two IRE-like hairpin-loop structures in mRNAs of TVCP4 and TVCP12 cysteine proteinases, have been identified in *T.vaginalis,* suggesting the existence of a post-transcriptional iron regulatory mechanism of critical genes by an IRE/IRP-like system in this protozoon.[149] DFO killed all *T.vaginalis* isolates with a minimum lethal concentration of 30 μM after 48 h of exposure, and a potent and persistent inhibitory effect of DFO on the parasite viability and growth was observed, with lower drug concentration and shorter time of exposure.[150]

Tritrichomonas foetus is a protozoan pathogen of cattle, and its growth and virulence is greatly influenced by the iron concentration of the culture medium. In iron-restricted media both, Lf and Tf support *T.foetus* growth. However, a specific binding to the outer parasitic membrane has been demonstrated only for Lf, whose uptake at 37^0 C is about 3.5-fold higher, a finding indicating a mechanism of receptor-mediated endocytosis. In contrast, Tf binding is nonspecific, and iron retrieval is achieved via extracellular release and siderophore assistance.[151] Many microbial siderophores can also support *T. foetus* growth under iron-limited conditions, providing iron to ferredoxin, the major siderophore of the parasite. Iron uptake is not mediated by previous extracellular reduction, although *T.foetus* possesses some ferrireductase activity. Siderophores are pinocytosed by the parasites in small vesicles, exhibiting a very acidic environment. Hemin also supports *T. foetus* growth, probably with the involvement of heme oxygenase.[152] Parasites grown in iron-depleted media exhibit reduced capability to destroy epithelial cell monolayers and reduced activity of several cysteine proteases, indicating that iron is an extracellular signal, modulating T.foetus' ability to interact with host epithelial cells.[153] In one study, mice inoculated intraperitoneally with a moderately- or a highly-virulent strain of *T.foetus* and treated with ferric citrate exhibited high mortality rate by the moderately-virulent strain up to the level of the highly-virulent strain. Peritoneal cultures showed that iron overload was associated with stimulation of parasite replication, which was strongly suppressed in untreated mice, and the less virulent strains showed lower efficiency for iron acquisition from Tf and other sources.[154]

The greatest experience about the influence of iron metabolism on parasite growth has emerged from the study of malaria infection. *Plasmodium* grows up fluently in the intraerythrocyte environment, where plenty of iron, contained in hemoglobin, can be easily accessed and uptaken. Since about 3 decades ago there has been emerging evidence that, iron deprivation might represent an important mechanism in the battle of man against malaria.[155] Asymptomatic parasitemia has been associated with the existence of hypochromic anemia, in the absence of a prominent acute phase reaction. These patients exhibit higher serum hepcidin concentration, higher ferritin, lower iron and transferrin levels, and lower transferrin saturation, and consequently have impaired intestinal iron absorption and dietary iron utilization. On the other hand malaria commonly coexists with a background of frank iron deficiency. Antimalarial treatment partly restores low-grade inflammation and decreases serum hepcidin, ferritin, and other indeces of inflammation, and should be preceded of any effort for anemia correction with iron. Clearance of parasitemia increases dietary iron absorption but did not affect systemic iron utilization. Therefore, in areas of high prevalence of malaria, since asymptomatic parasitemia has a protracted course, careful clinical evaluation of anemic patients is mandatory, because the unjustified or mistimed iron supplementation will be ineffective and may even be hazardous and render malaria symptomatic.[156, 157] Among pregnant women in areas with high malaria prevalence, malaria parasitemia, hookworm infection, gravidity and advanced gestational age were associated with lower hemoglobin and iron deficiency. Malaria parasitemia, *Ascaris lumbricodes* and *Trichuris trichiura* infections and older age were associated with lower serum ferritin levels.[158]

Intraerythrocytic malaria parasites digest hemoglobin to obtain the amino acids needed for their own protein synthesis. Hemoglobin degradation and total parasite protein content increase in parallel with parasite maturation, but the rate of hemoglobin degradation is higher, than the utilized amount of amino acids.[159] Hemoglobin degradation yields also large quantities of ferriprotoporphyrin IX and iron, which create a highly oxidative erythrocyte environment and high requirements for detoxification. Redox-active iron released inside the erythrocyte, mediate the conversion of H_2O_2 to hydroxyl radical $[HO]^-$ which is more reactive. Superoxide dismutase (SOD) and nitroxide SOD detoxifies the erythrocyte and acts similarly to the antimalarial drug 4-OH,2,2,6,6,tetramethyl piperidine-N-oxyl (Tempol) in *P.falciparum* growth. Tempol inhibits parasite growth, and induces accelerated mortality in a SOD-overexpressing mouse model of malaria.[160] SOD has therefore a protective role for the erythrocytes, and transgenic copper/zinc superoxide dismutase- - (CuZnSOD) mouse strains show higher sensitivity to infection by *Plasmodium berghei*. Moreover, treatment of infected erythrocytes, either SOD transgenic or normal, with oxidative stress inducers, reduces parasite viability. Therefore, CuZnSOD does not support plasmodium development, and impairment of its activity results in higher oxidative stress, favoring malaria growth.[161]

Iron deficiency modulates *Plasmodium yoelii* development in hepatocytes, by inactivating hepatic xanthine-oxidase. Iron-deficient mice infected with *Pl. yoelii* sporozoites, exhibited enhanced development of hepatic stage, resulting in the earlier appearance of blood parasites. An iron-starving diet increased penetration of sporozoites into liver cells, whereas inactivation of hepatic xanthine-oxidase inhibited both, sporozoite penetration and schizont maturation. Moreover, inhibition of heme synthesis also results in inhibition of parasite development.[162] Another mechanism, favorably influencing the clinical course of *Pl.falciparum* infection in iron deficient subjects, is the faster clearance of infected erythrocytes. Iron deficiency accelerates unifected erythrocyte death and enhances death and removal of infected erythrocytes by phagocytosis, which is evident from phosphatidylserine exposure. Indeed, parasitized iron deficient erythrocytes are more susceptible to phagocytosis in vitro, than normal erythrocytes.[163,164] The importance of iron in plasmodium growth has shifted antimalarial treatment strategies and research towards the identification and application of new drugs intervening with the parasite iron metabolism. More details on the topic are mentioned in the following paragraphs.

Trypanosomiasis or Chagas' disease has been associated with iron overload. *Trypanosoma* possesses a unique mechanism of adaptation and iron acquisition from the host environment. *Trypanosoma brucei* escapes destruction by the host immune system, by regularly replacing its *Variant Surface Glycoprotein* (VSG) coat. The VSG is expressed together with expression site associated genes, encoding the heterodimeric Tf receptor. There are about 20 VSG expression sites and trypanosomes can change the active site, according to environmental conditions. Since the various Tf receptor genes, localized in different expression sites, differ somewhat in sequence, expression site switching results in the production of a slightly different Tf receptor. Trypanosomes can adapt the expression site of its Tf receptor to achieve the highest affinity for the host Tf molecule.[165]

Hypochromic anemia is a dominant characteristic of this disease and its severity is correlated with the severity of trypanosomiasis. The parasite induces a strong type-I immune response, activating bone marrow and tissue macrophages and establishing an imbalance between erythropoiesis and erythrophagocytosis or erythroblastic apoptosis, which is the typical pathogenetic mechanism of anemia of chronic disease.[166] In a murine model of trypanosomiasis, erythrophagocytosis by cytokine-activated M1 macrophages was the main initial cause of aggressive anemia during the acute phase of infection. Persistence of type I cytokine production in the chronic phase of infection perpetuates and deteriorates anemia. Meanwhile, iron homeostasis is perturbed and there is increased iron sequestration by macrophages, resulting after upregulation of Fp, Tf and ceruloplasmin genes, indicating that iron export is reduced. In the chronic phase of trypanosomiasis, iron sequestration worsens, while the enhanced uptake of iron-containing molecules is maintained.[167]

Entamoeba histolytica trophozoites can grow in vitro within culture media, containing ferrous or ferric iron, and they can use hemoglobin, holotransferrin, hololactoferrin and ferritin as iron sources. Iron-binding proteins are specifically bound to the amoeba surface, are uptaken by endocytosis, traffick through the endosomal/lysosomal route and are degraded by neutral and acidic cysteine-proteases. Tf and ferritin are mainly uptaken as clathrin-coated vesicles. However, apolactoferrin bound to membrane lipids and cholesterol, induces cell death. In vivo trophozoites secrete products capable to destroy enterocytes, erythrocytes and hepatocytes, releasing Tf, hemoglobin, ferritin and other iron-containing proteins, which, together with Lf derived from neutrophils and acinar cells, can be used as iron supplies by amoebas.[168] Many biological functions and pathogenicity of the free-living amoeba *Naegleria fowleri* are dependent on the composition of the culture medium. The iron-containing porphyrins hemin or hematin or the iron-free protoporphyrin IX, can support *N.fowleri* growth in serum free media, whereas iron-binding proteins, including hemoglobin cannot.[169] Some growth-promoting factors for *Entamoeba* species are low molecular weight substances, found in cellular fractions of various cells, and are probably siderophores, such as ferredoxins and rubredoxin.[170]

Hookworm infection has been associated with growth delay and iron deficiency anemia. In a mouse model of this disease, infected animals, fed with a standard diet exhibited significant growth delay and reduced hemoglobin levels, compared to uninfected controls, whereas no significant difference in weight or hemoglobin concentration was observed between infected and uninfected animals, fed with an iron-restricted diet. Moreover, iron-restricted animals exhibited reduced intestinal worm burden, compared to animals fed with the standard diet. Finally, infected animals fed with intermediate-iron containing diet exhibited greater weight loss and anemia, than animals fed with iron-restricted- or high-iron diets. Mortality was also higher in the intermediate-iron containing diet. Therefore, severe dietary iron restriction impairs hookworm development, but moderate iron restriction enhances host susceptibility to severe disease.[171]

The human blood fluke *Schistosoma japonicum* is responsible for significant morbidity and mortality in tropical areas. For this fluke and some other invertebrates, an additional role for iron has been postulated, and this concerns the stabilization of the extracellular matrix. *Schistosoma* requires iron for its development and stores abundant iron in the vitelline (eggshell-forming) cells of the female system, in the form of yolk ferritin that is upregulated in females and is also expressed at low levels in egg-stages and adult males. Iron concentrations have been found higher in the female- than the male adult parasite, but also in the parasite eggs and purified eggshell, whose matrix is composed of heavily cross-linked eggshell precursor proteins.[172]

9. Clinical considerations - infections in iron overloaded patients

As previously noted, iron is crucial for the growth and proliferation of all microorganisms, due to its role in mitochondrial respiration and DNA synthesis. Iron starvation and oxidative stress are the hurdles that bacteria must overcome to establish an infection. In some cases there is excess iron available and specific infections are more common. Iron overload may be secondary to lysis of red cells from free heme compounds, as a result of trauma and due to altered metabolism (hemochromatosis, hepatic disease or post chemotherapy).

In the presence of hemolytic disorders, caused by malaria or *Bartonella bacilliformis* (in cases of Oroya fever) *salmonella* infections are noted.[173] The presence of free hemoglobin or heme may effectively impair or completely destroy the mechanism of natural resistance. Bullen et al. showed that ferric citrate, hematin hydrochloride, lysed guinea-pig red cells and crystalline human hemoglobin greatly enhanced *E. coli* virulence, when injected intraperitoneally into normal guinea-pigs.[174]

Blood transfusions may increase the free hemoglobin. Red blood cell transfusions should be used sparingly, keeping in mind the potential risks of infection and poor outcomes in critically ill patients. In a prospective, observational cohort study by Taylor et al. the posttransfusion nosocomial infection rate was 14.3% in 428 evaluable patients, significantly higher than that observed in nontransfused patients (5.8%; $p < 0.0001$).[175] In a multivariate analysis controlling for patient age, maximum storage age of red blood cells, and number of red blood cell transfusions, only the number of transfusions was independently associated with nosocomial infection (odds ratio 1.097; $p = 0.005$). In addition mortality and length of stay (in intensive care unit and hospital) were significantly higher in transfused patients, even when corrected for illness severity.[176] Secondary analysis of a multicentered, prospective observational study of transfusion practice in intensive care units in the United States showed that transfusion of packed red blood cells increases the risk of developing VAP (ventilator associated pneumonia). The effect of transfusion on late-onset VAP was more pronounced (odds ratio 2.16; 95% CI, 1.27-3.66) and demonstrated a positive dose-response relationship.[177] To determine whether blood transfusion influences infection after trauma, Agarwal et al. analyzed data on 5366 consecutive patients, hospitalized for more than 2 days. Even when patients were stratified by Injury Severity Score, the infection rate increased significantly with the higher numbers of transfused blood units. Blood transfusion in the injured patients is an important independent statistical predictor of infection. Its contribution cannot be attributed to age, sex, or the underlying mechanism of severity of injury.[178] Both, modified and native human hemoglobin may promote infection.[179] They showed that pyridoxalated polymerised human hemoglobin promotes fulminant *E. coli* septicemia in mice, which draws attention to the potential danger of such products in the clinic.

Hereditary hemochromatosis is the prototype disease for primary iron overload. *Vibrio vulnificus* has been linked to primary sepsis, which usually occurs in patients with underlying liver disease (cirrhosis or hemochromatosis).[180] Although this pathogen can be destroyed by human plasma, it multiplies rapidly when free iron is available. After eating raw sea food, like oysters, the patient develops high fever, prostration, hypotension and in most cases characteristic cutaneous manifestations (initially erythematous patches followed by ecchymoses, vesicles and bullae) with a mortality rate up to 50% without the prompt therapy. Primary hemochromatosis was the commonest underlying disease in patients with liver abscesses caused by *Yersinia enterocolitica*.[181] Some *Yersinia* strains are unable to synthesize siderophores but they can exploit host-chelated iron stores and the drug DFO. As a result, iron overload appears to be independent risk factor for *Y. enterocolitica* bacteremia, mainly by the serotypes O:3 and O:9. *Yersinia* bacteremia must be considered as an indicator of possible iron overload and *Yersinia* infection must be suspected in febrile hemochromatosic patients. In the past, patients with chronic renal failure, undergoing dialysis received multiple transfusions and frequent parenteral iron preparations. In a study by Boelaer *Yersinia* bacteremias (*Y. enterocolitica* and *Y. pseudotuberculosis*) were detected more often when ferritin levels were >500 ng/ml.[182] *Y. enterocolitica* has also been identified as a causative agent of posttransfusion septic shock. *Yersinia* bacteremias complicate the transfusions of blood that has been stored for more than 3 weeks.[183,184] The high-pathogenicity island (HPI), present in pathogenic *Yersinia* and encoding the siderophore yersiniabactin, has been found in *E. coli* pathotypes, responsible for bacteremias, neonatal meningitis and urosepsis.[185]

The spleen, an important part of the reticuloendothelial system, acts as a filter for circulating debris, including bacteria and as an important source of lymphoid cells and antibody production. Splenectomy may alter the ability to prevent or suppress some infections. There appears to be a high risk of severe bacterial infections when splenectomy is performed in patients with thalassaemia major, hepatitis, cirrhosis, histocytosis or inborn errors of metabolism.[186,187] Seventy three patients with β-thalassemia/HbE were studied 1-28 years after splenectomy. Serum ferritin levels in both, HbH and β-thalassemia/Hb E patients were higher than normal. They were higher in β-thalassemia/HbE than HbH disease. Most striking was the significantly higher serum ferritin levels in splenectomized patients with β-thalassemia/HbE disease than in the nonsplenectomized ones. After splenectomy, in patients with β-thalassemia/HbE disease, there was an increase of the Tf saturation in addition to increased circulating non-trasferrin bound iron.[188]

Levels of serum iron are elevated in patients undergoing hematopoietic stem cell transplantation (HSCT), as a result of disturbed iron metabolism, pre-transplantation blood transfusions, or cytotoxic therapy, for conditioning before HSCT. The complications of iron overload in HSCT patients include bacterial and fungal infections, mucositis, chronic liver disease (fibrosis progression), sinusoidal obstruction syndrome, and other regimen-related toxicities. Iron overload can be considered as an independent adverse prognostic factor in allogeneic HSCT. Screeneing for iron overload at various time points before and after transplantation may be beneficial especially in patients with thalassemia and myelodysplastic syndromes.[189]

Singh et al, assessed the role of hepatic explant iron overload as a risk factor for *Staph. aureus* bacteremia in liver transplant recipients. Noncarriers (patients without *S. aureus* nasal carriage) who developed *S. aureus* bacteremia were more likely to have hepatic iron overload. A quantifiable assessment of hepatic iron in patients without carriage at the time of transplantation can potentially identify those who may be at risk for early *S. aureus* bacteremia.[190] In healthy humans the lower respiratory tract as well as all mucosa, contains a very low free iron concentration (10^{-18} M), while in cystic fibrosis (CF) patients, sputum iron concentration is very high, showing a median value of 63×10^{-6} M. Accumulation of catalytic reactive iron contributes to subsequent clinical complications in the lung disorders by the production of ROS and increases bacterial growth and virulence. The iron-overload of the sputum of CF patients induces nonmotile forms, aggregation and biofilm formation both in *Pseudomonas aeruginosa* and *Burkholderia cenocepacia* which are the main pathogens in these patients, facilitating the penetration of host epithelial barriers and contributing to the establishment of infection, colonization, persistence and systemic spread of these pathogens.[191]

In human plasma, a fall in Eh (oxidation-reduction potential) or pH results in the abolition or marked reduction of its bactericidal properties. This is highly relevant to infection after trauma, where a fall in Eh and pH frequently accompanies tissue damage. Hypoxia interferes with the oxidative killing of many bacteria by polymorphonuclear leukocytes. In addition it produces a fall in tissue Eh and as a result free ferrous iron is produced, leading to overwhelming growth of bacteria. If the Eh is lowered, the ferric iron is reduced to the ferrous form, no longer bound to Tf.

The bactericidal power of fresh human plasma against *Klebsiella pneumoniae* and *E. coli* is extremely sensitive to changes in Eh and pH. At a high Eh (approx. +200 mV) the bacteria were destroyed, but rapid regrowth was observed when the Eh was lowered to -400 mV. Abolition of the bactericidal effect was also produced by adding ferric iron at a high Eh (approx. +200 mV). Lowering the pH to 6.5 reduced or prevented the bactericidal effect. Rising the Eh from -400 to +200 mV restored the bactericidal effect.[192] Some bacteria like *Cl. Perfringens* or *E. coli* have developed reducing systems. They may take advantage of a reduction in skin Eh and they are capable of lowering the Eh of tissue fluids to a level where Fe^{2+} is freely available. These results are probably related to the availability of iron for bacterial growth, and could be important for understanding the development of infection in injured or diseased tissue. Iron supplementation to treat anemia is controversial, since it may promote the progression of the underlying infectious disease but existing data are insufficient to support this hypothesis.[193]

10. Iron chelators as adjuvant treatment in systemic fungal and protozoan infections

It is self-evident if we take into consideration all the above, that an important weapon in the war against the various infectious microorganisms might be iron deprivation. Many efforts have been performed for this task, in targeting the appropriate microbial pathway, identifying the ideal compound for each microorganism, evaluating its efficacy, confirming its safety and testing its clinical usefulness. The usually acute clinical course of bacterial infections, the abundance of antibiotics and the relative satisfactory handling has restricted research programs testing iron chelators for fungal and protozoan infections and infestations.

Among fungal infections the most challenging is zygomycosis, for which effective treatment is still unavailable. Many studies, elaborating animal models for this disease have tried to address the efficacy of iron chelating agents, against this mycosis. In a mouse model of zygomycosis, animals were infected with *R. oryzae* spores, and 24 h later were treated with DFP at dose levels of 50, 100 or 200 mg/kg every day or every other day. The dose of 100 mg/kg every other day resulted in a significant survival advantage of DFP-treated mice, as compared with placebo-treated animals. The other dose schedules were either ineffective or toxic. The survival advantage was comparable to, although lower than, that of Liposomal Amphotericin-B (LAmB)-treated mice. Both drugs significantly reduced the brain fungal burden as compared with placebo. The beneficial effect of DFP was abrogated when animals were given ferric chloride.[133] In a similar mouse model of established zygomycosis, the administration of DFX was associated with comparable efficacy to that of LAmB. DFX has shown efficacy in neutropenic and diabetic ketoacidotic mice with zygomycosis. In these experiments, DFX at a daily dose of 20 mg/kg, starting 24 h after infection was synergistic with LAmB at a high-dose schedule of 15 mg/kg daily, in the reduction of fungal burden from the brain and the kidney. Moreover, the combination of the two drugs significantly improved survival time as compared with placebo or each drug separately.[134] Similar results have been obtained with the combination treatment in a mouse model of aspergillosis.[135]

The use of iron chelators as adjuvant treatment in systemic zygomycosis and other mycoses appears to be rational, and has been shown to be effective in sporadic cases. Reed et al. reported a case of a 40-year-old diabetic patient with aggressive rhinocerebral zygomycosis and progressive central nervous system involvement, despite combination treatment with high-dose LAmB plus caspofungin and surgical debridement. As brain magnetic resonance imaging (MRI) showed new parenchymal lesions and left cavernous sinus thrombosis, he was given a 7-day salvage treatment with DFX 1000 mg daily. A new brain MRI scan showed significant improvement, and treatment with LAmB was discontinued. The patient, 4 months later, remained in good condition without any neurological deficit. This is the first reported case of zygomycosis being successfully treated with a combination of classical antifungal treatment and an iron chelator.[194] We have recently treated two patients with acute lymphoblastic leukemia in remission (one of them following allogeneic transplantation) with zygomycosis (one with concurrent rhinocerebral and pulmonary form, the second with classical rhinocerebral form) with a combination of LAmB 10 mg/kg, posaconazole and DFX 20 mg/kg daily. Restricted intranasal and intrasinus surgical debridement was also applied repeatedly. Both patients responded very well, with rapid defervescence, resolution of pain and chymosis, and disappearance of the dense pulmonary and sinonasal infiltrates (unpublished data). Some more published cases have also shown encouraging results[195] however in other cases, iron chelation treatment was unsuccessful.[196]

Therefore, the possible benefit of iron chelation as adjuvant treatment in systemic mycoses, and particularly in zygomycosis, had to be tested in a prospective randomized trial. Such a clinical trial, the DEFEAT mucor study, investigated the existence of synergy between the classical treatment plus or minus DFX. Twenty patients with proven or probable zygomycosis were randomized to receive LAmB plus DFX (20 mg/kg/day for 14 days) or LAmB plus placebo. Surprisingly, death was more frequent in the DFX than in the placebo arm and global success was worse for the DFX arm, since patients of this arm had higher mortality rate at 90 days. This was attributed to population imbalances between the two arms, and therefore, make generalizable conclusions cannot be drawn.[197]

DFO, although is a xenosiderophore for *Zygomycetes*, may have direct and irreversible toxic effects on *P.carinii,* independently of iron chelation. This direct and irreversible damage of *P.carinii* by DFO was confirmed in vivo, in an animal model, in which a once-a-week aerosol treatment of PCP with DFO was effective in 100% of the animals, both as a prophylactic and as a curative treatment.[198]

All the available iron chelators can inhibit the growth of malaria parasites. Using a flow cytometric method for testing in vitro drug susceptibility of *Pl.falciparum* to hydroxypyridinone derivatives and to DFO, it has been found that both classes of chelators exhibited dose-dependent inhibition of parasite growth, but DFO demonstrated a stronger inhibitory effect. The MIC required for the parasite growth, correlated with observed abnormal microscopic morphology, and sensitivity to iron chelators was shown for both, chloroquine- and pyrimethamine-resistant parasites.[199] In another study, comparing the efficacy of DFO and DFX at 30 μM/l or 60 μM/l, added in cultures of *Pl. falciparum* in human erythrocytes, it was observed that DFX had marked antimalarial activity by 6 h after exposure, and over 48 h of culture, and although the IC50s were similar for DFX and DFO, malarial growth was significantly lower with DFX than with DFO at both concentrations (P=0.001).[200]

Dexrazoxane is an iron chelating prodrug, used for the protection of anthracyclin-induced cardiotoxicity, which must undergo intracellular hydrolysis to bind iron. Investigating the antimalarial properties of dexrazoxane on *Pl. falciparum* cultured in human erythrocytes, and on *P.yoelii* cultured in mouse hepatocytes, it was found that dexrazoxane inhibited *P. falciparum* growth, only at suprapharmacologic concentrations. In contrast, pharmacologic concentrations of dexrazoxane inhibited *P.yoelli* growth by 45-69%, implying the presence of a dexrazoxane-hydrolyzing enzyme in hepatocytes but not in erythrocytes or malaria parasites.[201] Novel aroylhydrazone and thiosemicarbazone iron chelators exhibit strong inhibitory activity on cultured tumor cells. These compounds were tested as antimalarials on chloroquine-sensitive- and -resistant strains of *Pl. falciparum*, and were significantly more active in both strains than DFO. The anti-malarial activity correlated with anti-proliferative activity against neoplastic cells. This class of lipophilic chelators may be potentially useful agents as anti-malarials.[202] Among various other synthetic siderophores the most promising profile (low MIC for plasmodia and minimum toxicity to mammalian cells) was demonstrated by an acylated monocatecholate or a triscatecholate as substituent.[203] To examine the site of action of antimalarial iron chelators, Loyevsky et al. have shown that specific fluorescence indicating the presence of iron chelators was observed within the parasites, implying that iron chelators bind labile iron within the plasmodium.[204]

The antimalarial activity of zinc-desferrioxamine (Zn-DFO) was found to be superior to that of DFO in vitro. A possible explanation is that the complex Zn-DFO might be more easily permeable into parasitized erythrocytes, exchange zinc for ferric ions due to higher affinity and deprive iron from the parasite. Parasites treated with Zn-DFO were less likely to recover at a later stage, in comparison to parasites treated with DFO, therefore, the complex Zn-DFO, which is more effective in vitro, should be examined for its in vivo activity.[205]

Many iron chelators are very effective in the treatment of trypanosomiasis and almost as effective as benznidazole, the classical drug used for the treatment of this disease. Some of them inhibit *T.Cruzi* growth at very low concentrations, thanks to their ability to interfere with and disrupt essential steps of epimastigote iron, copper or zinc metabolism at intracellular sites.[206] Eleven out of 13 other iron chelators inhibited trypanosoma growth in vitro, but many of these chelators were also cytotoxic for human HL-60 cells and therefore were not further tested. Newer, more specific, lipophilic iron-chelators may serve as lead compounds for novel anti-trypanosomal drug development.[207] Bloodstream forms of *T.brucei* are 10 times more sensitive than mammalian cells to iron depletion, and treatment with DFO inhibits parasite proliferation, inducing inhibition of DNA synthesis and decrease in oxygen consumption, findings implying that DFO impairs ribonucleotide reductase and alternative oxidase activity, apparently by chelating cellular iron and preventing its incorporation into the newly synthesized apoproteins. DFO treatment for 24 h has no effect on superoxide dismutase activity.[208] Three compounds of an aminothiol family of iron chelators were tested against *Trypanosoma Cruzi*. BAT-TE completely arrested the growth of trypomastigote forms in mouse blood, while BAT-TM arrested growth in *T.cruzi*-infected mice. These results render BAT derivatives potential candidates for the clearing of donated blood from trypomastigotes in endemic areas.[209]

11. References

[1] Thelander L, Graslund A, Thelander M. Continual presence of oxygen and iron required for mammalian ribonucleotide reduction: Possible regulation mechanism. Biochem Biophys Res Commun 1983; 110:859-865.

[2] Weiss G. Modification of iron regulation by the inflammatory response. Best Pract Res Clin Haematol 2005; 18: 183-201.

[3] Aisen P, Enns C, Wessling-Resnick M. (2001) Chemistry and biology of eukaryotic iron metabolism. Int. J. Biochem. Cell Biol. 2001; 33:940-959.

[4] Imlay JA, Chin SM, Linn S. Toxic DNA damage by hydrogen peroxide through the Fenton reaction in vivo and in vitro. Science 1988; 240:640-642.

[5] Gazitt Y, Reddy SV, Alcantara O, Yang J, Boldt DH. A new molecular role for iron in regulation of cell cycling and differentiation of HL-60 human leukemia cells: iron is required for transcription of p21(WAF1/CIP1) in cells induced by phorbol myristate acetate. J Cell Physiol. 2001; 187(1):124-135.

[6] Alcantara O, Kalidas M, Baltathakis I, Boldt DH. Expression of multiple genes regulating cell cycle and apoptosis in differentiating hematopoietic cells is dependent on iron. Exp Hematol. 2001; 29(9):1060-1069.

[7] Dong Fu, Richardson DR. Iron chelation and regulation of the cell cycle: 2 mechanisms of inhibitor p21CIP1/WAF1 by iron depletion post-transcriptional regulation of the universal cyclin-dependent kinase. Blood 2007; 110: 752–761.

[8] Kehrer JP. The Haber-Weiss reaction and mechanisms of toxicity. Toxicology 2000; 149(1):43-50.

[9] Shaw GC, Cope JJ, Li L, Corson K, Hersey C, Ackermann GE et al. Mitoferrin is essential for erythroid iron assimilation. Nature 2006; 440:96-100.

[10] Hentze MW, Muckenthaler MU, Andrews NC. Balancing acts: Molecular control of mammalian iron metabolism. Cell 2004; 117:285-297.

[11] Hentze MW, Kuhn LC. Molecular control of vertebrate iron metabolism: mRNA-based regulatory circuits operated by iron, nitric oxide, and oxidative stress. Proc Natl Acad Sci USA 1996; 93:8175-82.

[12] Napier I, Ponka P, Richardson DR. Iron trafficking in the mitochondrion: Novel pathways revealed by disease. Blood 2005; 105:1867-1874.

[13] Renton FJ, Jeitner TM. Cell cycle-dependent inhibition of the proliferation of human neural tumor cell lines by iron chelators. Biochem Pharmacol 1996; 51:1553-61.

[14] Gao J, Richardson DR. The potential of iron chelators of the pyridoxal isonicotinoyl hydrazone class as effective antiproliferative agents, IV: The mechanisms involved in inhibiting cell-cycle progression. Blood 2001; 98:842-50.

[15] Darnell G, Richardson DR. The potential of analogues of the pyridoxal isonicotinoyl hydrazone class as effective antiproliferative agents, III: the effect of the ligands on molecular targets involved in proliferation. Blood. 1999; 94:781-792.

[16] Kulp KS, Green SL, Vulliet PR. Iron deprivation inhibits cyclin-dependent kinase activity and decreases cyclin D/CDK4 protein levels in asynchronous MDA-MB-453 human breast cancer cells. Exp Cell Res 1996; 229:60-8.

[17] Nurtjahja-Tjendraputra E, Fu D, Phang JM, Richardson DR. Iron chelation regulates cyclin D1 expression via the proteasome: A link to iron deficiency-mediated growth suppression. Blood 2007; 109:4045-54.

[18] Wang G, Miskimins R, Miskimins WK. Regulation of p27(Kip1) by intracellular iron levels. Biometals. 2004; 17(1):15-24.

[19] Lee SH, Pyo CW, Hahm DH, Kim J, Choi SY. Iron-saturated lactoferrin stimulates cell cycle progression through PI3K/Akt pathway. Mol Cells. 2009; 28(1):37-42.

[20] Le NT, Richardson DR. The role of iron in cell cycle progression and the proliferation of neoplastic cells. Biochim Biophys Acta. 2002; 1603(1):31-46.

[21] Triantafyllou A, Liakos P, Tsakalof A, Chachami G, Paraskeva E, Molyvdas PA, Georgatsou E, Simos G, Bonanou S. The flavonoid quercetin induces hypoxia-

inducible factor-1alpha (HIF-1alpha) and inhibits cell proliferation by depleting intracellular iron. Free Radic Res. 2007; 41(3):342-56.
[22] Schauen M, Spitkovsky D, Schubert J, Fischer JH, Hayashi J, Wiesner RJ. Respiratory chain deficiency slows down cell-cycle progression via reduced ROS generation and is associated with a reduction of p21CIP1/WAF1. J Cell Physiol. 2006; 209(1):103-12.
[23] Ashizuka M, Fukuda T, Nakamura T, Shirasuna K, Iwai K, Izumi H et al. Novel translational control through an iron-responsive element by interaction of multifunctional protein YB-1 and IRP2. Mol Cell Biol. 2002; 22(18):6375-6383.
[24] Nevitt T. War-Fe-re: iron at the core of fungal virulence and host immunity. Biometals. 2011; 24(3):547-558.
[25] Berlutti F, Pantanella F, Natalizi T, Frioni A, Paesano R, Polimeni A, Valenti P. Antiviral properties of lactoferrin-a natural immunity molecule. Molecules. 2011; 16(8):6992-7018.
[26] Yen CC, Shen CJ, Hsu WH, Chang YH, Lin HT, Chen HL, Chen CM. Lactoferrin: an iron-binding antimicrobial protein against Escherichia coli infection. Biometals. 2011; 24(4):585-94.
[27] Kruzel ML, Actor JK, Radak Z, Bacsi A, Saavedra-Molina A, Boldogh I: Lactoferrin decreases LPS-induced mito-chondrial dysfunction in cultured cells and in animal endotoxemia model. Innate Immun. 2010; 16(2):67-79.
[28] Sandrini SM, Shergill R, Woodward J, Muralikuttan R, Haigh RD, Lyte M, Freestone PP. Elucidation of the mechanism by which catecholamine stress hormones liberate iron from the innate immune defense proteins transferrin and lactoferrin. J Bacteriol. 2010; 192(2):587-594.
[29] Actor JK, Hwang SA, Kruzel ML. Lactoferrin as a natural immune modulator. Curr Pharm Des. 2009; 15:1956-1973
[30] Legrand D, Mazurier J. A critical review of the roles of host lactoferrin in immunity. Biometals. 2010; 23(3):365-376.
[31] Hayworth JL, Kasper KJ, Leon-Ponte M, Herfst CA, Yue D, Brintnell WC et al: Attenuation of massive cytokine response to the staphylococcal enterotoxin B superantigen by the innate immunomodulatory protein lactofer-rin. Clin Exp Immunol. 2009; 157(1):60-70.
[32] Nielsen SM, Hansen GH, Danielsen EM. Lactoferrin targets T cells in the small intestine. J Gastroenterol. 2010; 45(11):1121-1128.
[33] Macedo MF, de Sousa M, Ned RM, Mascarenhas C, Andrews NC, Correia-Neves M. Transferrin is required for early T-cell differentiation. Immunology 2004; 112(4):543-549.
[34] Lucas JJ, Szepesi A, Domenico J, Takase K, Tordai A, Terada N, Gelfand EW. Effects of iron-depletion on cell cycle progression in normal human T lymphocytes: selective inhibition of the appearance of the cyclin A-associated component of the p33cdk2 kinase. Blood. 1995; 86(6):2268-2280.
[35] Gharagozloo M, Khoshdel Z, Amirghofran Z. The effect of an iron (III) chelator, silybin, on the proliferation and cell cycle of Jurkat cells: a comparison with desferrioxamine. Eur J Pharmacol. 2008; 589(1-3):1-7.
[36] Gupta A, Zhuo J, Zha J, Reddy S, Olp J, Pai A. Effect of different intravenous iron preparations on lymphocyte intracellular reactive oxygen species generation and subpopulation survival. BMC Nephrol. 2010; 11:16.
[37] Kang JL, Lee HS, Jung HJ, Kim HJ. Iron tetrakis (N-methyl-4'-pyridyl) porphyrinato inhibits proliferative activity of thymocytes by blocking activation of p38 mitogen-

activated protein kinase, nuclear factor-kappaB, and interleukin-2 secretion. Toxicol Appl Pharmacol. 2003; 191(2):147-155.
[38] Gira AK, Casper KA, Otto KB, Naik SM, Caughman SW, Swerlick RA. Induction of interferon regulatory factor 1 expression in human dermal endothelial cells by interferon-gamma and tumor necrosis factor-alpha is transcri-ptionally regulated and requires iron. J Invest Dermatol. 2003; 121(5):1191-1196.
[39] Johnson EE, Sandgren A, Cherayil BJ, Murray M, Wessling-Resnick M. Role of ferroportin in macrophage-mediated immunity. Infect Immun. 2010; 78(12):5099-5106.
[40] Pinto JP, Dias V, Zoller H, Porto G, Carmo H, Carvalho F, de Sousa M. Hepcidin messenger RNA expression in human lymphocytes. Immunology. 2010; 130(2):217-230.
[41] Corna G, Campana L, Pignatti E, Castiglioni A, Tagliafico E, Bosurgi L et al. Polarization dictates iron handling by inflammatory and alternatively activated macrophages. Haematologica 2010; 95(11):1814-1822.
[42] Appelberg R. Macrophage nutriprive antimicrobial mechanisms. J Leukoc Biol. 2006; 79(6):1117-1128.
[43] Kuvibidila SR, Porretta C. Differential effects of iron deficiency on the expression of CD80 and CD86 co-stimulatory receptors in mitogen-treated and untreated murine spleen cells. J Cell Biochem. 2002; 86(3):571-582.
[44] Yildirim K, Karatay S, Melikoglu MA, Gureser G, Ugur M, Senel K. Associations between acute phase reactant levels and disease activity score (DAS28) in patients with rheumatoid arthritis. *Ann Clin Lab Sci* 2004; 34:423-426.
[45] Lim MK, Lee CK, Ju YS, Cho YS, Lee MS, Yoo B, Moon HB. Serum ferritin as a serological marker of activity in systemic lupus erythematosus. *Rheumatol Int* 2001; 20:89-93.
[46] Sfagos C, Makis AC, Chaidos A, Hatzimichael EC, Dalamaga A, Kosma K, Bourantas KL. Serum ferritin, transferrin and soluble transferring receptor levels in multiple sclerosis patients. *Mult Sclerosis* 2005; 11:272-275.
[47] Izawa T, Yamate J, Franklin RJ, Kuwamura M.Abnormal iron accumulation is involved in the pathogenesis of the demyelinating dmy rat but not in the hypomyelinating mv rat. Brain Res. 2010; 1349:105-114.
[48] Hulet SW, Powers S, Connor JR. Distribution of transferring and ferritin binding in normal and multiple sclerotic human brains. J Neurol Sci 1999; 165:48-55.
[49] Levine SM, Maiti S, Emerson MR, Pedchenko TV. Apoferritin attenuates experimental allergic encephalomyelitis in SJL mice. Dev Neurosci 2002; 24:177-183.
[50] Sakata S, Nagai K, Maekawa H, Kimata Y, Komaki T, Nakamura S, Miura K. Serum ferritin concentration in subacute thyroiditis. Metabolism 1991; 40:683-688.
[51] Tran TN, Eubanks SK, Schaffer KJ, Zhou CY, Linder MC. Secretion of ferritin by rat hepatoma cells and its regulation by inflammatory cytokines and iron. Blood 1997; 90(12): 4979-4986.
[52] Fervenza FC, Croatt AJ, Bittar CM, Rosenthal DW, Lager DJ, Leung N et al. Induction of heme oxygenase-1 and ferritin in the kidney in warm antibody hemolytic anemia. Am J Kidney Dis. 2008; 52(5):972-977.
[53] Blancou P, Tardif V, Simon T, Rémy S, Carreño L, Kalergis A, Anegon I. Immunoregulatory properties of heme oxygenase-1. Methods Mol Biol. 2011; 677:247-268.

[54] Habel ME, Lemieux R, Jung D. Habel M, Lemieux R, Jung D. Iron specific growth inhibition of Burkitt's lymphoma cells in vitro, associated with a decrease in translocated c-myc expression. J Cell Physiol. 2005; 203(1):277-285.

[55] Kakhlon O, Gruenbaum Y, Cabantchik ZI. Repression of ferritin expression increases the labile iron pool, oxidative stress, and short-term growth of human erythroleukemia cells. Blood 2001; 97(9):2863-2871.

[56] Kadner R. Regulation by Iron: RNA rules the rust. J Bacteriol 2005; 187(20): 6870-6873

[57] Stauff DL, Skaar EP. The heme sensor system (HssRS) of Staphylococcus Aureus. Contrib Microbiol 2009;16: 210-135.

[58] Argandoña M, Nieto JJ, Iglesias-Guerra F, Calderón MI, García-Estepa R, Vargas C. Interplay between iron homeostasis and the osmotic stress response in the halophilic bacterium Chromohalobacter salexigens. Appl Environ Microbiol. 2010; 76(11):3575-3589.

[59] Neiland JB. Siderophores: structure and function of microbial iron transport compounds. J Biol Chem 1995; 270: 26723-26726.

[60] Ferguson AD, Chakraborty R, Smith BS, Esser L, van der Helm D, Deisenhofer J. Structural basis of gating by the outer membrane transporter FecA. Science 2002;295:1715-1719

[61] Ferguson A, Deisenhofer J. Metal import through microbial membrane.Cell 2004; 116: 15-24.

[62] Krewulak KD, Vogel HJ. Structural biology of bacterial iron uptake. Biochim Biophys Acta. 2008 ;1778(9):1781-804.

[63] Clarke TE, Ku SY, Dougan DR, Vogel HJ, Tari LW. The structure of the ferric siderophore binding protein FhuD complexed with gallichrome. Nat Struct Biol 2000; 7: 287-291.

[64] Goetz M, Bubert A, Wang G, Chico-Calero I, Vazquez-Boland JA, Beck M et al. Microinjection and growth of bacteria in the cytosol of mammalian host cells. Proc Natl Acad Sci U S A. 2001; 98(21):12221-12226.

[65] Borreqaard N, Cowland JB. Neutrophil gelatinase-associated lipocalin, a siderophore-binding eukaryotic protein. Biometals 2006; 19:211-215.

[66] Flo TH, Smith KD, Sato S, Rodriguez DJ, Holmes MA, Strong RK, Akira S, Aderem A. Lipocalin 2 mediates an innate immune response to bacterial infection by sequestrating iron. Nature 2004; 432:917-921.

[67] Fischbach MA, Lin H, Liu DR, Walsh CT. How pathogenic bacteria evade mammalian sabotage in the battle for iron. Nat Chem Biol 2006;2: 132-138.

[68] Müller SI, Valdebenito M, Hantke K. Salmochelin, the long-overlooked catecholate siderophore of Salmonella. Biometals 2009; 22(4):691-695.

[69] Wandersman C, Delepelaire P. Bacterial iron sources: from siderophores to hemophores. Annu Rev Microbiol 2004; 58:611-647.

[70] Perkins-Balding D, Ratliff-Griffin M, and Stojiljkovic I. Iron Transport Systems in *Neisseria meningitides*. Microbiol Mol Biol Rev 2004; 68(1):154-171.

[71] Nielsen MJ, Møller HJ, Moestrup SK. Hemoglobin and heme scavenger receptors. Antioxid Redox Signal. 2010; 12(2):261-273.

[72] Cescau S, Cwerman H, Létoffé S, Delepelaire P, Wandersman C, Biville F. Heme acquisition by hemophores. Biometals 2007; 20:603-613.

[73] Létoffé S, Redeker V, Wandersman C. Isolation and characterization of an extracellular haem-binding protein from Pseudomonas aeruginosa that shares function and sequence similarities with the Serratia marcescens HasA haemophore. Mol Microbiol. 1998; 28(6):1223-1234.

[74] Gray-Owen SD, Schryvers AB. Bacterial transferrin and lactoferrin receptors. Trends Microbiol 1996; 4:185-191.

[75] Baysse C, De Vos D, Naudet Y, Vandermonde A, Ochsner U, Meyer JM et al. Vanadium interferes with siderophore-mediated iron uptake in Pseudomonas aeruginosa. Microbiology 2000; 146 (Pt 10):2425-2434.

[76] Mossialos D, Meyer JM, Budzikiewicz H, Wolff U, Koedam N, Baysse C, Anjaiah V, Cornelis P. Quinolobactin, a new siderophore of Pseudomonas fluorescens ATCC 17400, the production of which is repressed by the cognate pyoverdine. Appl Environ Microbiol. 2000; 66(2).487-492.

[77] Huston WM, Jennings MP, McEwan AG. The multicopper oxidase of Pseudomonas aeruginosa is a ferroxidase with a central role in iron acquisition. Mol Microbiol. 2002; 45(6):1741-1750.

[78] Balado M, Osorio CR, Lemos ML. Biosynthetic and regulatory elements involved in the production of the siderophore vanchrobactin in Vibrio anguillarum. Microbiology 2008; 154(Pt 5): 1400-1413.

[79] Bellmann-Weiler R, Martinz V, Kurz K, Engl S, Feistritzer C, Fuchs D et al. Divergent modulation of Chlamydia pneumoniae infection cycle in human monocytic and endothelial cells by iron, tryptophan availability and interferon gamma. Immunobiology 2010; 215(9-10):842-848.

[80] Mair SM, Nairz M, Bellmann-Weiler R, Muehlbacher T, Schroll A, Theurl I et al. Nifedipine affects the course of Salmonella enterica serovar Typhimurium infection by modulating macrophage iron homeostasis. J Infect Dis. 2011; 204(5):685-694.

[81] López-Goñi I, Moriyón I. Production of 2,3-dihydroxybenzoic acid by *Brucella* species. Curr. Microbiol 1995; 31:291-293.

[82] González-Carreró MI, Sangari FJ, Agüero J, García Lobo JM. *Brucella abortus* 2308 produces *brucebactin*, a highly efficient catecholic siderophore. Microbiology 2002; 148:353-360.

[83] Halling SM, Peterson-Burch BD, Bricker BJ, Zuerner RL, Zing Z, Li LL, Kapur V, Alt DP, Olsen SC. Completion of the gene sequence of *Brucella abortus* and comparison to the highly similar genomes of *Brucella melitensis* and *Brucella suis*. J Bacteriol 2005; 187:2715-2726.

[84] Mills M, Payne SM. Identification of *shuA*, the gene encoding the heme receptor of *Shigella dysenteriae*, and analysis of invasion and intracellular multiplication of a *shuA* mutant. Infect Immun 1997; 65:5358-5363.

[85] Paulley JT, Anderson ES, Martin Roop II R. *Brucella abortus* requires the heme transporter BhuA for maintenance of chronic infection in BALB/c Mice Infect Immun 2007; 75:5248-5254.

[86] Hentze MW, Muckenthaler MU, AndrewsNC. Balancing acts: molecular control of mammalian iron metabolism. Cell 2004; 117:285-297.

[87] Nemeth E, Tuttle MS, Powelson J, Vaughn MB, Donovan A, Ward DM, Ganz T, Kaplan J. Hepsidin regulates cellular iron efflux by binding to ferroportin and inducing its internalisation. Science 2004; 306:2090-2093.

[88] Appelberg R. Macrophage nutriprive antimicrobial mechanisms. J Leukoc Biol 2006; 79:1117-1128.

[89] Ratledge C. Iron, mycobacteria and tuberculosis.Tuberculosis 2004; 84:110-130.

[90] Rodriguez GM, Voskuil MI, Gold B, Schoolnik GK, Smith I. *ideR*, an essential gene in *Mycobacterium tuberculosis*: role of IdeR in iron-dependent gene expression, iron metabolism, and oxidative stress response. *Infect Immun 2002;* 70:3371-3381.

[91] Ludwiczek S, Aigner E, Theuri I, Weiss G. Cytokine-mediated regulation of iron transport in human monocyte cells. Blood 2003; 101:4148-4154.
[92] Gomes MS, Boelaert JR, Appelberg R. Role of iron in experimental Mycobacterium avium infection. J Clin Virol. 2001; 20:117-122.
[93] Kahnert A, Seiler P, Sein M, et al. Alternativeactivation deprives macrophages of a coordinated defense program to *Mycobacterium tuberculosis.* Eur J Immunol 2006; 36:631-647.
[94] Sow FB, Florence WC, Satoskar AR, Schlesinger LS, Zwilling BS, Lafuse WP. Expression and localization of hepcidin in macrophages: a role in host defense against tuberculosis. J Leukoc Biol 2007; 82:934-945.
[95] Sow FB, Alvarez GR, Gross RP, Satoskar AR, Schlesinger LS, Zwilling BS, Lafuse WP. Role of STAT1, NF-kappaB and C/EBPbeta in the macrophage transcriptional regulation of hepsidin by mycobacterial infection and IFN-gamma. J Leukoc Biol 2009;86: 1247-1258.
[96] Weinberg ED. Iron availability and infection. Biochim Biophys Acta. 2009; 1790(7):600-605.
[97] Andersson Y, Lindquist S, Lagerqvist C, Hernell O. Lactoferrin is responsible for the fungistatic effect of human milk. Early Hum Dev 2000; 59: 95-105.
[98] Bullen JJ, Griffiths E. Iron binding proteins and host defence. In: Bullen JJ, Griffiths E, eds. 'Iron and infection.' Molecular, physiological and clinical aspects, 2nd ed. Chichester: Wiley, 1999; 327-368.
[99] Halliwell B, Aruoma OI, Mufti G, Bomford A. Bleomycin detectable iron in serum from leukaemic patients before and after chemotherapy. FEBS Lett 1988; 241: 202–204.
[100] Alexander J, Limaye AP, Ko CW, Bronner MP, Kowdley KV. Association of hepatic iron overload with invasive fungal infection in liver transplant recipients. Liver Transpl 2006; 12: 1799–1804.
[101] de Locht M, Boelaert JR, Schneider YJ. Iron uptake from ferrioxamine and from ferrirhizoferrin by germinating spores of Rhizopus microsporus. Biochem Pharmacol 1994; 47: 1843–1850.
[102] Nyilasi I, Papp T, Tako´ M, Nagy E, Vagvolgyi C. Iron gathering of opportunistic pathogenic fungi. A mini review. Acta Microbiol Immunol Hung 2005; 52: 185–197.
[103] Ramanan N, Wang Y. A high-affinity iron permease essential for Candida albicans virulence. Science 2000; 288: 1062–1064.
[104] Hsu PC, Yang CY, Lan CY. Candida albicans Hap43 is a repressor induced under low-iron conditions and is essential for iron-responsive transcriptional regulation and virulence. Eukaryot Cell. 2011; 10(2):207-225.
[105] Nevitt T, Thiele DJ. Host iron withholding demands siderophore utilization for Candida glabrata to survive macrophage killing. PLoS Pathog. 2011; 7(3):e1001322.
[106] Tangen KL, Jung WH, Sham AP, Lian T, Kronstad JW. The iron- and cAMP-regulated gene SIT1 influences ferrioxamine B utilization, melanization and cell wall structure in C. neoformans. Microbiology 2007; 153(Pt 1): 29–41.
[107] Hissen AHT, Wan AN, Warwas ML, Pinto LJ, Moore MM. The Aspergillus fumigatus siderophore biosynthetic gene sidA, encoding L-ornithine N5-oxygenase, is required for virulence. Infect Immun 2005; 73:5493–5503.
[108] Hissen AH, Chow JM, Pinto LJ, Moore MM. Survival of Aspergillus fumigatus in serum involves removal of iron from transferrin: the role of siderophores. Infect Immun 2004; 72:1402–1408.

[109] Schrett M, Beckmann N, Varga J, Heinekamp T, Jacobsen ID, Jöchl C et al. HapX-mediated adaption to iron starvation is crucial for virulence of Aspergillus fumigatus. PLoS Pathog. 2010 Sep 30;6(9):e1001124.
[110] Schrett M, Bignell E, Kragl C et al. Distinct roles for intra- and extracellular siderophores during Aspergillus fumigatus infection. PLoS Pathog 2007; 3: 1195–1207.
[111] Timmerman MM, Woods JP. Potential role for extracellular glutathione-dependent ferric reductase in utilization of environmental and host ferric compounds by Histoplasma capsulatum. Infect Immun 2001; 69: 7671–7678.
[112] Nyhus K, Wilborn AT, Jacobson ES. Ferric iron reduction by Cryptococcus neoformans. Infect Immun 1997; 65: 434–438.
[113] Anand VK, Alemar G, Griswold JA Jr. Intracranial complications of mucormycosis: an experimental model and clinical review. Laryngoscope 1992; 102: 656-662.
[114] Petrikkos G, Skiada A, Sambatakou H et al. Mucormycosis: ten-year experience at a tertiary-care center in Greece. Eur J Clin Microbiol Infect Dis 2003; 22: 753-756.
[115] Maertens J, Demuynck H, Verbeken EK et al. Mucormycosis in allogeneic bone marrow transplant recipients: report of five cases and review of the role of iron overload in the pathogenesis. Bone Marrow Transplant 1999; 24: 307-312.
[116] Spellberg B, Edwards JJ, Ibrahim A. Novel perspectives on mucormycosis: pathophysiology, presentation, and management. Clin Microbiol Rev 2005; 18: 556-569.
[117] Symeonidis A. The role of iron and iron chelators in zygomycosis. Clin Microbiol Infect. 2009; 15(s5): 26-32.
[118] Artis WM, Fountain JA, Delcher HK, Jones HE. A mechanism of susceptibility to mucormycosis in diabetic ketoacidosis: transferrin and iron availability. Diabetes 1982; 31: 1109-1114.
[119] McNab AA, McKelvie P. Iron overload is a risk factor for zygomycosis. Arch Ophthalmol 1997; 115: 919-921.
[120] Kubota N, Miyazawa K, Shoji N et al. A massive intraventricular thrombosis by disseminated mucormycosis in a patient with myelodysplastic syndrome during deferoxamine therapy. Haematologica 2003; 88: EIM13.
[121] Miyata Y, Kajiguchi T, Saito M, Takeyama H. Development of arterial thrombus of Mucorales hyphae during deferoxamine therapy in a patient with aplastic anemia in transformation to myelodysplastic syndrome [in Japanese]. Rinsho Ketsueki 2000; 41: 129-134.
[122] Fu Y, Lee H, Collins M et al. Cloning and functional characterization of the Rhiz. oryzae high affinity iron permease (rFTR1) gene. FEMS Microbiol Lett 2004; 235: 169-176.
[123] Nyilasi I, Papp T, Csernetics A, Krizsa´n K, Nagy E, Va´gvlgyi C. High-affinity iron permease (FTR1) gene sequence-based molecular identification of clinically important Zygomycetes. Clin Microbiol Infect 2008; 14: 393-397.
[124] Ibrahim AS, Gebremariam T, Lin L, Luo G, Husseiny MI, Skory CD et al. The high affinity iron permease is a key virulence factor required for Rhizopus oryzae pathogenesis. Mol Microbiol. 2010; 77(3):587-604.
[125] Boelaert JR, Fenves AZ, Coburn JW. Deferoxamine therapy and mucormycosis in dialysis patients: report of an international registry. Am J Kidney Dis 1991; 18: 660–667.

[126] Kaneko T, Abe F, Ito M, Hotchi M, Yamada K, Okada Y. Intestinal mucormycosis in a hemodialysis patient treated with desferrioxamine. Acta Pathol Jpn 1991; 41: 561-566
[127] Boelaert JR, de Locht M, van Cutsem J et al. Mucormycosis during deferoxamine therapy is a siderophore mediated infection: in-vitro and in-vivo animal studies. J Clin Invest 1993; 91: 1979-1986.
[128] Verdonck AK, Boelaert JR, Gordts BZ, Van Landuyt HW. Effect of ferrioxamine on the growth of Rhizopus. Mycoses 1993; 36: 9-12.
[129] Boelaert JR, Van Cutsem J, de Locht M, Schneider YJ, Crichton RR. Deferoxamine augments growth and pathogenicity of Rhizopus, while hydroxypyridinone chelators have no effect. Kidney Int 1994; 45: 667-671.
[130] Verpooten GA, D'Haese PC, Boelaert JR, Becaus I, Lamberts LV, De Broe ME. Pharmacokinetics of aluminoxamine and ferrioxamine and dose finding of deferrioxamine in haemodialysis patients. Nephrol Dial Transplant 1992; 7: 931-938.
[131] Neufeld EJ. Oral chelators deferasirox and deferiprone for transfusional iron overload in thalassemia major: new data, new questions. Blood 2006; 107: 3436-3441.
[132] Symeonidis A. The role of iron and iron chelators in zygomycosis. Clin Microbiol Infect. 2009; 15(s5): 26-32.
[133] Ibrahim AS, Edwards JE Jr, Fu Y, Spellberg B. Deferiprone iron chelation as a novel therapy for experimental mucormycosis. J Antimicrob Chemother 2006; 58: 1070-1073.
[134] Ibrahim AS, Gebermariam T, Fu Y et al. The iron chelator deferasirox protects mice from mucormycosis through iron starvation. J Clin Invest 2007; 117: 2649-2657.
[135] Ibrahim AS, Gebremariam T, French SW, Edwards JE Jr, Spellberg B. The iron chelator deferasirox enhances liposomal amphotericin B efficacy in treating murine invasive pulmonary aspergillosis. J Antimicrob Chemother. 2010; 65(2):289-292.
[136] Pope CD, O'Connell W, Cianciotto NP. Legionella pneumophila mutants, that are defective for iron acquisition and assimilation and intracellular infection. Infect Immun. 1996; 64(2):629-636.
[137] Peracino B, Balest A, Bozzaro S. Phosphoinositides differentially regulate bacterial uptake and Nramp1-induced resistance to Legionella infection in Dictyostelium. J Cell Sci. 2010; 123(Pt 23): 4039-4051.
[138] Pollok RC, Farthing MJ, Bajaj-Elliott M, Sanderson IR, McDonald V. Interferon-γ induces enterocyte resistance against infection by the intracellular pathogen Cryptosporidium parvum. Gastroenterology 2001; 120(1):99-107.
[139] Dziadek B, Dytnerska-Dzitko K, Długońska H. The modulation of transferrin receptors level on mouse macropha-ges and fibroblasts by Toxoplasma gondii. Pol J Microbiol. 2004; 53 Suppl:75-80.
[140] Halonen SK, Weiss LM. Investigation into the mechanism of gamma interferon-mediated inhibition of Toxoplasma gondii in murine astrocytes. Infect Immun. 2000; 68(6):3426-3430.
[141] Ye B, Zheng YQ, Wu WH, Zhang J. Iron chelator daphnetin against Pneumocystis carinii in vitro. Chin Med J (Engl). 2004; 117(11):1704-1708.
[142] Das NK, Biswas S, Solanki S, Mukhopadhyay CK. Leishmania donovani depletes labile iron pool to exploit iron uptake capacity of macrophage for its intracellular growth. Cell Microbiol. 2009; 11(1):83-94.

[143] Bisti S, Konidou G, Papageorgiou F, Milon G, Boelaert JR, Soteriadou K. The outcome of Leishmania major expe-rimental infection in BALB/c mice can be modulated by exogenously delivered iron. Eur J Immunol. 2000; 30(12):3732-3740.
[144] Plewes KA, Barr SD, Gedamu L. Iron superoxide dismutases targeted to the glycosomes of Leishmania chagasi are important for survival. Infect Immun. 2003; 71(10):5910-5920.
[145] Anstead GM, Chandrasekar B, Zhao W, Yang J, Perez L, Melby PC. Malnutrition alters the innate immune response and increases early visceralization following Leishmania donovani infection. Infect Immun 2001; 69(8):4709-4718.
[146] Malafaia G, Marcon Lde N, Pereira Lde F, Pedrosa ML, Rezende SA. Leishmania chagasi: effect of the iron deficiency on the infection in BALB/c mice. Exp Parasitol. 2011; 127(3):719-723.
[147] Huynh C, Sacks DL, Andrews NW. A Leishmania amazonensis ZIP family iron transporter is essential for parasite replication within macrophage phagolysosomes. J Exp Med. 2006; 203(10):2363-2375.
[148] Alderete JF, Nguyen J, Mundodi V, Lehker MW. Heme-iron increases levels of AP65-mediated adherence by Trichomonas vaginalis. Microb Pathog. 2004; 36(5):263-271.
[149] Torres-Romero JC, Arroyo R. Responsiveness of Trichomonas vaginalis to iron concentrations: evidence for a post-transcriptional iron regulation by an IRE/IRP-like system. Infect Genet Evol. 2009; 9(6):1065-1074.
[150] Mahmoud MS. Effect of the iron chelator deferoxamine on Trichomonas vaginalis in vitro. J Egypt Soc Parasitol. 2002; 32(3):691-704.
[151] Tachezy J, Kulda J, Bahníková I, Suchan P, Rázga J, Schrével J. Tritrichomonas foetus: iron acquisition from lactoferrin and transferrin. Exp Parasitol. 1996; 83(2):216-228.
[152] Sutak R, Chamot C, Tachezy J, Camadro JM, Lesuisse E. Siderophore and haem iron use by Tritrichomonas foetus. Microbiology. 2004; 150(Pt 12):3979-3987.
[153] Melo-Braga MB, da Rocha-Azevedo B, Silva-Filho FC. Tritrichomonas foetus: the role played by iron during parasite interaction with epithelial cells. Exp Parasitol. 2003; 105(2):111-120.
[154] Kulda J, Poislová M, Suchan P, Tachezy J. Iron enhancement of experimental infection of mice by Tritrichomonas foetus. Parasitol Res. 1999; 85(8-9):692-699.
[155] Weinberg ED, Moon J. Malaria and iron: history and review. Drug Metab Rev. 2009; 41(4):644-662.
[156] de Mast Q, Syafruddin D, Keijmel S, Riekerink TO, Deky O, Asih PB et al. Increased serum hepcidin and alterations in blood iron parameters associated with asymptomatic P.falciparum and P.vivax malaria. Haematologica 2010; 95(7):1068-1074.
[157] Cercamondi CI, Egli IM, Ahouandjinou E, Dossa R, Zeder C, Salami L et al. Afebrile Plasmodium falciparum parasitemia decreases absorption of fortification iron but does not affect systemic iron utilization: a double stable-isotope study in young Beninese women. Am J Clin Nutr. 2010; 92(6):1385-1392.
[158] Ndyomugyenyi R, Kabatereine N, Olsen A, Magnussen P. Malaria and hookworm infections in relation to hemoglobin and serum ferritin levels in pregnancy in Masindi district, western Uganda. Trans R Soc Trop Med Hyg. 2008; 102(2):130-136.
[159] Krugliak M, Zhang J, Ginsburg H. Intraerythrocytic Plasmodium falciparum utilizes only a fraction of the amino acids derived from the digestion of host cell cytosol for the biosynthesis of its proteins. Mol Biochem Parasitol. 2002; 119(2):249-256.
[160] Schwartz E, Samuni A, Friedman I, Hempelmann E, Golenser J. The role of superoxide dismutation in malaria parasites. Inflammation 1999; 23(4):361-370.

[161] Golenser J, Peled-Kamar M, Schwartz E, Friedman I, Groner Y, Pollack Y. Transgenic mice with elevated level of CuZnSOD are highly susceptible to malaria infection. Free Radic Biol Med. 1998; 24(9):1504-1510.
[162] Goma J, Renia L, Miltgen F, Mazier D. Effects of iron deficiency on the hepatic development of Plasmodium yoelii. Parasite 1995; 2(4):351-356.
[163] Koka S, Föller M, Lamprecht G, Boini KM, Lang C, Huber SM, Lang F. Iron deficiency influences the course of malaria in Plasmodium berghei infected mice. Biochem Biophys Res Commun. 2007; 357(3):608-614.
[164] Matsuzaki-Moriya C, Tu L, Ishida H, Imai T, Suzue K, Hirai M et al. A critical role for phagocytosis in resistance to malaria in iron-deficient mice. Eur J Immunol. 2011; 41(5):1365-1375.
[165] Gerrits H, Mussmann R, Bitter W, Kieft R, Borst P. The physiological significance of transferrin receptor variations in Trypanosoma brucei. Mol Biochem Parasitol. 2002; 119(2):237-247.
[166] Weiss G, Goodnough LT. Anaemia of chronic disease. N Eng J Med 2005; 352:1011-1023.
[167] Stijlemans B, Vankrunkelsven A, Brys L, Magez S, De Baetselier P. Role of iron homeostasis in trypanosomiasis-associated anemia. Immunobiology 2008; 213(9-10):823-835.
[168] López-Soto F, León-Sicairos N, Reyes-López M, Serrano-Luna J, Ordaz-Pichardo C, Piña-Vázquez C, Ortiz-Estrada G, de la Garza M. Use and endocytosis of iron-containing proteins by Entamoeba histolytica trophozoites. Infect Genet Evol. 2009; 9(6):1038-1050.
[169] Bradley SG, Toney DM, Zhang Y, Marciano-Cabral F. Dependence of growth, metabolic expression, and pathogenicity of Naegleria fowleri on exogenous porphyrins. J Parasitol. 1996; 82(5):763-768.
[170] Khalifa SA, Imai E, Kobayashi S, Haghighi A, Hayakawa E, Takeuchi T. Growth-promoting effect on iron-sulfur proteins on axenic cultures of Entamoeba dispar. Parasite 2006; 13(1):51-58.
[171] Held MR, Bungiro RD, Harrison LM, Hamza I, Cappello M. Dietary iron content mediates hookworm pathogenesis in vivo. Infect Immun. 2006; 74(1):289-295.
[172] Jones MK, McManus DP, Sivadorai P, Glanfield A, Moertel L, Belli SI, Gobert GN. Tracking the fate of iron in early development of human blood flukes. Int J Biochem Cell Biol. 2007; 39(9):1646-1658.
[173] Mabey DCW, Brown A, Greenwood BM. *Plasmodium falciparum* malaria and *Salmonella* infections in Gambian children. J Infect Dis 1987; 155:1319-1321.
[174] Bullen JJ, Leigh LC, Rogers HJ. The effect of iron compounds on the virulence of *Escherichia coli* for guinea-pigs. Immunology 1986; 15:581-588.
[175] Taylor RW, Manganaro L, O'Brien J, Trottier SJ, Parkar N, Veremakis C. Impact of allogenic packed red blood cell transfusions on nosocomial infection rates in the critically ill patient. Crit Care Med 2002; 30:2249-2254.
[176] Taylor RW, O'Brien J, Trottier SJ, Manganaro L, Cytron M, Lesko MF et al. Red blood cell transfusions and nosocomial infections in critically ill patients Crit Care Med. 2006;34(9): 2302-2308.
[177] Shorr, AF, Duh MS, Kelly KM, Kolief MH. Red blood cell transfusion and ventillator-associated pneumonia, a potential link? Crit Care Med 2004; 32:666-674.
[178] Agarwal N, Murphy JG, Cayten CG Stahl WM. Blood transfusion increases the risk of infection after trauma. Arch Surg 1993; 128:171-176.

[179] Griffiths E, Cortes A, Gilbert N, Stevenson P, MacDonald S, Pepper D. Haemoglobin-based blood substitutes and sepsis. Lancet 1995; 345:158-160.
[180] Chart H, Griffiths E. The availability of iron and the growth of *Vibrio vulnificus* in sera from patients with haemochromatosis. FEMS Microbiol Lett 1985; 26:227-231
[181] Vadillo M, Corbella X, Pac V, Fernandez-Viladrich P, Pujol R. Multiple liver abscesses due to *Yersinia enterocolitica* discloses primary hemo chromatosis: three case reports and review. Clin Infect Dis 1994; 18: 938-941.
[182] Boelaert JR, van Landuyt HW, Valcke YJ, et al. The role of iron overload in *Yersinia enterocolitica* and *Yersinia pseudotuberculosis* bacteremia in hemodialysis patients. J Infect Dis 1987; 156:384-387.
[183] Leclercq A, Martin L, Vergnes ML, Ounnoughene N, Laran JF, GiraudP, Carniel E. Fatal Yersinia enterocolitica biotype 4 serovar O:3 sepsis after red blood cell transfusion. Transfusion 2005; 45:814-818.
[184] Beresford AM. Transfusion reaction due to Yersinia enterocolitica and review of other reported cases. Pathology 1995; 27(2):133-135.
[185] Clermont O, Bonacorsi S, Bingen E. The Yersinia high-pathogenicity island is highly predominant in virulence-associated phylogenetic groups of Escherichia coli. FEMS Microbiol Lett. 2001; 196:153-157.
[186] Eraklis AJ, Brammer SR, Diamond LK, Gross RE. Hazard of overwhelming infection after splenectomy in childhood. N Engl J Med 1967; 267:1225-1229.
[187] Bishard N, Omari H, Lavi I Raz R. Risk of infection and death among post-splenectomy patients. J Infect 2001; 43(3):182-186.
[188] Pootrakul P, Rugkiatsakul R, Wasi P. Increased transferrin iron saturation in splenectomized thalassaemic patients. Br J Haematol. 1980; 46(1):143-145.
[189] de White T. The role of iron in patients after bone marrow transplantation. Blood Rev 2008; 22(suppl2): S22-28.
[190] Singh N, Wannstedt C, Keyes L, Mayher D, Tickerhoof L, Akoad M et al. Hepatic iron content and the risk of Staphylococcus aureus bacteremia in liver transplant recipients. Prog Transplant 2007; 17(4):332-336.
[191] Berlutti F, Morea C, Battistoni A, Sarli S, Cipriani P, Superti F et al. Iron availability influences aggregation, biofilm, adhesion and invasion of Pseudomonas aeruginosa and Burkholderia cenocepacia. Int J Immunopathol Pharmacol 2005; 18(4): 661-670.
[192] Bullen JJ, Spalding PB, Ward CG, Rogers HJ. The role of Eh, pH, and iron in the bactericidal power of human plasma. FEMS Microbiol Lett 1992; 94: 47-52.
[193] Weiss G. Modification of iron regulation by the inflammatory response. Best Pract Res Clin Haematol 2005;18: 183-201.
[194] Reed C, Ibrahim A, Edwards JE Jr, Walot I, Spellberg B. Deferasirox, an iron-chelating agent, as salvage therapy for rhinocerebral mucormycosis. Antimicrob Agents Chemother 2006; 50: 3968-3969.
[195] Ting JY, Chan SY, Lung DC, Ho AC, Chiang AK, Ha SY et al. Intra-abdominal Rhizopus microsporus infection successfully treated by combined aggressive surgical, antifungal, and iron chelating therapy. J Pediatr Hematol Oncol. 2010; 32(6):e238-240.
[196] Soummer A, Mathonnet A, Scatton O et al. Failure of deferasirox, an iron chelator agent, combined with antifungals in a case of severe zygomycosis. Antimicrob Agents Chemother 2008; 52:1585-1586.
[197] Spellberg B, Ibrahim AS, Chin-Hong PV, Kontoyiannis DP, Morris MI, Perfect JR et al. The Deferasirox-AmBisome Therapy for Mucormycosis (DEFEAT Mucor) study: a

randomized, double-blinded, placebo-controlled trial. J Antimicrob Chemother. 2011 (in press).
[198] Clarkson AB Jr, Turkel-Parrella D, Williams JH, Chen LC, Gordon T, Merali S. Action of deferoxamine against Pneumocystis carinii. Antimicrob Agents Chemother. 2001; 45(12):3560-3565.
[199] Pattanapanyasat K, Thaithong S, Kyle DE, Udomsangpetch R, Yongvanitchit K, Hider RC, Webster HK. Flow cytometric assessment of hydroxypyridinone iron chelators on in vitro growth of drug-resistant malaria. Cytometry 1997; 27(1):84-91.
[200] Goudeau C, Loyevsky M, Kassim OO, Gordeuk VR, Nick H. Assessment of antimalarial effect of ICL670A on in vitro cultures of Plasmodium falciparum. Br J Haematol. 2001; 115(4):918-923.
[201] Loyevsky M, Sacci JB Jr, Boehme P, Weglicki W, John C, Gordeuk VR. Plasmodium falciparum and Plasmodium yoelii: effect of the iron chelation prodrug dexrazoxane on in vitro cultures. Exp Parasitol. 1999; 91(2):105-114.
[202] Walcourt A, Loyevsky M, Lovejoy DB, Gordeuk VR, Richardson DR. Novel aroylhydrazone and thiosemicarbazone iron chelators with anti-malarial activity against chloroquine-resistant and -sensitive parasites. Int J Biochem Cell Biol. 2004; 36(3):401-407.
[203] Rotheneder A, Fritsche G, Heinisch L, Möllmann U, Heggemann S, Larcher C, Weiss G. Effects of synthetic siderophores on proliferation of Plasmodium falciparum in infected human erythrocytes. Antimicrob Agents Chemother. 2002; 46(6):2010-2013.
[204] Loyevsky M, John C, Dickens B, Hu V, Miller JH, Gordeuk VR. Chelation of iron within the erythrocytic Pl. falciparum parasite by iron chelators. Mol Biochem Parasitol. 1999; 101(1-2):43-59.
[205] Chevion M, Chuang L, Golenser J. Effects of zinc-desferrioxamine on Plasmodium falciparum in culture. Antimicrob Agents Chemother. 1995; 39(8):1902-1905.
[206] Rodrigues RR, Lane JE, Carter CE, Bogitsh BJ, Singh PK, Zimmerman LJ et al. Chelating agent inhibition of Trypanosoma cruzi epimastigotes in vitro. J Inorg Biochem. 1995; 60(4):277-288.
[207] Merschjohann K, Steverding D. In vitro growth inhibition of bloodstream forms of Trypanosoma brucei and Trypanosoma congolense by iron chelators. Kinetoplastid Biol Dis. 2006; 5:3.
[208] Breidbach T, Scory S, Krauth-Siegel RL, Steverding D. Growth inhibition of bloodstream forms of Trypanosoma brucei by the iron chelator deferoxamine. Int J Parasitol. 2002; 32(4):473-479.
[209] Deharo E, Loyevsky M, John C, Balanza E, Ruiz G, Muñoz V, Gordeuk VR. Aminothiol multidentate chelators against Chagas disease. Exp Parasitol. 2000; 94(3):198-200.

4

Cytotoxicity of *Aspergillus* Fungi as a Potential Infectious Threat

Agnieszka Gniadek
Department of Medical and Environmental Nursing, Faculty of Health Sciences, Jagiellonian University Medical College, Kraków, Poland

1. Introduction

Moulds constitute the largest group of bacteria, prevailing both in the indoor and outdoor air. Approximately 200 000 species of moulds have been identified so far, where only a small group of around 200 may present a threat to human health. Fungi from *Aspergillus* species are among the moulds considered to be most pathogenic. They also constitute the group of most pathogenic moulds most frequently isolated from the environment. Over 250 types of this species are known; about 50 of them were precisely described before the year 2000 (Klich, 2009). Pathogenicity, due to their toxicity, was also documented in other species: *Aspergillus fumigatus, Aspergillus flavus, Aspergillus ochraceus, Aspergillus niger, Aspergillus versicolor, Aspergillus parasiticus. Aspergillus nidulans, Aspergillus ustus, Aspergillus glaucus, Aspergillus clavatus, Aspergillus sydowii* and *Aspergillus terreus*. Their taxonomic identification is still an open topic because of their morphological variability and ability to produce metabolites; new species which exhibit adverse health effects to humans are constantly being detected. *Aspergillus lentulus* is one of the recently detected species of considerable clinical importance; it reveals similarity to *Aspergillus fumigatus*, one of the most pathogenic fungus for humans (Balajee et al., 2005).Table 1 presents the classification of species of fungi pathogenic to humans from the *Aspergillus* species. The list has been created by the authors of "Atlas Grzybów Chorobotwórczych Człowieka" ("Atlas of Fungi Pathogenic to Humans") (Krzyściak et al., 2011).

2. Fungal metabolites of *Aspergillus* species present a threat for human health

In their metabolic process, moulds produce mycotoxins. Those natural products, poisonous to humans and animals, are created as the result of a secondary metabolic process of fungi, when grown on organic substrates. Chemical structure of these metabolites varies, however, they are largely of small molecular mass, which conditions their varied toxic characteristics. So far over 400 metabolites produced by moulds have been identified from different genus of fungi: *Aspergillus* sp., *Penicillium* sp., *Fusarium* sp., *Alternaria* sp. *Trichothecium* sp. or *Stachybotrys* sp. Secondary metabolites of fungi from *Aspergillus* species are: ochratoxin A, aflatoxin B1, aflatoxins G1 and M1, trichothecenes, sterigmatosystin, patulins, gliotoxins or cyclopiazonic acid. Table 2 presents metabolites produced by the selected, most pathogenic

Subtype	Section	Teleomorph	Species linked to infections in humans
Aspergillus	*Aspergillus*	*Eurotium*	*A. chevalieri (Eurotium chavalieri)* *A. glaucus (Eurotium herbariorum)* *A. hollandicus (Eurotium amstelodami)* *A. reptans (Eurotium repens)* *A. rubrobrunneus (Erotium rubrum)* *A. sejunctus*
	Restricti		*A. caesiellus* *A. conicus* *A. pencilliodes* *A. restrictus*
Fumigati	*Fumigati*	*Neosartorya*	*A. fischerianus (Neosartorya fischeri)* *A. fumigatus* *A. fumisynnematus* *A. lentulus* *A. spinosus (Neosartorya spinosa)* *A. thermomutans (Neosartorya pseudofischeri)* *A. viridinutans* *Neosartorya coreana* – no confirmation of pathogenicity in humans *Neosartorya fennelliae* - no confirmation of pathogenicity in humans *Neosartorya hiratsukae* *Neosartorya udagawae*
	Cervini		
Ornati	*Ornati*	*Neocarpentels*	
Clavati	*Clavati*	n.n.	*A. clavatoanicus* *A. clavtus*
Nidulantes	*Usti*		*A. calidoustus* *A. deflectus* *A. ustus*
	Versicolores		*A. granulosus* *A. janus* *A. sydowii* *A. versicolor*
	Terrei	*Fennellia*	*A. alabamensis* *A. terreus*
	Flavipedes	*Fennellia*	*A. carneus* *A. flavipes* *A. niveus (Fennellia nivea)*
	Nidulantes	*Emericella*	*A. nidulans (Emericella nidulans)* *A. quadrilineata A. tetrazonus (Emericella quadrilineata)* *A. unguius (Emericella unguis)*
Circumdati	*Circumdati*	*Neopetrmyces*	*A. alutaceus* (isolated from sputum, pathogenicity not confirmed in humans) *A. ochraceus* *A. sclerotiorum*
	Flavi	*Petromyces*	*A. alliaceus* *A. avenaceus* *A. beijingensis*

			A. flavus var. *oryzae (A. oryzae* teleomorph: *Eurotium oryzae)* *A. flavus* *A. tamarii*
	Nigri	*Petromyces, Saitoa*	*A. (niger* var.*) awamori* *A. aculeatus* *A. atroviolaceus* *A. japonicus* *A. niger*
	Candidi		*A. candidus*
	Wentii	*Chaetosartorya*	
	Cremei		
	Sparsi		*A. wangduanlii*
Stilbothamnium			
Ochraceoroseus			
n.n.	*n. n.*		*A. qizutongii* *A. ochraceopetaliformis*

Table 1. Classification of pathogenic to humans *Aspergillus* species.

to humans *Aspergillus* species . (Krzyściak et al., 2011; Bräse et al., 2009; Skaug et al., 2001; Pitt et al., 2000; Smith et al., 1995)

No	Species	Metabolites
1	*Aspergillus fumigatus*	gliotoxin, verruculogen, fumitremorgin A and B, fumitoxin, tryptoguivaline, fumigallin, helvolic acid , sphingofungins, brevianamide A, coumarin
2	*Aspergillus flavus*	kojic acid, 3-nitropropionic acid, cyclopiazonic acid, aflatoxin B1, B2, G1, G2, aspergillic acid, violaxanthin, aspertoxin
3	*Aspergillus niger*	naphto-g-pyrones, malformin, ochratoxin A, toxic oxalates, violaxanthin
4	*Aspergillus ochraceus*	penicillic acid, ochratoxin A and B, xanthomeganin, viomellein, violaxanthin, circumdatin A, B, C
5	*Aspergillus versicolor*	sterigmatocystin, nidulotoxin, antrachinons, anthraquinoid
6	*Aspergillus candidus*	kojic acid, terphenyllin, candidulin, xanthoascin, beta nitropropionic acid
7	*Aspergillus terreus*	terreic acid, patulin, citrinin, citreoviridin, lovastatin, gliotoxin, terrain, patulin
8	*Aspergillus nidulans*	sterigmatocystin, penicillin, cotanin, nidulotoxin
9	*Aspergillus clavatus*	patulin, cytochalasin E, tryptoguivaline, kojic acid, clavatol, kotanin
10	*Aspergillus lentulus*	gliotoxin, cyclopiazonic terreic acid, neosartorin, auranthine and pyripyropenes A, E
11	*Aspergillus parasiticus*	Aflatoxins A1, B1, G1, G2

Table 2. Metabolites of selected species of *Aspergillus* fungi.

Natural metabolites produced by fungi are for the most part cytotoxic to different cellular structures and depress their key processes such as RNA and DNA synthesis (Burr, 2001). Mycotoxins differ with respect to their nature, action towards target cells, cellular structures and their internal processes. Best described mycotoxins produced by fungi of the *Aspergillus* species are aflatoxins and ochratoxins. Aflatoxins are highly saturated heterocyclic compounds which contain elements of furan. Ochratoxins constitute a group of poliketides derived from isocoumarin, related to L-phenylalanine. Degradation of ochratoxin A within the human body produces (4-R)-4 hydroxyochratoxin A and ochratoxin α, which create an albumin bond in the plasma. Creation of such bond facilitates the substances` persistence in the human body for an extended period of time (Budak, 1998).

Influence on the health in exposed individuals exerted by secondary metabolites includes carcinogenic, teratogenic, mutagenic, hepatotoxic and nephrotoxic action (it particularly concerns aflatoxin A_1 and ochratoxin A) (Fischer & Dott 2003;Burr, 2001). Sterigmatocystin is one of the aflatoxin precursors on its biosynthesis pathway and its carcinogenic action is only slighly lower than that of aflatoxin itself. Gliotoxin is considered to be responsive to immunosuppression and cellular apoptosis; it is also a likely virulence factor in mycoses caused by *A. fumigatus*. Gliotoxin is a very frequently detected toxin in the serum of patients suffering from aspergillosis. (Bok et al., 2005). This toxin is present in the serum of animals with a natural *A. fumigatus* infection and in cancer patients with invasive aspergillosis (Lewis et al., 2005).

This was confirmed in the findings obtained by Kupfahl, in which analysis of gliotoxin was performed in 158 *Aspergillus* strains (100 *A. fumigatus*) originating from patients with invasive aspergillosis and from the environment. During analysis of the strains and their ability to produce gliotoxin he discovered that gliotoxin was detected in the majority of *A. fumigatus* strains isolated both from clinical materials and from the environment (98% and 96% respectively) (Kupfahl et al., 2008).

The variety of metabolites produced by fungi of the *Aspergillus* species (*A. fumigatus* produces as well fumigallin, helvolic acid, tryptoguivaline, *A. candidus* kojic acid, terphenyllin, *A. ochraceus* penicillic acid or viomellein, while *A. niger* produces malformin) equips the fungi with multiple options of invading the host`s body, at the same time limiting the therapeutic options resulting from targeted prophylaxis. As it turns out, applying targeted chemoprophylaxis does not always prove to be effective, as the medicine does not affect all of the metabolites produced just by one strain of fungi (Bräse et al., 2009; Domsch et al, 2007; Ribeiro et al., 2005; Raper & Fennell, 1965).

3. Epidemiology of infection and clinical health outcome, as caused by fungi of the *Aspergillus* species

Fungi of the *Aspergillus* species are typical isogenic opportunistic bacteria, which for the most part fail to trigger an infection with a healthy person; however, they constitute a threat predominantly to persons with immunity disorders. Factors which facilitate the conditions necessary for a fungal invasion are: disturbances in the functions of T lymphocytes, phagocytes as well as the reticuloendothelial system, chemo- and radiotherapy, skin incisions related surgery, therapy or care. Risk factors for developing an invasive aspergillosis are chronic neutropenia (exceeding 3 weeks), corticosteroid treatment, hematological neoplasms, cytotoxic treatment, AIDS- Acquired Immune Deficiency Syndrome and bone marrow transplant. Certain influence has also been attributed to cytomegalovirus (CMV) contraction. Treatment with infliximab, a monoclonal antibody against tumour necrosis (TNFα), has been described in literature as being a determining factor for aspergillosis. Mechanisms, through which the predisposition factors intensify invasiveness of fungi of the *Aspergillus* species, act through or directly at the host, or the fungus, or both. Factors which determine pathogenicity of the *Aspergillus* fungi are multiple polar or neutral lipids, phenolic compounds and heterocyclic toxins (mycotoxins). An additional factor intensifying the pathogenicity of the *Aspergillus* fungi is their capacity to produce various proteolytic enzymes e.g. protease, which assist fungal colonisation in the infected host tissues (Türel, 2011; Kurnatowski &Miśkiewicz, 2009; Macura, 1998).

A source of infection with *Aspergillus* fungi may be another infected person, in whose body the fungal process develops, but primarily it is the hospital environment: air, water pipe system, ventilation system, hospital food as well as the medical equipment. For isogenic fungi of the *Aspergillus* type the obvious portal of entry is the respiratory system of a sick person, as well as skin with lesions, e.g. a burn or damaged cornea. Infection within the respiratory system develops as a result of inhalation of the fungal spores present in the air. Very often, prior to development of aspergillosis, a patient`s oronasal cavity is subject to fungal spore colonization. A developing fungus located in the lungs (incubation period spans between 2 days to 3 months) results in haemorrhagic infarctions, which cause a further transmission of the infection through the bloodstream to the brain, liver, spleen, kidneys, pericardium or skin (Mortensen, 2011; Garczewska, 2008)

For patients with lymphopenia - where the number of CD4 cells is lower than 0.2 x 10e9/l - most of the cases where the respiratory tract is colonized with *Aspergillus,* aspergillosis may develop as a result. With immunosuppressed patients, e.g. those suffering from hematological neoplasms, the most predominant form of fungal infection is invasive aspergillosis in 70% of cases caused by *A. fumigatus*. A variant of aspergillosis a little less common is general aspergillosis which affects central nervous system, sinuses, kidneys, skin or bones. Observational studies (a five year period of observation carried out on 3228 patients who underwent HSCT (haematopoietic stem cell transplant) at 11 transplant wards in Italy, where fungal infection prophylaxis was implemented by means of use of fluconazole, fungal infections were observed in 121 patients (3.7%), where 75% of cases were invasive aspergillosis, mostly of *Aspergillus* aetiology (Asano-Mori, 2010; Pagano, 2007). Unfortunately, *Aspergillus* fungal infections display a high mortality rate. In untreated aspergillosis, mortality rate can soar as high as 100%, and in the cases where treatment is introduced it drops only slightly down to 60%. One of the patient groups highly susceptible to invasive fungal infections caused by *Aspergillus* is the hematooncologic patients, where mortality rate with chemotherapy patients is as high as 49.3%, and with patients who underwent a haematopoietic stem cell transplant it reaches 86.7%. It was also shown that invasive aspergillosis is prevalent more often with the allogeneic bone marrow transplant patients (2.9-16.0%), rather than with those who underwent the autologous bone marrow transplant (0.3-1.1%) (Butrym et al., 2011; Fraquet et al., 2004). Uncharacteristic symptoms and diagnostic difficulties represent a key reason for delayed diagnosis of the infections caused by the fungi of *Aspergillus* species and deferred commencement of adequate treatment. Chamilos et al. in their research showed that as many as 75% of fungal infection cases confirmed in post mortem analysis were not diagnosed when the patients were still alive (Chamilos et al., 2008). Very often symptoms of fungal infections caused by moulds, are misdiagnosed as bacterial infections. A success case of a 47-year old woman suffering from sarcoidosis, who had been treated with steroids, and for two years had a confirmed lung cavity, indicates that a successful treatment of aspergillosis is possible. In that case, major symptoms of the disease were high fever, chronic cough with sputum, weight loss and hemoptysis. After an ineffective course of antibiotic therapy, the patient was diagnosed with candidiasis and semi-invasive aspergillosis. A computer tomography (CT) scan revealed a mycetoma in the lung cavity, culture of the sputum revealed an *Aspergillus* infection, and a significant improvement after antifungal treatment confirmed the diagnosis of aspergillosis caused by fungi from *A. niger* (Kosacka et al., 2010).

At present, the most sensitive test able to confirm aspergillosis is a high resolution CT scan in conjunction with the galactomannan test, which detects the antigen peculiar to *Aspergillus*. Other molecular recognition techniques based on PCR reaction are also used in detecting nosocomial aspergillosis. Genetic material of a fungus in clinical materials can be isolated by certain starters, e.g. from the sequence of alkaline proteinase or on the basis of 26SrRNA (Kriengkauykiat et al., 2011; Garczewska, 2008, Kędzierska et al., 2007)

Most common forms of nosocomial infections with moulds from the *Aspergillus* species are as follows:

- aspergilloma located in the lungs, usually after tuberculosis
- invasive aspergilloma (usually the pulmonary variation - in immunocompromised patients, leukaemia and post-transplant patients, in children suffering from chronic granulomatous disease)
- paranasal sinus aspergillosis (in immunocompromised patients)
- central nervous system aspergillosis (accompanies its disseminated version or as a result of sinusitis)
- *Aspergillus* endocarditis and cardiac aspergillosis - (follow an open-heart surgery)
- eye aspergillosis, endophtalmitis (in patients with endocarditis and following an organ transplant, often as the result of eye injury or transmission via bloodstream)
- aspergillosis of the bone marrow (bone marrow aspergillosis) - in children with granulomatous disease
- disseminated aspergillosis - as oesophageal infection, infection of the intestines, or organ infection: liver, spleen or kidneys.
- chronic necrotising pulmonary aspergillosis - in patients with pulmonary diseases
- skin aspergillosis - in patients with catheters or as the result of transmission via bloodstream.
- allergic bronchopulmonary aspergillosis (asthma) - inhaling spores of fungus by persons allergic to its antigens (Garczewska, 2008).

As previously mentioned, fungi from *Aspergillus fumigatus* species bear most significant clinical relevance for humans. This fungal species may cause acute and chronic inhalatory respiratory tract infections (aspergillosis, aspergilloma) as well as infections of the hematopoietic system, digestive system, genitourinary tract, skeletal muscles, and nervous system. The primary focus of infection in such cases is usually located in the lungs. Another pathogenic species which causes infections of the respiratory system and which also may cause allergic aspergillosis is *Aspergillus flavus*. This fungus is also responsible for cases of chronic invasive sinusitis as well as deep fungal infections (of the kidneys, endocardium, and central nervous system). *Aspergillus ochraceus* may be the cause behind antromycosis, pulmonary invasion and onychomycosis. Fungi of the *Aspergillus niger* species may also cause infections of the inner and outer ear (otomycosis) as well as pulmonary aspergillosis. Similarly to other species of the *Aspergillus species*, it rarely is responsible for surface aspergillosis. *Aspergillus versicolor* may constitute an etiological factor for otomycosis, osteomylitis, skin lesions or pulmonary diseases. Recently, clinical significance has been attributed to infections caused by *Aspergillus terreus*. Its spores may cause an allergic reaction or invasive aspergillosis of the respiratory system, as well as infections of the skin, eye or liver. Aspergillosis in patients with compromised immunity has been attributed more frequently to this species. In retrospective research spanning over 10 years, carried out in Austria (Medical University Hospital of Innsbruck), for 67 cases of invasive aspergillosis, nearly half (32) were infections caused by *A. terreus*, while the remaining cases were attributed to other species of *Aspergillus* (Lass-Flörl et al., 2005).

4. Environmental factors facilitating development of fungi of the *Aspergillus* species

Environmental parameters adding up to microclimate of rooms which affect people`s physical state comprise: air temperature, relative humidity, airflow in the people zone, purity of the air - both with respect to chemical and microbiological cleanliness, intensity of smells, light and noise levels. Indoors, microclimate is made up of the following factors: outdoor climate, heating and ventilation, people in the room, technological processes which take place inside, thermal characteristics of the room (Kaiser, 2011).

Indoor environment is an active ecosystem which evolves as the time progresses, with changes in humidity, temperature, presence of other microorganisms. Humidity in the rooms designated for people should be between 30-70%. Excessively humid air encourages multiplication of microorganisms (bacteria, mould), decomposition and water condensation, which increases microbiological contamination of the air. Depending on their designation, temperature in hospital rooms is maintained at different levels, usually falling into the 22-25°C temperature brackets.

Moulds grow mainly in the environment where air humidity exceeds 45%, temperature is within the range of 5°C 35°C (optimum 18°-27°C), and water activity a_w exceeds 0.8. Such environment is conducive to production of secondary metabolites - mycotoxins. *Penicillium* and *Aspergillus* are dominating mould species in the rooms where water activity is around 0.85 (Jarviss, 2003). Coefficient of hygroscopic expansion a_w for fungi is lower than for bacteria, for the latter the prerequisite for development is the 0.99 to 0.995 range. Fungi of the *A.flavus* type belong to the group of fungi which require higher air and soil humidity. It requires a 0.902 a_w level, which constitutes an extremely humid environment (Zyska, 1999).

Development of fungi may be affected by light in many different ways. Depending on the species, light may inhibit spore development or cause its abundant growth. It has been found that with one of the *Alternaria* species light of wavelength of 0.415xm-0.49xm completely blocks spore development, while wavelength below 0.39xm and exceeding 0.5xm stimulates spore growth (Zyska, 2001).

Influence of hydrostatic pressure on fungi growth has not been adequately researched. Fungi show no sensitivity to hyperbaria. Fungal endospores display a unique resilience to high pressure. Osmotic pressure inside hyphae of some species may be as high as 4255 hPa (Kurnatowska, 1998). Mould conidia of *A.niger* do not show sensitivity to pressure of 1000MPa. Growth of most yeast is halted, however, at pressure levels of as little as 0.8 MPa. A considerable drop in the hydrostatic pressure - hypobaria, or even deep vacuum, do not pose a threat to cells of many types of fungi. Deep vacuum had little or no impact on fungal vegetative forms and endospores, e.g. those from the *Cheatomium globosum, Aspergillus oryzae,* and *Aspergillus terreus* species (Piotrowska, 2000).

From among external environmental chemical factors, the most important is acidity or alkalinity, which is measured in pH parameters. Lowest and highest values on the pH scale, within the boundaries of growth of a fungus, represent the scope characteristic for a given species. This factor ranging between 5 to 6 is appropriate for most fungi. As in the majority of cases fungi favour pH below 7, most may be labelled acidophilic. Many species of *Aspergillus, Penicillium,* and *Fusarium* may grow at pH close to 2. At the same time, species like *Penicillium variabilis i Fusarium oxysporum* thrive in the environment where pH reaches 11. It should also be added that fungi trigger a shift in pH levels in the soil they grow in (Haasum & Nielsen, 1998).

Fungi belong to aerobes or facultative anaerobes. An oxygen increase in the environment lowers the mycelium mass and starts a degenerative process, however, it does not destroy the fungus. An increase in carbon dioxide content also halts the growth of a fungus (Kurnatowska, 1998).

From among moulds, fungi of the *Aspergillus* species demonstrate highest pathogenicity; however, despite their prevalence in the environment, they produce fewer mycotoxins than the less prevalent mould of *Stachybotrys*. It is not a rule of the thumb for all fungi of the *Aspergillus* species, as sterigmatocystin produced by *Aspergillus versicolor* may produce approximately 1% of the total biomass of fungi from this species, with water activity at level 1. This fungus is rarely obtained from indoor environment, as the species occurs in colder regions, in mountain and polar climatic zones. Fungi most often isolated from the indoor air belong to *A. fumigatus* and *A. niger* species (Fog Nielsen, 2003).

Among all the microorganisms present in the indoor air, moulds are most prevalent, however, it is crucial to remember, that live microorganisms (bacteria and fungi) make up only 10% of the total microorganism mass. Survivability of bacteria and moulds in the air is contingent upon peculiar to species susceptibility to desiccation and to the impact of ultraviolet rays. Most susceptible to desiccation are the vegetative forms of bacteria, while the most resilient are fungal spores. Fungal spores measure between 1.5 to 20 µm. One of the largest spores are: *Rhizopus* 4- 6 µm, *Mucor* 4-8 µm, *Fusarium* 2.4-3.5 µm, *A. niger* 2.5-3.5 µm, *A. flavus* 3.5-4.5 µm, while the smallest spores belong to the most pathogenic species of the *Aspergillus* species: (*A. terreus* 1.5 - 2.5 µm, *A. fumigatus* 2.5 - 3 µm, or *A. versicolor* 2 -3.5 µm) (Krzyściak at al., 2011). Figures 1-3 present a scanning microscope image, showing conidiophores of fungi of the following species: *A. candidus, A. niger* and *A. flavus*. Images from author`s own collection.

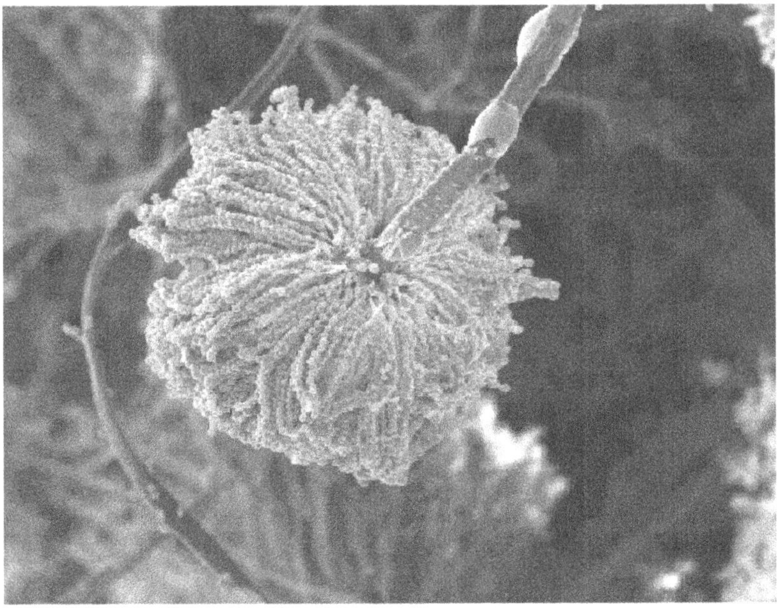

Fig. 1. *Aspergillus candidus* as seen under the scanning microscope; magnified by 1500x.

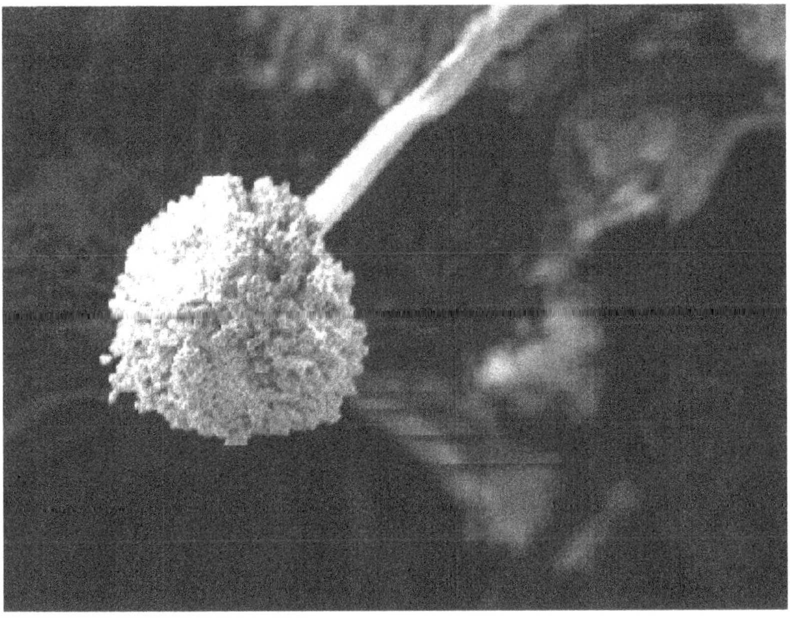

Fig. 2. *Aspergillus niger* as seen under the scanning microscope; magnified by 1000x.

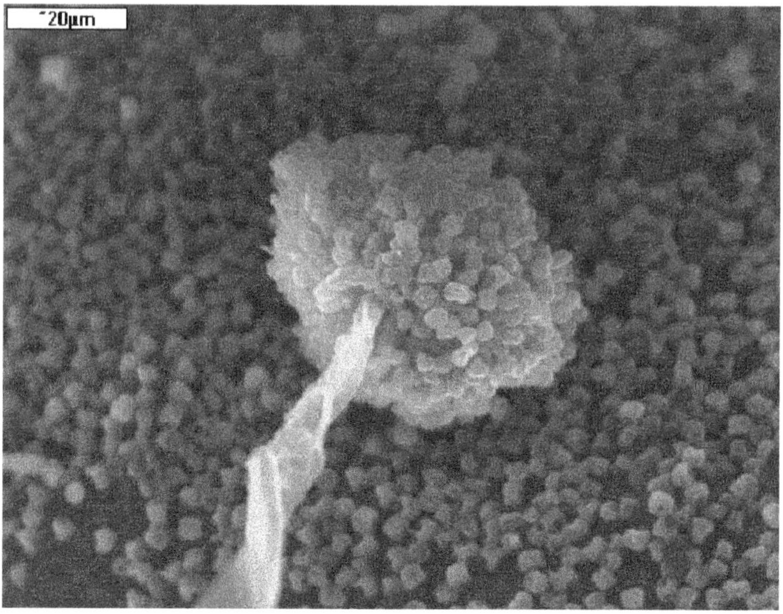

Fig. 3. *Aspergillus flavus* as seen under the scanning microscope; magnified by 1000x.

In contained rooms, not equipped with specialist ventilation systems and adequate air filtration, fungi and certain bacteria colonize places favourable to their development. Such areas are usually polluted places with increased humidity levels: ventilation shafts, air filters, noise reducing filters, insulation layers, air coolers, humidifier systems. Infected areas of such systems present a secondary source of microbiological contamination of the air. Ventilation and air-conditioning systems are more responsible for polluting the air with fungi than with bacteria. Most serious air infections happen in places where condensation is present. The risk increases if the systems are not properly utilised and if the air contains significant amounts of pollutants (Kaiser, 2011).

Required cleanliness level of air provided for indoors is achieved by filtration by means of air conditioning systems and ventilation equipped with proper filters. For indoor spaces with high hygienic standards it is crucial to implement the use of multi-tier filtration systems. A modern air-conditioning system contains a laminar flow ceiling cabinet. Such system for operating rooms (hospital rooms with high standards of microbiological cleanliness) should provide the necessary amount of fresh air and an adequate frequency of airflow changes per hour. A factor that may limit the occurrence of infections with patients who undergo surgery is creating an environment free from bacteria as well as keeping the surgery time as short as possible (Kremer et al., 2010). Knochen et al. in a study that compared environments of operating theatres, where floors were routinely disinfected after each surgery, with those where theatres were cleaned only when visible dirt appeared, and concluded that none of the procedures influences the number of infections occurring in patients undergoing surgery. Utilizing a laminar flow ceiling cabinet proves to be a sufficient bacteria limiting method (Knochen et al., 2010).

The problem of providing microbiological cleanliness inside hospital rooms is not exclusively related to observing the principles of air filter exchange in air conditioning systems according to manufacturer`s instructions. According to Kaiser (Kaiser, 2004), periodical ventilation of the air-conditioning system is necessary as well as drying the ventilation pipes and elements of the equipment. He also states that air-conditioning system should not be completely shut off . On the contrary, Dettenkofer et al. suggest that shutting off the ventilation systems in the operating rooms when they are not in use probably does not increase microbiological contamination of the indoor air shortly after the system is switched back on (Dettenkofer et al., 2003).

Proper utilisation of operating rooms also entails isolation of the inner environment from any possibility of contamination access from outside, by maintaining a pressure difference between the inner and outer rooms. Where proper ventilation systems are unavailable, limiting microbiological contamination from staff may result in an approximate twofold reduction in infections. Conclusions of research carried out by Lidwell suggest that with a drop in microbiological contamination concentration of the air below 10 c.f.u/m^3, the drop in risk of infection is minor (Lidwell, 1982). With such low levels of concentration of bacteria in the air, transmission of infectious pathogenic microorganisms this way becomes a less serious cause of infection.

4.1 Influence of physical and chemical factors on cytotoxicity of fungi

Fungi are not cytotoxic unless there are circumstances enabling them to produce metabolites. The factors conducive to toxin production include: culture medium, life cycle of the fungi, availability of nutrients, environmental conditions and/or the simultaneous presence of other moulds [Kelman et al., 2004; Pitt et al.,2000). It has been established that in laboratory settings fungal monocultures lose their toxin production potential (Jarvis & Miller, 2005). Environmental conditions considerably influence the synthesis of fungal virulence factors. When fungal receptors receive variations in such factors as moisture, temperature, water activity and the presence of nitrogen, a signal transduction cascade that controls effector genes expression may be activated, which results in toxin production. The processes of sporulation and mycotoxin production in the *Aspergillus* fungi are regulated by the protein G transduction signals pathway (Singh & Del Poeta, 2011). The investigations carried out by Watanabe et al. gave evidence that good environmental conditions, in this case oxygenation, stimulated the *A. fumigatus* fungi to gliotoxin production and were conducive to the increase of their general cytotoxicity (Watanabe et al., 2004).

The presence of the *Aspergillus* fungi in the human environment does not necessarily cause infection in risk group patients. Those fungi are opportunistic bacteria and are cleared away by means of natural defence mechanisms in healthy individuals, however, they produce severe invasive infections in immunosuppressed patients. So far, the threshold value establishing a requisite for opportunistic infection has not been determined. Therefore, the goal of preventive action should be to eliminate *Aspergillus* fungi from human environment. Such aim, however, is hard to attain as, obviously, among all bacteria in the air, moulds are most numerous. Methods of absolute elimination of mould spores from the environment have been known, though. Nevertheless, from a practical point of view it is not feasible. Bearing in mind immunosuppressed patients, the Airinspace Technologies system was created. It is based on creating a protective chamber around a patient, where air exchange takes place 60 times per hour, with the use of plasma as a bacteria killing agent, it is still very difficult to provide a patient with ultra-sterile air (Poirot et al., 2007).

Our own study on mycological cleanness of hospital rooms indoor air revealed that the *Aspergillus* species amounted to 20-38% of all of the moulds isolated, and the most frequently identified species was *A. fumigatus* [Gniadek et al., 2010; Gniadek et al., 2009). Domination of this species in the indoor air may be tantamount to a high risk of infection. The risk may be confirmed by the findings of *Aspergillus* cytotoxicity evaluation in such sites as adult intensive therapy ward, intensive neonatal care unit and chemotherapy and radiotherapy wards. The analysis was performed using an MTT test (3-(4.5-dimethylthiazol-2-yl) 2.5 diphenyltetrazolium bromide) in which general cytotoxicity was tested on swine kidney cells (SK), sensitive to most mycotoxins. The test is based on the reduction of yellow MTT tetrazolium salt to violet formazan, insoluble in water. The reduction occurs in the presence of intact SK, not damaged by mycotoxins. The intensity of reaction is proportional to the amount of metabolically active SK. When the SK are infected with moulds producing mycotoxins, their mitochondria fail to reduce tetrazolium salt into formazan. Therefore, when the SK are damaged by mycotoxins, the reaction is less intensive or does not occur, which can be measured photometrically as more or less intensive change of colour. Thus, the reduction or the absence of the reaction gives evidence of cytotoxicity of the fungal strain tested (Hanelt et al., 1994).

The analysis comprised the evaluation of a test sample (Petri dish with the moulds on Czapek medium) and a control sample (Petri dish with Czapek medium). The SK were grown in medium containing antibiotics (penicillin and streptomycin, Sigma Aldrich) and calf fetal serum (Sigma Aldrich) in the Hera Cell incubator with carbon dioxide, manufactured by Heraeus (5% CO2, 37°C, 98% humidity). The number of SK was 2.2×105. The ranges of testing concentrations were prepared in the ratio 1:2 and amounted from 31.251 to 0.061 cm^2/l. The value was expressed in terms of cm^2/ml, where the area of the Petri dish from which the moulds were extracted together with the medium, was measured in square centimetres.

The quantitative evaluation of cytotoxicity was performed using a microslide spectrophotometer (Elisa Digiscan reader, Asys Hitech GmbH, Austria) and the programme MikroWin 2000 (Mikrotek Laborsysteme GmbH, Germany). The readings were made at the wave-length of 510 nm. All of the absorption values below 50% of the threshold activity were considered as toxic. So, the borderline toxic concentration was evaluated on the basis of the dilution i.e. the mean inhibitory concentration IC50 was equal to the smallest sample (in cm2/ml) which was toxic to the SK. The cytotoxicity was considered as low (+) when the values were within the range of 31.251>15.625>7.813 [cm^2/ml], intermediate (++) for the values >3.906>1.953>0.977 [cm^2/ml], and high (+++) for >0.488>0.244>0.122>0.061. The lack of cytotoxicity was reported when the absorption value exceeded 31.251 [cm^2/ml] (Gareis, 1994).

In own researches for 57 isolated strains - *A. fumigatus, A. ochraceus, A. niger, A. flavus, A. versicolor* and *A. ustus*, as many as 48 (84%) were cytotoxic. It was also established that the *A. niger* species was considerably less cytotoxic than *A. ochraceus* and *A. fumigatus* ($p<0.05$) (Fig 4).

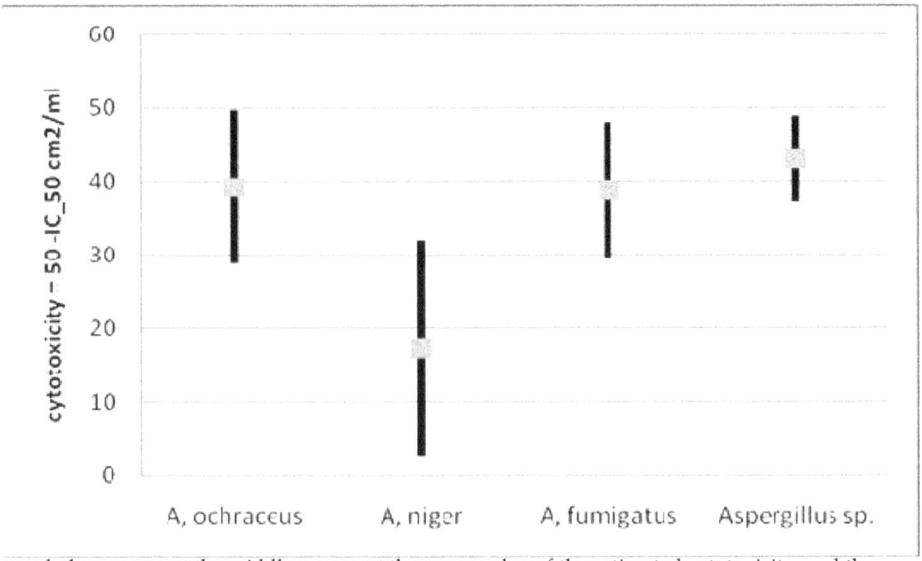

Legend: the squares at the middle represent the mean value of the estimated cytotoxicity, and the vertical lines represent the size of the confidence interval of the estimated cytotoxicity.

Fig. 4. Intervals of confidence 95% CI and mean value of *Aspergillus* cytotoxicity estimated as difference between reference level equal to 50 and measured value of IC 50 cm^2/ml.

Research has shown that among all of the examined strains the strains of *A. fumigatus*, but not of other species, were either of intermediate or high cytotoxicity (Gniadek et al., 2011). Particularly, eight out of nine strains isolated from indoor air in adult intensive care unit were cytotoxic. High cytotoxicity was found in the following species: *A. fumigatus, A. ochraceus* and *A. flavus,* while the cytotoxivity of *A. niger* was intermediate or lacked cytotoxicity altogether (Gniadek et al., 2009). A further confirmation of those findings was brought by another study in which the highest fungal virulence towards murine macrophages was found in *A. fumigatus,* while the lowest in *A. niger* and *A. terreus* (Kamei et al., 2002).

The considerable cytotoxicity of fungi isolated from the environment where immunocompromised patients are present encourages intensifying observations concerning the influence of environmental mycobiota on human health. Cases of aspergillosis caused by airborne infections were observed (a patient with aspergilosis infected two other patients in the same intensive therapy unit by airborne route). Recent literature does not provide evidence what level of exposure to toxin producing fungi may be dangerous to the health (Pegues et al., 2002). Nevertheless, there is a common opinion that moulds present indoors may be dangerous and the environmental conditions must be improved. The measurements of environmental occurrence of fungi indoors should include an evaluation of their cytotoxicity when the fungi are known to be toxic. Those measures should be habitual and preventive because evaluation after occurrence of infection will only reflect estimaton of risk at the initial stage of the disease and may not reflect the exposure to harmful substances in the course of the disease. It seems a fair policy that as preventive treatment for patients with compromised immunity, in order to contain the exposure, the mycological cleanliness of hospital environment should be monitored, inclusive of marking the cytotoxicity of fungi commonly labelled pathogenic.

5. Conclusion

From the epidemiological point of view, the results of exposure to a mix of mycotoxins and other noxious substances present in the air we breathe indoors remain unknown. Therefore, the adverse effect of fungi to human health may be evaluated by means of finding the relationship between the disease (predisposition) and exposure level (detection of pathogenic spores) in relation to symptoms typical for experimental conditions caused by myotoxins.

6. References

Asano-Mori, Y. (2010). Fungal infections after hematopoietic stem cell transplantation. *International Journal Hematology*, Vol. 91, No. 4, pp. 576-587, ISSN 0925-5710

Balajee, S.; Gribskov, J.; Hanley, E.; Nickle, D. & Marr K. (2005). *Aspergillus lentulus* sp. nov., a new sibling species of A. fumigatus. *Eukaryotic Cell*, Vol. 4, No. 3, pp. 625–632, ISSN 1535-9778

Bok, J.; Balajee, S.; Marr, K.; Andes, D.; Nielsen, K.; Frisvad, J. & Keller, N. (2005). LaeA, a regulator of morphogenetic fungal virulence factors. *Eukaryotic Cell*, Vol.4, No. 9, pp. 1574–1582, ISSN:1535-9778.

Bräse, S.; Encinas, A.; Keck, J. & Nising, C. (2009). Chemistry and biology of mycotoxins and related fungal metabolites. *Chemical Reviews*, Vo. 109, No. 9, pp. 3903-3990, ISSN 0009-2665

Budak, A. (1998). Mikotoksyny, In *Zarys mikologii lekarskiej*, E. Baran, (Ed.), 533 - 538,Volumed, ISBN 83- 85564-17-9, Wrocław, Poland

Burr, M. (2001). Health effects of indoor moldes. *Reviews on Environmental Health*, Vol. 16, No. 2, pp. 97-103, ISSN 0048-7554

Butrym, A.; Zywar, K.; Dzietczenia, J. & Mazur G. (2011). Invasive fungal infections in patients with hematological malignancies. *Mykologia Lekarska*, Vol. 18, No. 1, pp. 47-53, ISSN 1232-986X

Chamilos, G.; Luna, M.; Lewis, R.; Bodey, G.; Chemaly, R.; Tarrand, J.; Safdar, A.; Raad, I. & Kontoyiannis, D. (2006). Invasive fungal minfections in patients with hematologic malignancies in a tertiary care center: an autopsy study over a 15 year period (1989-2003). *Hematologica*, Vol. 91, No. 7, pp. 986-989, ISSN 0390-6078

Dettenkofer, M.; Scherrer, M.; Hoch, V.; Glaser, H.; Schwarzer, G.; Zentner, J. & Daschner, E. (2003). Shutting down operating theater ventilation when the theater is not in use: infection control and environmental aspects. *Infection Control Hospital Epidemiology, Vol.* 24, No. 8, pp.596-600, ISSN 0899-823X

Domsch, K.; Gams, W. &, Anderson, T. (2007). *Compedium of soli fungi* ed.2., IHW-Verlag, ISBN 978-3-930167-69-2, Eching, Germany

Fischer, G. & Dott, W. (2003). Relevance of airborne fungi and their secondary metabolites for environmental, occupational and indoor hygiene. *Archives of Microbiology*, Vol. 179, No. 2, pp. 75-82, ISSN 0302-8933

Fischer, G.; Müller, T.; Schwalbe, R.;Ostrowski,R. & Dott, W. (2000). Species-specific profiles of mycotoxins produced in cultures and associated with conidia of airborne fungi derived from biowaste. *International Journal of Hygiene and Environmental Health*, Vol. 203, No. 2, pp. 105 - 116, ISSN 1438-4639

Fog Nielsen, K. (2003). Mycotoxin production by indoor molds. *Fungal Genetics and Biology*, Vol. 39, No. 2, pp. 103-117, ISSN 1087-1845

Fraquet, T.; Gimenez, A. & Hidalgo, A. (2004). Imaging of opportunistic fungal infections in immunocompromised patient. *European Journal of Radiology*, Vol. 51, No. 2, pp. 130-138, ISSN 0720-048X

Garczewska, B. (2008). Szpitalne zakażenia grzybicze, In: *Zakażenia szpitalne*, D. Dzierżanowska, (Ed.), 409-425, α- medica press, ISBN 978-83-7522-022-3, Bielsko-Biała, Poland

Gareis, M. (1994). Cytotoxicity testing of samples originating from problem buildings, In: *Fungi and Bacteria in Indoor Air Environments: Health Effects, Detection and Remediation*, E. Johanning, (Ed.), 139 - 144, Eastern New York Occupational Health Program, Saratoga Springs, ISBN 0964730707, New York, USA,

Gniadek, A.; Macura, A.B.; Twarużek, M. & Grajewski, J. (2010). Cytotoxicity of Aspergillus strains isolated from the neonatal intensive care unit environment. *Advances in Medical Sciences*, Vol. 55, No. 2, pp. 242-249, ISSN 1896-1126

Gniadek, A.; Macura, A.B. & Twarużek, M. (2009). Characteristics fungi present in the intensive care unit environment. Part 2. Cytotoxicity of the isolated *Aspergillus* fungi. *Mikologia Lekarska*, Vol.16, No.1, pp. 15-18, ISSN 1232-986X

Gniadek, A.; Macura, A,B. & Górkiewicz, M. (2011). Cytotoxicity of *Aspergillus* fungi isolated from hospital environment. *Polish Journal of Microbiology*, Vol.60, No.1, pp. 59-63, ISSN 1733-1331

Haasum, I. & Nielsen, P. (1998). Ecophysiological characterization o common food -borne fungi in relation to pH and water activity under various atmospheric compositions. *Journal of Applied Microbiology*, Vol.84, No.3, pp. 451 - 460, ISSN 1364-5072

Hanelt, M.; Gareis, M. & Kollarczik, B.(1994). Cytotoxicity of mycotoxins evaluated by the MTT-cell culture assay. *Mycopathologia*, Vol. 128, No. 3, pp. 167 - 174, ISSN 0301-486X

Jarvis, B. (2003). Analysis for mycotoxins: the chemist's perspective. *Archives of Environmental Health*, Vo. 58, No. 8, pp. 479-483, ISSN 0003-9896

Jarvis, B. & Miller, J. (2005). Mycotoxins as harmful indoor air contaminants. *Applied Microbiology and Biotechnology*, Vol.66, No.4, pp. 367-372, ISSN 0175-7598

Kaiser, K. (2004). Wpływ zanieczyszczenia instalacji wentylacyjnych i klimatyzacyjnych podczas ich używania na jakość powietrza w obiektach szpitalnych. *Technika Chłodnicza i Klimatyzacyja* Vol. 98, pp.116-124, ISSN 1231-188X

Kaiser, K. (2011). Jakość powietrza wewnętrznego w szpitalach, In: *Profilaktyka zakażeń szpitalnych – bezpieczeństwo środowiska szpitalnego*, A. Pawińska, (Ed.), 57-87, α-medica press, ISBN 978-83-7522-068-1, Bielsko-Biała, Poland

Kamei, K.; Watanabe, A.; Nishimura, K. & Miyaji, M. (2002). Cytotoxicity of *Aspergillus fumigatus* culture filtrate against macrophages. *Nihon Ishinkin Gakkai Zasshi*, Vol.43, No.1, pp. 37-41, ISSN 0916-4804

Kelman, B.; Robbins, C.; Swenson, L. & Hardin, B. (2004). Risk from inhaled mycotoxins in indoor office and residential environments. *International Journal of Toxicology*, Vol.23, No.1, pp. 3-10, ISSN 1091-5818

Kędzierska, A.; Kochan, P.; Pietrzyk, A. & Kędzierska, J. (2007). Current status of fungal cell wall components in the immunodiagnostics of invasive fungal infections in humans: galactomannan, mannan and (1-->3)-beta-D-glucan antigens. *European Journal of Clinical Microbiology & Infectious Diseases*, Vol. 26, No. 11, pp. 755-766, ISSN 0934-9723

Klich, M. (2009). Health effects of *Aspergillus* in food and air. *Toxicology and Industrial Health*, Vol.25, No. 9-10, pp. 657-667, ISSN 0748-2337

Knochen, H.; Hübner, N.; Below, H.; Assadian, O.; Külpmann, R.; Kohlmann, T.; Hildebrand, K.; Clemens, S.; Bartels, C. & Kramer, A. (2010). Influence of floor disinfection on microbial and particulate burden measured under low turbulance air flow in ophthalmological operation theatres. *Klinische Monatsblätter für Augenheilkunde*, Vol. 227, No.11, pp.871-878, ISSN 0023-2165

Kosacka, M.; Nawrot, U.; Porębska, I.; Gostkowska A.; Dyła, T. & Jankowska R. (2010). The case of pulmonary semi-invasive aspergillosis and candidiasis of bronchi in patient with sarcoidosis. *Mikologia Lekarska*, Vol.17, No.4, pp. 244-247, ISSN 1232-986X

Kramer, A.; Külpmann, R.; Wille, F.; Christiansen, B.; Exner, M.; Kohlmann, T.; Heidecke, C.; Lippert, H.; Oldhafer, K.; Schilling, M.; Below, H.; Harnoss, J. & Assadian, O. (2010). Importance of displacement ventilation for operations and small surgical procedures from the infection preventive point of view. *Zentralblatt fur Chirurgie*, Vol.135, No. 1, pp.11-17, ISSN 0044-409X

Kriengkauykiat, J.; Ito, J. & Dadwal, S. (2011). Epidemiology and treatment approaches in management of invasive fungal infections. *Clinical Epidemiology*, Vol. 3, pp. 175–191, ISSN 1179-1349

Krzyściak, P.; Skóra, M. & Macura A.B. (2011). *Atlas grzybów chorobotwórczych człowieka*, MedPharm POLSKA, ISBN 978-83-60466-80-3, Wrocław, Poland

Kupfahl, C.; Michalka, A.; Lass-Flörl, C.; Fischer, G.; Haase, G.; Ruppert, T.; Geginat, G. & Hof, H. (2008). Gliotoxin production by clinical and environmental *Aspergillus fumigatus* strains. *International Journal of Medical Microbiology*, Vol. 298, No. 3-4, pp.319-327, ISSN 1438-4221

Kurnatowska, A. (1998). Biologia i ekologia grzybów chorobotwórczych, In: *Zarys mikologii lekarskiej*, E. Baran, (Ed.), 21 - 35,Volumed, ISBN 83-85564-17-9, Wrocław, Poland

Kurnatowski, P. & Miśkiewicz, S. (2009). Invasive aspergillosis among patients undergoing an transplantation. *Mikologia Lekarska*, Vol. 16, No.1, pp. 50-53, ISSN 1232-986X

Lass-Flörl, C.; Griff, K.; Mayr, A.; Petzer, A.; Gastl, G.; Bonatti, H,; Freund, M.; Kropshofer, G.; Dierich, M. & Nachbaur, D. (2005). Epidemiology and outcome of infections due to *Aspergillus terreus*: 10-year single centre experience. *British Journal of Haematology*, Vol. 131, No. 2, pp. 201-207, ISSN 0007-1048

Lewis, R.; Wiederhold, N.; Chi, J.; Han, X.; Komanduri, K.; Kontoyiannis, D. & Prince, R. (2005). Detection of gliotoxin in experimental and human aspergillosis. *Infection and Immunity*, Vol. 73, No. 1, pp. 635–637, ISSN 0019-9567

Lidwell, O.; Lowbury, E.; Whyte, W.; Blowers, R.; Stanley, S. & Lowe, D. (1982). Effect of ultraclean air in operating rooms on deep sepsis in the joint after total hip or knee replacement: a randomised study. *British Medical Journal* (*Clinical Research* ed), Vol. 285, No. 3, pp.10-14, ISSN 0267-0623

Macura, A.B. (1998). Czynniki sprzyjające zakażeniom grzybiczym. In *Zarys mikologii lekarskiej*, E. Baran, (Ed.), 289 - 295,Volumed, ISBN 83-85564-17-9, Wrocław, Poland

Mortensen, K.; Johansen, H.; Fuursted, K.; Knudsen, J.; Gahrn-Hansen, B.; Jensen, R.;. Howard, S. & Arendrup, M. (2011). A prospective survey of *Aspergillus* spp. in respiratory tract samples: prevalence, clinical impact and antifungal susceptibility. *European Journal of Clinical Microbiology & Infectious Diseases*, Epub ahead of print, DOI 10.1007/s10096-011-1229-7, ISSN 1435-4373

Pagano, L.; Caira, M.; Nosari, A.; Van Lint, M.; Candoni, A.; Offidani, M.; Aloisi, T.; Irrera, G.;Bonini, A.; Picardi, M.; Caramatti, C.; Invernizzi, R.; Mattei, D.; Melillo, L.; de Waure, C.; Reddiconto, G.; Fianchi, L.; Valentini, C.; Girmenia, C.; Leone, G. & Aversa, F. (2007). Fungal infections in recipients of hematopoietic stem cell transplants: results of the SEIFEM B-2004 study - Sorveglianza Epidemiologica Infezioni Fungine Nelle Emopatie Maligne. *Clinical Infectious Diseases*, Vol. 45, No.9, pp. 1161-1170, ISSN 1058-4838

Pegues, D.; Lasker, B.; McNeil, M.; Hamm, P.; Lundal, J. & Kubak, B. (2002). Cluster of cases on invasive aspergillosis in a transplant intensive care unit: evidence of person - to - person airborne tranmission. *Clinical Infectious Diseases*, Vol. 34, No. 3, pp. 412-416, . ISSN 1058-4838

Piotrowska, M. (2000). Grzyby strzępkowe, In: *Mikrobiologia techniczna*, Z. Libudzisz &., K. Kowal, (Ed.), 63-85, Politechnika Łódzka, ISBN 83-87198-5-1, Łódź, Polska

Pitt, J.; Basilico, J.; Abarca, M. & López L. (2000). Mycotoxins and toxigenic fungi. *Medical Mycology*, Vol. 38 (Suppl. 1), pp. 41-46, ISSN 1369-3786

Raper, K. & Fennell D. (1965). *The Genus Aspergillus*. The Williams & Wilkins Company. ISBN 978-1-904455-53-0, Baltimore, USA.

Ribeiro, S.; Santana, A,; Arriagada, G.; Martins, J. & Takagaki, T. (2005). A novel cause of invasive pulmonary infection in an immunocompetent patient: *Aspergillus candidus*. *The Journal of Infection*, Vol.51, No. 4, pp. 195-197, ISSN 0163-4453

Richardson, M. (2005). Changing patterns and trends in systemic fungal infections. *The Journal of Antimicrobial Chemotherapy*, Vol.56, Suppl. 1, pp. 5-11, ISSN 0305-7453

Poirot, J.; Gangneux, J.; Fischer, A.; Malbernard, M.; Challier, S.; Laudinet, N. & Bergeron, V. (2007). Evaluation of a new mobile system for protecting immune-suppressed patients against airborne contamination. *American Journal of Infection Control*, Vol.35, No. 7 pp.460-466, ISSN 0196-6553

Shelton, B., Kirkland, K.; Flanders, W. & Morris G. (2002). Profiles of airborne fungi in buildings and outdoor environments in the United States. *Applied and Environmental Microbiology*, Vol.68, No. 4, pp. 1743–1753, ISSN 0099-2240

Singh, A. & Del Poeta, M. (2011). Lipid signalling in pathogenic fungi. *Cellular Microbiology*, Vol.13, No. 2, pp.177-185, ISSN 1462-5814

Skaug, M.; Eduard, W. & Stormer, F. (2001). Ochratoxin A in airborne dust and fungal conidia. *Mycopathologia*, Vo. 151, No. 2, pp. 93-98, ISSN 0301-486X

Smith, J.; Solomons, G.; Lewis, C. & Anderson, J. (1995). Role of mycotoxins in human and animal nutrition and health. *Natural Toxins*, Vol. 3, No. 4, pp.187-192, ISSN 1056-9014

Türel, O. (2011). Newer antifungal agents. *Expert Review of Anti-Infective Therapy*, Vol. 9, No. 3, pp.325-338, ISSN 1478-7210

Watanabe, A.; Kamei, K.; Sekine, T.; Higurashi, H.; Ochiai, E.; Hashimoto, Y. & Nishimura, K. (2004). Cytotoxic substances from *Aspergillus fumigatus* in oxygenated or poorly oxygenated environment. *Mycopathologia*, Vol. 158, No. 1, pp. 1-7, ISSN 0301-486X

Zyska, B. (1999). *Zagrożenia biologiczne w budynku*, Arkady, ISBN 83-213-4117-9, Warszawa, Poland

Zyska, B. (2001). *Katastrofy, awarie i zagrożenia mikrobiologiczne w przemyśle i budownictwie*, Politechnika Łódzka, ISBN 83-7283-018-5, Łódź, Poland

5

Expression and Characterization of Bovine Milk Antimicrobial Proteins Lactoperoxidase and Lactoferrin by Vaccinia Virus

Tetsuya Tanaka[1], Xuenan Xuan[2], Kozo Fujisaki[1] and Kei-ichi Shimazaki[3]
[1]*Laboratory of Emerging Infectious Diseases, Department of Frontier Veterinary Science, Faculty of Agriculture, Kagoshima University, Korimoto, Kagoshima,*
[2]*National Research Center for Protozoan Diseases, Obihiro University of Agriculture and Veterinary Medicine, Obihiro, Hokkaido,*
[3]*Laboratory of Dairy Food Science, Research Faculty Agriculture, Hokkaido University, Sapporo, Hokkaido,*
Japan

1. Introduction

Lactoperoxidase (LPO), a heme-containing oxidation-reduction enzyme present in milk and saliva, is part of an antimicrobial system, and converts thiocyanate to hypothiocyanate in a hydrogen peroxide-dependent reaction. The molecular weight of LPO is approximately 78 kDa, and the carbohydrate moiety comprises about 10% of the total weight (Mansson-Rahemtulla et al., 1988). LPO, myeloperoxidase (MPO), eosinophil peroxidase (EPO) and thyroid peroxidase (TPO) belong to the homologous mammalian peroxidase family and share 50 to 70% identity. Even higher homology can be found among their active site-related residues. These peroxidases can catalyze oxidation of halides and pseudohalides such as thiocyanate by hydrogen peroxide to form potent oxidant and bactericidal agents. MPO has been shown to inactivate influenza virus (Yamamoto et al., 1991) and HIV-1 virus (Klebanoff & Kazazi, 1995). Human recombinant MPO has been shown to have a virucidal effect on HIV-1 virus (Moguilevsky et al., 1992; Chochola et al., 1994) and cytomegalovirus (EI Messaoudi et al., 2002). However, few studies have examined whether LPO inhibits virus infection *in vitro* and *in vivo*.

Lactoferrin (LF), also called lactotransferrin, is an iron-binding protein present in milk, saliva, tears, mucus secretions and secondary granules of neutrophils. Each LF molecule can bind 2 Fe (III) ions tightly but reversibly. This binding is dependent on concomitant binding of anions such as bicarbonate and carbonate, which play an essential role in holding the metal firmly (Masson et al., 1968). Thus, LF can exist in an iron-free (apo) or iron-bound (holo) state. LF is a prominent antimicrobial component of mucosal surfaces prone to attack by microbial pathogens. LF is actively secreted by neutrophils in the inflammatory response (Gutteberg et al., 1984). As an anti-microbial component of colostrum and milk, LF may play significant roles in protection of neonates from infectious diseases (García-Montoya et al., 2011). The importance of LF in host defense is underlined by findings indicating that patients with congenital or acquired defects of LF production exhibit an abnormal predisposition to recurrent infections by bacteria, fungi and parasites (Venge et al., 1984; Tanaka et al., 1996). Patients with acute viral illnesses such as chickenpox, measles, rubella, hepatitis or Epstein-Barr virus infection have reduced plasma LF concentrations, although their total neutrophil numbers are similar to those of non-infected subjects (Bayners et al., 1986).

Vaccinia virus belongs to the family of poxviridae, and is the most intensively studied member of the poxvirus family (Moss et al., 1990). Poxviruses replicate in the cytoplasm of infected cells without using nuclear enzymes of the host cells for transcription or DNA synthesis. Vaccinia virus has circumvented the need for nuclear enzymes by encoding or packaging a complete enzyme system for transcription (Moss et al., 1990) and DNA synthesis, including a DNA-dependent DNA polymerase (Moss & Cooper, 1982), DNA topoisomerase (Shuman et al., 1987) and DNA ligase (Kerr et al., 1989). Consequently, the vaccinia virus is widely used as an expression system in molecular biotechnology. Recombinant vaccinia virus has been demonstrated to be an effective antigen delivery system for infectious diseases in many species, with rabies and rinderpest being notable examples (Ertl and Xiang, 1996; Tsukiyama et al., 1989). In addition recombinant vaccinia virus can give rise to long-term immunity (Inui et al., 1995). In previous studies, recombinant vaccinia virus has been used produce cytokines (e.g., IFN-β, IFN-γ) (Kohonen-Corish et al., 1989, 1990; Peplinski et al., 1996; Nishikawa et al., 2000, 2001), but it has not yet been used for expression of bovine LPO (bLPO) or bovine LF (bLF). In the present study, we constructed recombinant vaccinia viruses that express bLPO and bLF with antiviral activity, and characterized production of bLPO and bLF and replication of the recombinant virus. The present results indicate that expression of bLPO and bLF by recombinant vaccinia virus may be useful for treatment of infectious diseases in humans or animals (Tanaka et al., 2006).

2. Materials and methods

2.1 Cells and viruses

Rabbit kidney (RK13) cells were cultured in Eagle's minimum essential medium (EMEM, Sigma Chemicals Co., St. Louis, MO, USA) supplemented with 8% heat-inactivated fetal bovine serum (FBS). Vaccinia virus LC16mO (mO) strain and its recombinant were propagated in RK13 cells in EMEM supplemented with 8% FBS.

2.2 Construction of recombinant vaccinia virus that expresses bLPO and bLF

bLPO or bLF cDNA was amplified from mammary gland cells, using reverse polymerase chain reaction (RT-PCR) with primers designed from bLPO or bLF cDNA (Dull et al., 1990; Nakamura et al., 2001). The PCR products were blunted by T4 DNA polymerase and ligated with the vaccinia virus transfer vector pAK8 (Yasuda et al., 1990), which was cut with *Sal* I and then blunted. The plasmid (pAK/bLPO or pAK/bLF) was transfected into RK13 cells using a lipofectin reagent (Life Technologies Japan, Tokyo, Japan) for 1 h after infection with the mO strain. After 2 days of incubation, culture medium was collected. We isolated recombinant virus (vv/bLPO or vv/bLF) produced by homologous recombination between pAK8 and viral thymidine kinase (TK-) cells in the presence of 100 μg/ml 5-bromo-2′-deoxyuridine, selecting TK- viruses by plaque isolation.

2.3 Immunofluorescence test (IFAT)

RK13 cells were infected with mO, vv/bLPO and vv/bLF (5 plaque-forming units [PFU]/cell, 48 h), and subjected to indirect immunofluorescence assay test (IFAT). The infected RK13 cells were fixed with acetone, and incubated with mouse anti-bLPO monoclonal antibody (anti-bLPO mAb) or mouse anti-bLF monoclonal antibody (anti-bLF mAb); these antibodies were produced by the present authors (Shimazaki et al., 1998; Watanabe et al., 1998). The cells were then stained with fluorescein-conjugated goat anti-mouse antibody (Southern Biotechnology Associates Inc., Birmingham, AL, UK) or fluorescein-conjugated sheep anti-rabbit antibody (Waco Pure Chemical, Osaka, Japan). The cells were observed using fluorescence microscopy.

2.4 Sodium dodecylsulfate-polyacrylamide gel electrophoresis (SDS-PAGE) and western blot analysis

RK13 cells in tissue culture (colony diameter, 15 mm) were infected with the mO strain or the recombinant vaccinia virus at a multiplicity of infection (moi) of 5 for 1 h at 37°C. Then, the cells were washed with EMEM and cultured in 500 μl of EMEM at 37°C for 48 h. The cell extracts and culture supernatants were subjected to SDS-PAGE (Laemmli, 1970) under reducing conditions, followed by electrical transfer of proteins to a PVDF membrane (Osmonics Inc., Westborough, MA, USA). The membrane was immersed in blocking buffer (phosphate-buffered saline [PBS] containing 3% bovine serum albumin) at 4°C overnight, incubated with rabbit anti-bLPO polyclonal antibody (anti-bLPO Ab) or anti-bLF mAb (diluted in the blocking buffer) at 37°C for 1 h, washed 3 times with PBS, and then incubated with alkaline phosphatase-conjugated goat anti-rabbit IgG antibodies (Promega Co., Madison, WI, USA) or horseradish peroxidase-conjugated goat anti-mouse IgG antibodies (Waco Pure Chemical, Osaka, Japan) (diluted in the blocking buffer) at 37°C for 1 h. The membrane was visualized by incubation with BCIP/NBT color substrate (Promega Co.) or 0.5 mg/ml diaminobenzidine and 0.005% H_2O_2.

2.5 Tunicamycin treatment

Recombinant vaccinia virus-infected RK13 cells (5 PFU/cell) were incubated in EMEM containing 1 μg/ml tunicamycin (Sigma Chemical Co.), which prevents synthesis of N-linked sugars, for 1 to 48 h post-infection (pi). The cells were then harvested, and the cell lysate was subjected to Western blot analysis to assay for expression of recombinant proteins.

2.6 Virus growth analysis

RK13 cells were infected with mO or recombinant viruses at a moi of 5 PFU/cell. After 1 h, the infected cells were washed with EMEM and cultured for 12-72 h after viral infection. Virus titers were determined by plaque titration according to Nishikawa et al. (2000). Data from this experiment were evaluated using Student's t-test. The 95% level of significance was used in the analysis.

3. Results

3.1 Expression of bLPO and bLF by recombinant vaccinia virus in RK13 cells

Vaccinia virus mO strain and pAK/bLPO or pAk/bLF were allowed to infect RK13 cells, and virus-containing medium of the infected RK13 cells was collected and analyzed by IFAT or Western blotting for the presence of recombinant bLPO or bLF. A recombinant bLPO or bLF-expressing clone was selected by the plaque-assay technique. vv/bLPO-infected cells were examined by IFAT and reacted with anti-bLPO mAb (Fig. 1B). Anti-bLF mAb reacted with vv/bLF-infected RK13 cells (Fig. 1C). mO-infected cells served as negative reference and were labeled with both antibody reagents (Fig. 1A). Recombinant bLPO and bLF were detected in cell extracts by Western blot analysis using anti-bLPO Ab and anti-bLF mAb (Fig. 2A, C lane 4). Recombinant bLPO and bLF were secreted into supernatants, as indicated by recombinant bLPO bands at 88 and 90 kDa and bLF band at 80 kDa (Fig.2B, D lane 4). The apparent molecular weight of these recombinant bLPO molecules (88 and 90 kDa) was greater than that of native bLPO (78 kDa), but apparent molecular weight of the bLF molecules (80 kDa) was equal to that of native bLF (80 kDa). To test whether the increase of molecular weights in recombinant bLPO was due to glycosylation, the infected cells were treated with tunicamycin. As a result, no protein was secreted into the supernatant by infected cells treated with tunicamycin (data not shown). In the cell extracts, the apparent molecular weight of bLPO was reduced to 80 kDa (Fig. 3 lane 4), indicating that recombinant bLPO were modified by N-linked sugars. The 90 kDa molecule would be a proprotein. Recombinant bLF was not detected in cell extracts from infected cells treated with tunicamycin, suggesting that tunicamycin treatment completely abolished production of recombinant bLF (data not shown).

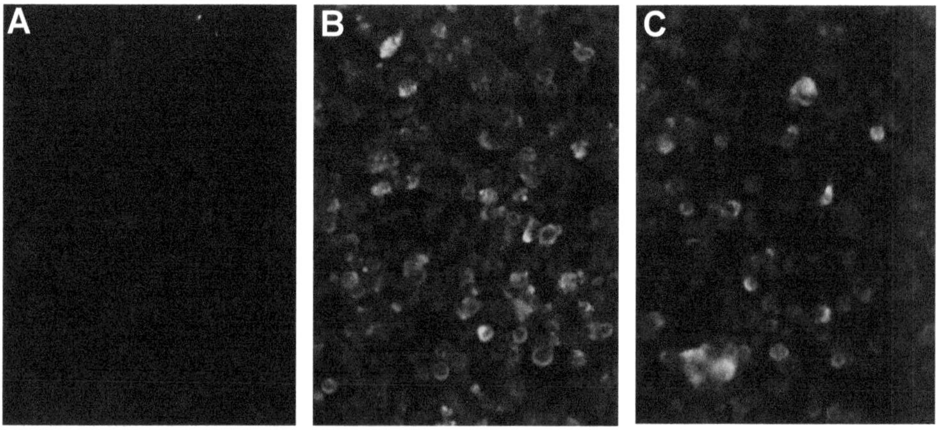

Fig. 1. Immunofluorescence analysis of vv/bLPO and vv/bLF expressed in RK 13 cells. (A) mO-infected RK13 cells reacted with anti-bLPO mAb and anti-bLF mAb. (B) vv/bLPO-infected RK13 cells reacted with anti-bLPO mAb. (C) vv/bLF-infected RK13 cells reacted with anti-bLF mAb.

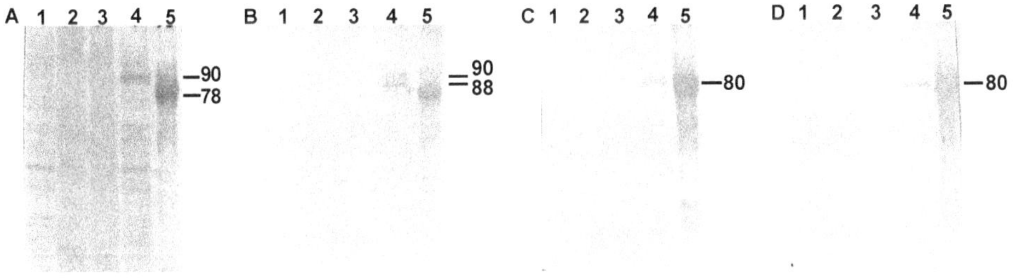

Fig. 2. Western blot analysis of bLPO (A, B) and bLF (C, D) in RK13 cells. Cell extracts (A, C) and culture supernatants (B, D) of RK13 cells infected with recombinant vaccinia virus were analyzed using anti-bLPO Ab or anti-bLF mAb. Lane 1, RK13 cells; lane 2, mO-infected RK13 cells; lane 3, vv/green florescence protein-infected RK13 cells; lane 4, vv/bLPO- or vv/bLF-infected RK13 cells; lane 5, native bLPO or bLF (2 μg). Molecular weights of marker proteins are given in kDa.

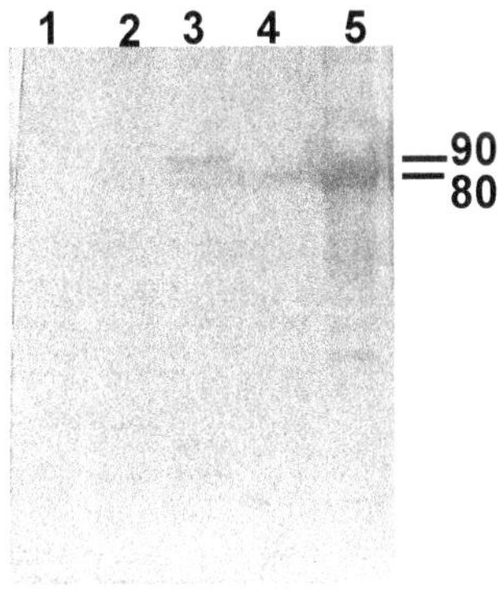

Fig. 3. Western blot analysis of bLPO in RK13 cells treated with tunicamycin. Cell extracts of RK13 cells infected with recombinant vaccinia virus were analyzed using anti-bLPO Ab. Lane 1, mO-infected RK13 cells; lane 2, mO-infected RK13 cells treated with tunicamycin; lane 3, vv/bLPO-infected RK13 cells; lane 4, vv/bLPO-infected RK13 cells treated with tunicamycin; lane 5, native bLPO (2 μg). Molecular weights of marker proteins are given in kDa.

3.2 Time course of bLPO and bLF production in the recombinant vaccinia virus system

To analyze the kinetics of expression of bLPO and bLF gene products, culture supernatants from RK13 cells infected with vv/bLPO and vv/bLF were collected from 12-72 h pi. Recombinant bLPO and bLF were first detectable in culture supernatant at 24 h pi (Fig. 4 lane 2). The amount of recombinant bLPO and bLF increased from 36 to 48 h pi, and reached plateau levels by 72 h pi (Fig. 4 lane 3-6).

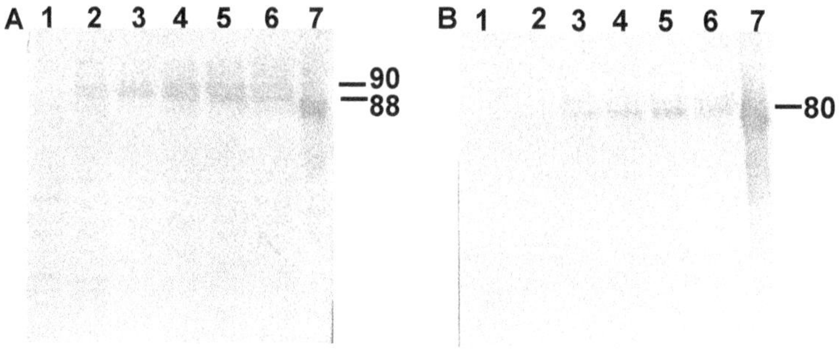

Fig.4. Kinetics of rbLPO (A) and rbLF (B) synthesis. RK13 cells were infected with recombinant vaccinia virus and harvested at 12 (lane 1), 24 (lane 2), 36 (lane 3), 48 (lane 4), 60 (lane 5) and 72 hours pi (lane 6). Lane 7, native bLPO or bLF (2 μg). Culture supernatants of infected RK13 cells were analyzed by Western blotting using anti-bLPO Ab or anti-bLF mAb. Molecular weights of marker proteins are given in kDa.

3.3 Growth analysis of vv/bLPO and vv/bLF in RK13 cells

The growth curves of mO, vv/bLPO and vv/bLF are compared in Fig. 5. Peak titers (reached at 48 h pi) of mO, vv/bLPO and vv/bLF were 1.6×10^5, 1.6×10^5 and 0.2×10^5 PFU/ml, respectively. These results indicate that bLF, but not bLPO, inhibits growth of recombinant virus in infected RK13 cells. There were no significant differences in growth between mO and vv/bLPO until 72 h pi ($P>0.05$, Student's t test mO vs. vv/bLPO). However, there were significant differences in growth between mO and vv/bLPO on one side and vv/bLF on the other side 48h pi through 72 h pi ($P<0.05$, Student's t test mO or vv/bLPO vs. vv/bLF).

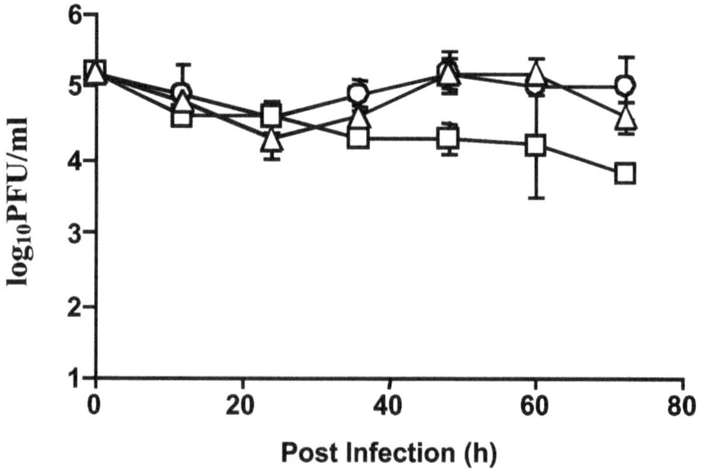

Fig. 5. Virus growth analysis. RK13 cells were infected with mO (○), vv/bLPO (△) and vv/bLF (□) at a moi of 5. Samples were harvested at the indicated time points, and progeny virus of RK13 cells was titered in triplicate.

4. Discussion

The expression systems using recombinant baculovirus or Chinese hamster ovary cells have been used to express bLPO (Tanaka et al., 2003; Watanabe et al., 1998). However, there have been no previous reports of use of vaccinia virus to express bLPO and bLF. The available evidence suggests that growth of vaccinia virus is inhibited by expression of bLPO and bLF. In the present study, recombinant vaccinia viruses expressing bLPO or bLF (vv/bLPO and vv/bLF, respectively) were constructed. RK13 cells were infected with vv/bLPO or vv/bLF, and we characterized virus growth and post-translation modifications of the resultant product.

Recombinant bLPO extracted from cell extracts and culture supernatants had an apparent molecular weight of 88 and 90 kDa, which is greater than that of native bLPO (78 kDa) in Western blot analysis. These size differences may be due to a difference in glycosylation level and differences in processing between RK13 cells and the mammary gland. When the infected RK13 cells were treated with tunicamycin, the apparent molecular weight of recombinant bLPO in the cells was 80 kDa, suggesting that recombinant bLPO is modified by N-linked glycosylation. Tunicamycin treatment completely abolished secretion of bLPO, indicating that N-linked glycosylation is essential for bLPO secretion. Therefore, recombinant bLPO was differentially processed during synthesis and secretion from RK13 cells compared with the mammary gland. A similar situation was previously reported for recombinant bLPO expressed in insect cells (Tanaka et al., 2003). Interestingly, the molecular weight of recombinant bLPO produced in RK13 cells was higher than that expressed in insect cells. The carbohydrate structure analysis of purified recombinant bLPO expressed in insect cells and native bLPO found different reactivity with PHA-E4, PNA, and RCA120 by using lectin assay (Tanaka et al., 2003). Therefore, the glycosylation level of recombinant protein might also be different between RK13 cells and insect cells. Most of the bLPO extracted from milk showed Asp-101 as the N-terminal amino acid residue (Dull et al., 1990; Watanabe et al., 2000). However, Watanabe et al. (2000) found also that different preparations of bLPO showed a different N-terminal amino acid residue. These variations may result from differences in the disk-electrophoresis and ion-exchange chromatography methods used for analysis (Carlström, 1969). Thus, it might be possible that the 90 kDa form of recombinant bLPO did not undergo proteolysis, whereas the 88 kDa form of recombinant bLPO be the result of proteolysis of some N-terminal amino acid residues during synthesis and secretion by RK 13 cells as observed for bLPO synthesized by the mammary gland.

Bovine Lactoferrin is a 80 kDa iron-binding glycoprotein found in physiological fluids of mammals. bLF has also an antimicrobial activity as bLPO, and presumably contributes to the protective functions of milk against infectious diseases. In RK13 cells infected with vv/bLF, recombinant bLF was detected in both cell extracts and culture supernatants. However, the replication of vv/bLF at a moi of 5 PFU/cell was inhibited by the antiviral activity of recombinant bLF, suggesting that vv/bLF has an antiviral effect against vaccinia virus. On the other hand, the expression of bLPO was also detected in cell extracts and culture supernatants of the vv/bLPO-infected cells as well as vv/bLF-infected cells. However, the replication of vv/bLPO at a moi of 5 PFU/cell was not inhibited by antiviral activity of recombinant bLPO, because LPO catalyzes oxidation of endogenous thiocyanate

(SCN^-) to produce hypothiocyanate ($OSCN^-$) only in the presence of hydrogen peroxide (H_2O_2). These products have a broad-spectrum antimicrobial and antiviral activity (Shin et al., 2001, 2005). Therefore due to the absence of thiocyanate (SCN^-) and/or hydrogen peroxide (H_2O_2) the replication of recombinant virus is not inhibited by recombinant bLPO.

Studies indicate that gene therapy using viral vectors containing the bLPO gene can produce anti-microbial and anti-tumor activity (Odajima et al., 1996; Stanislawski et al., 1989). The major problem with such viral vectors is their attenuation. The recombinant vaccinia viruses in this report are TK- in phenotype that may reduce pathogenicity *in vivo* (Buller et al., 1985) because of insertion of the bLPO gene into the TK gene. Our results demonstrate the attenuation of the viral pathogenicity by introduction of the bLPO gene into vaccinia virus. Thus fine tuning of bLPO activity, may allow the control of virulence of vaccinia virus vector necessary for medical and veterinary applications *in vivo*.

5. Conclusion

Lactoperoxidase (LPO) is a 78 kDa heme-containing oxidation-reduction enzyme present in milk, and lactoferrin (LF) is an 80 kDa iron-binding glycoprotein found in physiological fluids of mammals. LPO and LF have antimicrobial activity, and presumably contribute to the protective functions of milk against infectious diseases. In this study, recombinant vaccinia viruses expressing bovine lactoperoxidase (vv/bLPO) or bovine lactoferrin (vv/bLF) were constructed. In rabbit kidney (RK13) cells infected with vv/bLPO or vv/bLF, recombinant bLPO or bLF was detected in both cell extracts and supernatants. Growth of vv/bLPO at a multiplicity of infection was not inhibited by antiviral activity of recombinant bLPO, indicating that this recombinant virus could be used as a suicide viral vector. Unfortunately, growth of vv/bLF at a multiplicity of infection was inhibited by antiviral activity of recombinant bLF, suggesting that vv/bLF has an antiviral effect against vaccinia virus. These results indicate that a combination of bLPO and vaccinia virus vector may be useful for medical and veterinary applications *in vivo*.

6. Acknowledgments

This work was supported by grants from the Hokuto Foundation and the Food Science Institute Foundation (Ryoshoku-kenkyukai, Odawara). The first author is supported by Postdoctoral Fellowships for Research Abroad of the Japan Society for the Promotion of Science.

7. References

Baynes, R.; Bezwoda, W.; Bothwell, T.; Khan, Q. & Mansoor, N. (1986). The non immune inflammatory response: serial changes in plasma iron, iron binding capacity, lactoferrin, ferritin and C reactive protein. *Scandinavian Journal of clinical and Laboratory Investigation,* Vol.46, No.7, (November 1986), pp.695-704, ISSN 0036-5513

Buller, RM.; Smith, GL.; Cremer, K.; Notkins, AL. & Moss, B. (1985). Decreased virulence of recombinant vaccinia virus expression vectors is associated with thymidine kinase-negative phenotype. *Nature,* Vol.317, No.6004, (October 1985), pp.813-815, ISSN 0028-0836

Carlström, A. (1969). Lactoperoxidase. Identification of multiple molecular forms and their interrelationships. *Acta Chemica Scandinavica,* Vol. 23, No.1, (1969), pp.171-184, ISSN 0001-5393

Chochola, J.; Yamaguchi, Y.; Moguilevsky, N.; Bollen, A.; Strosberg, D.A. & Stanislawski, M. (1994). Virucidal effect of myeloperoxidase on human immunodeficiency virus type-1 infected cells. *Antimicrobial Agents and Chemotherapy,* Vol.38, No.5, (May 1994), pp.969-972, ISSN 0066-4804

Dull, TJ.; Uyeda, C.; Strosberg, AD.; Nedwin, G. & Seilhamer, J.J. (1990). Molecular cloning of cDNA encoding bovine and human lactoperoxidase. *DNA and Cell Biology,* Vol.9, No.7, (September 1990), pp.499-509, ISSN 1557-7430

El Messaoudi, K.; Verheyden, AM.; Thiry, L.; Fourez, S.; Tasiaux, N.; Bollen, A. & Moguilevsky, N. (2002). Human recombinant myeloperoxidase antiviral activity on cytomegalovirus. *Journal of Medical Virology,* Vol.66, No.2, (February 2002), pp.218-223, ISSN 1096-9071

Ertl, HC. & Xiang, Z. (1996). Novel vaccine approaches. *Journal of Immunology,* Vol. 156, No.10 , (May 1996), pp.3579-3582, ISSN 0022-1767

García-Montoya, IA.; Cendón, TS.; Arévalo-Gallegos, S. & Rascón-Cruz, Q. (2011) Lactoferrin a multiple bioactive protein: An overview. *Biochim Biophys Acta (BBA) - General Subjects,* (In press), ISSN 0304-4165

Gutteberg, T.; Haneberg, B. & Jorgenson, T. (1984). Lactoferrin in relation to acute phase proteins in sera from newborn infants with severe infections. *European Journal of Pediatrics,* Vol.142, No.1, (April 1984), pp.37-39, ISSN 0340-6199

Inui, K.; Barrett, T.; Kitching, RP. & Yamanouchi, K. (1995). Long-term immunity in cattle vaccinated with a recombinant rinderpest vaccine. *Veterinary Record,* Vol.137, No.26 , (December 1995), pp.669-670, ISSN 0042-4900

Kerr, SM. & Smith, GL. (1989). Vaccinia virus encodes a polypeptide with DNA ligase activity. *Nucleic Acids Research,* Vol.17, No.22, (November 1989), pp.9039-9050, ISSN 0305-1048

Klebanoff, SJ. & Kazazi, F. (1995). Inactivation of human immunodeficiency virus type 1 by the amine oxidase-peroxidase system. *Journal of Clinical Microbiology,* Vol.33, No.8 , (August 1995), pp.2054-2057, ISSN 0095-1137

Kohonen Corish, MR.; Blanden, RV. & King, N. (1989). Induction of cell surface expression of HLA antigens by human IFN-gamma encoded by recombinant vaccinia virus. *Journal of Immunology,* Vol.143, No.2 , (July 1989), pp.623-627, ISSN 0022-1767

Kohonen-Corish, MR.; King, NJ.; Woodhams, CE. & Ramshaw, IA. (1990). Immunodeficient mice recover from infection with vaccinia virus expressing interferon-gamma. *European Journal of Immunology,* Vol.20, No.1, (January 1990), pp.157-161, ISSN 1521-4141

Laemmli, UK. (1970). Cleavage of structural proteins during the assembly of the head of bacteriophage T4. *Nature,* Vol.227, No.5259, (August 1970), pp.680-685, ISSN 0028-0836

Masson, PL. & Heremans, JF. (1968). Presence of an iron binding protein (lactoferrin) in the genital tract of the female. I. its immunohistochemical localization in the endometrium. *Fertility and Sterility* Vol.19, No.5, (September 1968), pp.679-689, ISSN 0015-0282

Mansson-Rahemtulla, B.; Rahemtulla, F.; Baldone, DC.; Pruitt, KM. & Hjerpe, A. (1988). Purification and characterization of human salivary peroxidase. *Biochemistry,* Vol.27, No.1, (January 1988), pp.233-239, ISSN 0006-2960

Moguilevsky, N.; Steens, M.; Thiriart, C.; Prieels, J. P.; Thiry, L. & Bollen, A. (1992). Lethal oxidative damage to human immunodeficiency virus by human recombinant myeloperoxidase. *FEBS Letter,* Vol.302, No.3, (May 1992), pp.209-212, ISSN 0014-5793

Moss, B. (1990). Regulation of vaccinia virus transcription. *Annual Review of Biochemistry,* Vol.59, (July 1990), pp.661-688, ISSN 1545-4509

Moss, B. & Cooper, N. (1982). Genetic evidence for vaccinia virus-encoded DNA polymerase: isolation of phosphonoacetate-resistant enzyme from the cytoplasm of cells infected with mutant virus. *Journal of Virology,* Vol.43, No.2, (August 1982), pp. 673-678, ISSN 0022-538X

Nakamura, I.; Watanabe, A.; Tsunemitsu, H.; Lee, N-Y.; Kumura, H.; Shimazaki, K. & Yagi, Y. (2001). Production of recombinant bovine lactoferrin N-lobe in insect cells and its antimicrobial activity. *Protein Expression and Purification,* Vol.21, No.3, (April 2001), pp.424-431, ISSN 1046-5928

Nishikawa, Y.; Iwata, A.; Katsumata, A.; Xuan, X.; Nagasawa, H.; Igarashi, I.; Fujisaki, K.; Otsuka, H. & Mikami, T. (2001). Expression of canine interferon-γ by a recombinant vaccinia virus and its antiviral effect. *Virus Research,* Vol.75, No.2, (June 2001), pp.113-121, ISSN 0168-1702

Nishikawa, Y.; Iwata, A.; Xuan, X.; Nagasawa, H.; Fujisaki, K.; Otsuka, H. & Mikami, T. (2000). Expression of canine interferon-β by a recombinant vaccinia virus. *FEBS Letters,* Vol.466, No.1, (January 2000), pp.179-182, ISSN 0014-5793

Odajima, T.; Onishi, M.; Hayama, E.; Motoji, N.; Momose. Y. & Shigematsu, A. (1996). Cytolysis of B-16 melanoma tumor cells mediated by the myeloperoxidase and lactoperoxidase systems. *Biological Chemistry,* Vol.377, No.11, (November 1996), pp.689-693, ISSN 1431-6730

Peplinski, G.R.; Tsung, K.; Meko, J.B. & Norton, J.A. (1996). Prevention of murine breast cancer by vaccination with tumor cells modified by cytokine-producing recombinant vaccinia viruses. *Annals of Surgical Oncology,* Vol.3, No.1, (January 1996), pp.15-23, ISSN 1068-9265

Shimazaki, K.; Kamio, M.; Nan, M.S.; Harakawa, S.; Tanaka, T.; Omata, Y.; Saito, A.; Kumura, H.; Mikawa, K.; Igarashi, I. & Suzuki, N. (1998). Structure and immunochemical studies on bovine lactoferrin fragments. *Advances in Experimental Medicine and Biology,* Vol.443, (1998), pp. 41-48, ISSN 0065-2598

Shin, K.; Hayasawa, H. & Lönnerdal, B. (2001). Inhibition of *Escherichia coli* respiratory enzymes by the lactoperoxidase-hydrogen peroxidase-thiocyanate antimicrobial system. *Journal of Applied Microbiology,* Vol.90, No.4, (April 2001), pp.489-493, ISSN 1365-2672

Shin, K.; Wakabayashi, H.; Yamauchi, K.; Teraguchi, S.; Tamura, Y.; Kurokawa, M. & Shiraki, K. (2005). Effects of orally administered bovine lactoferrin and lactoperoxidase on influenza virus infection in mice. *Journal of Medical Microbiology,* Vol.54, No.8, (August 2005), pp.717-723, ISSN 0022-2615

Shuman, S. & Moss, B. (1987). Identification of a vaccinia virus gene encoding a type I DNA topoisomerase. *Proceedings of the National Academy of Sciences of the United States of America,* Vol.84, No.21, (November 1987), pp.7478-7482, ISSN 1091-6490

Stanislawski, M.; Rousseau, V.; Goavec, M. & Ito, H. (1989). Immunotoxins containing glucose oxidase and lactoperoxidase with tumoricidal properties: In vitro killing effectiveness in a mouse plasmacytoma cell model. *Cancer Research,* Vol.49, No.20, (October 1989), pp.5497-5540, ISSN 0008-5472

Tanaka, T.; Murakami, S.; Kumura, H.; Igarashi, I. & Shimazaki, K. (2006). Parasiticidal activity of bovine lactoperoxidase against *Toxoplasma gondii. Biochemstry and Cell Biology,* Vol.84, No.5, (October 2006), pp.774-779, ISSN 0829-8211

Tanaka, T.; Omata, Y.; Saito, A.; Shimazaki, K.; Igarashi, I. & Suzuki, N. (1996). Growth inhibitory effects of bovine lactoferrin to *Toxoplasma gondii* parasites in murine somatic cells. *The Journal of Veterinary Medical Science,* Vol.58, No.1, (January 1998), pp.61-65, ISSN 0916-7250

Tanaka, T.; Sato, S.; Kumura, H. & Shimazaki, K. (2003). Expression and characterization of bovine lactoperoxidase by recombinant baculovirus. *Bioscience Biotechnology and Biochemistry,* Vol.67, No.10, (October 2003), pp.2254-2261, ISSN 1347-6947

Tsukiyama, K.; Yoshikawa, Y.; Kamata, H.; Imaoka, K.; Asano, K.; Funahashi, S.; Maruyama, T.; Shida, H.; Sugimoto, M. & Yamanouchi, K. (1989). Development of heat-stable recombinant rinderpest vaccine. *Achieves Virology,* Vol.107, No.3-4, (September 1989), pp.225-235, ISSN 0304-8608

Venge, P.; Foucard, T.; Henrickson, J.; Hakansson, L. & Kreuger, A. (1984). Serum-levels of lactoferrin, lysozyme and myeloperoxidase in normal, infection-prone and leukemic children. *Clinica Chimica Acta,* Vol.136, No.2-3, (January 1984), pp.121-130, ISSN 0009-8981

Watanabe, S.; Murata, S.; Kumura, H.; Nakamura, S.; Bollen, A.; Moguilevsky, N. & Shimazaki, K. (2000). Bovine lactoperoxidase and its recombinant: comparison of structure and some biochemical properties. *Biochemical and Biophysical Research Communications,* Vol.274, No.3, (August 2000), pp.756-761, ISSN 0006-291X

Watanabe, S.; Varsalona, F.; Yoo, Y. C.; Guillaume, JP.; Bollen, A.; Shimazaki, K. & Moguilevsky, N. (1998). Recombinant bovine lactoperoxidase as a tool to study the heme environment in mammalian peroxidases. *FEBS Letters,* Vol.441, No.3, (December 1998), pp.476-479, ISSN 0014-5793

Yamamoto, K.; Miyoshi-Koshio, T.; Utsuki, Y.; Mizuno, S. & Suzuki, K. (1991). Virucidal activity and viral protein modification by myeloperoxidase: a candidate for defense factor of human polymorphonuclear leukocytes against influenza virus infection. *Journal of Infectious Diseases,* Vol.164, No.1, (July 1991), pp.8-14, ISSN 0022-1899

Yasuda, A.; Kimura-Kuroda, J.; Ogimoto, M.; Miyamoto, M.; Sata, T.; Sato, T.; Takamura, C.; Kurata, T.; Kojima, A. & and Yasui, K. (1990). Induction of protective immunity in animals vaccinated with recombinant vaccinia viruses that express PreM and E glycoproteins of Japanese encephalitis virus. *Journal of Virology*, Vol.64, No.6, (June 1990), pp.2788-2795, ISSN 0022-538X

Part 2

Molecular Epidemiology and Mitigation Strategy

6

Diphtheria Toxin and Cytosolic Translocation Factors

Ryan C. Ratts[1] and John R. Murphy[2]
[1]*Dartmouth Medical School*
[2]*Boston University School of Medicine*
USA

1. Introduction

Diphtheria Toxin (DT) was the first investigated bacterial protein toxin. As one of the most extensively studied bacterial protein toxins, it has served as a model system for the analysis of other protein toxins (Pappenheimer, 1977). As reviewed by Pappenheimer, Loeffler identified *Corynebacterium diphtheriae* as the causative agent of diphtheria in 1884, and the toxin was first described in the culture medium of *C. diphtheriae* by Roux and Yersin in 1888. The gene for DT is encoded by a family of closely related corynebacteriophages (Uchida et al., 1971; Greenfield et al., 1983), and is expressed only under conditions of iron deprivation (Pappenheimer, 1977). Regulation of DT expression is under control of the iron-activated diphtheria toxin repressor, DTxR, which is encoded in the *C. diphtheriae* genome and inhibits transcription of DT in the presence of iron and other transition metal ions (Love and Murphy, 2000).

DT is translated with a 25 amino acid signal peptide and is co-translationally secreted as a single 535 amino acid residue polypeptide chain with a molecular weight of 58 kDa (Smith, 1980; Kaczorek et al., 1983). Biochemical analysis of DT demonstrated that proteolytic 'nicking' of the toxin *in vitro* results in two fragments, A and B, which remain covalently attached by an inter-chain disulfide bond (Gill and Pappenheimer, 1971). Fragment A contains the enzymatic activity (Collier and Kandel, 1971), whereas Fragment B mediates binding to cell surface receptors and facilitates the cytosolic entry of fragment A (Drazin et al., 1971). X-ray crystallographic analysis, at a resolution of 2.5 Å, demonstrated that DT is composed of three structural domains: the amino terminal catalytic (C) domain corresponds to fragment A (21 kDa), and the transmembrane (T) and carboxy terminal receptor binding (R) domains comprise fragment B (37 kDa) (Figure 1) (Choe et al., 1992). A disulfide bond between Cys186 and Cys201 subtends a 14 amino acid protease sensitive loop and connects fragment A with fragment B (Gill and Pappenheimer, 1971). Furin mediated cleavage within this loop and retention of the disulfide bond have been shown to be pre-requisites for intoxication of eukaryotic cells (Ariansen et al., 1993; Tsuneoka et al., 1993).

Once delivered into cytosol, the C-domain catalyzes the NAD+-dependent ADP-ribosylation of elongation factor 2 (EF-2). EF-2 is a soluble translocase involved in protein synthesis, and is the only known substrate for the DT C domain in eukaryotic cells (Pappenheimer, 1977). Transfer of the ADP-ribosyl moiety of NAD^+ to a modified histidine residue in EF-2 (diphthamide) results in the irreversible arrest of chain elongation during protein synthesis (Collier and Cole, 1969), leading to cell death by apoptosis.

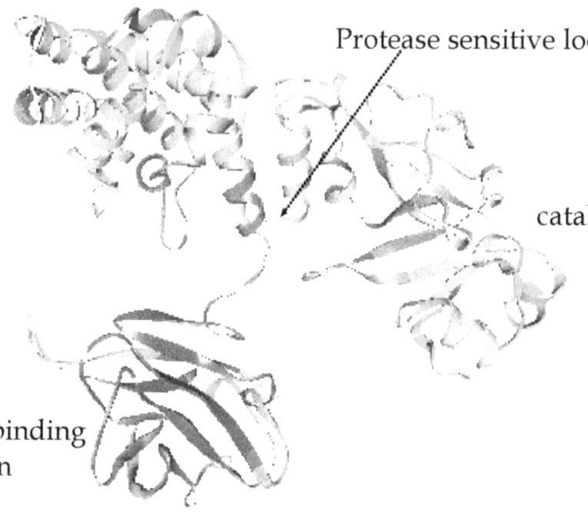

Fig. 1. X-Ray Crystallographic Structure of Diphtheria Toxin. PDB 1 MDT. Modified from Choe et al., 1992.

2. Receptor binding

Intoxication by DT involves an ordered sequence of events in which each structural domain of the toxin plays a precise and essential role and begins with toxin binding to cells expressing the heparin binding epidermal growth factor-like precursor (Figure 2) (Naglich et al., 1992). The sensitivity of targeted cells to intoxication by DT is roughly related to the number of receptors present on the cell surface, and is also enhanced by the diphtheria toxin receptor associated protein 27, DTRAP 27, which is the primate homologue of human CD9 (Mitamura et al., 1992). Human CD9 antigen, which is associated with the DT receptor but not DT itself, enhances sensitivity to DT through an unknown mechanism (Brown et al, 1993; Iwamoto et al., 1994),. In contrast to other AB toxins - such as abrin, ricin, and cholera - neither gangliosides nor galactosides have any effect on DT binding and intoxication (Pappenheimer, 1977).

In 1896, Paul Ehrlic coined the phrase "Zauberkugeln", or "magic bullet," for specifically targeting cells causing disease. This dream was realized almost a hundred years later by Murphy et al. (1986) with the design and synthesis of DT based fusion protein toxins that were targeted toward specific eukaryotic cell receptors. Substitution of the native R domain with a surrogate ligand results in the formation of a fusion protein toxin construct that targets cells expressing the appropriate cell surface receptor. The first genetically engineered fusion protein toxin, $DAB_{486}MSH$, consisted of DT fragment A and a portion of fragment B fused to α-melanocyte stimulating hormone (α-MSH) (Murphy et al., 1986). While this fusion protein toxin construct was prone to degradation, human interleukin 2 (IL-2) was selected as the next surrogate receptor binding domain and $DAB_{486}IL$-2 was next constructed (Williams et al., 1987). $DAB_{486}IL$-2 proved resistant to degradation, was

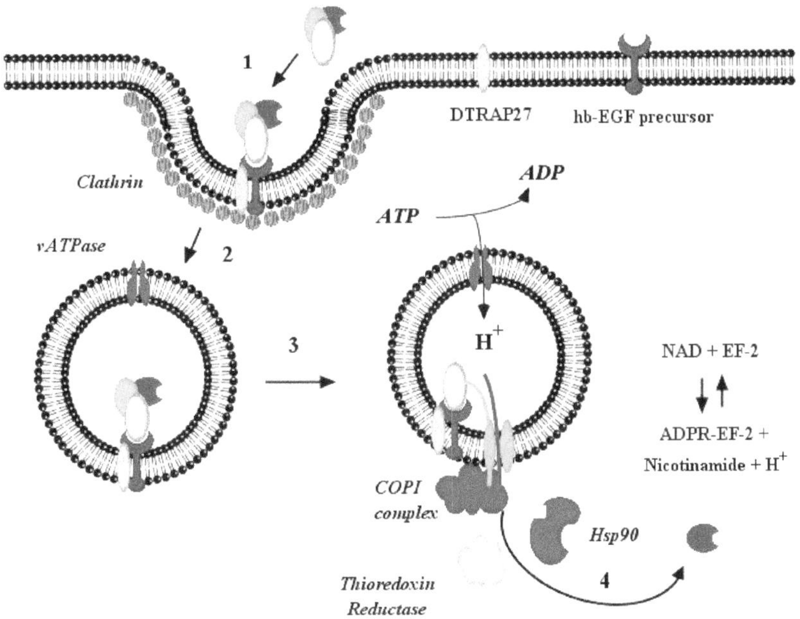

Fig. 2. Schematic Overiew of DT Intoxication. (1) DT binds to its cell surface receptor (2) Internalization of clathrin coated pits into early endosomal vesicles (3) Acidification of the endosomal lumen induces DT T domain insertion and pore formation (4) Translocation and cytosolic release of the DT C domain is facilitated by COPI complex, Thioredoxin Reductase and Hsp90. Refolded DT C domain catalyzes the ADP-ribosylation of EF-2. Diphtheria toxin: yellow = receptor binding (R) domain; green = transmembrane (T) domain; red = catalytic (C) domain. Reproduced from Murphy (2011).

remarkably potent (IC_{50} of 1 x 10^{-11} M), and was specifically targeted to cells only expressing high affinity IL-2 receptors (Bacha et al., 1980; Williams et al., 1990). Subsequent in-frame deletion analysis of the carboxy terminal residues in the DT portion of DAB_{486}IL-2 demonstrated that incorporation of a smaller portion of the diphtheria toxin fragment B, DAB_{389}IL-2, resulted in a chimeric toxin that was 10-fold more cytotoxic (Williams et al., 1990).

In the case of DAB_{389}IL-2, only the high affinity and intermediate affinity IL-2 receptor - toxin complexes are internalized (Waters et al., 1990). The specific expression of the high affinity IL-2 receptor on only activated and proliferating T-cells made DAB_{389}IL-2 a potential therapeutic agent for the treatment of both T-cell mediated malignancies and autoimmune diseases (Ratts and vanderSpek, 2002). In 1999, DAB_{389}IL-2 (ONTAK®) was the first fusion protein toxin construct approved by the U.S. Food and Drug Administration for clinical use in humans, and is currently used for the treatment of CD25 positive refractory cutaneous T cell lymphoma (Ratts and vanderSpek,2002). In designing fusion protein constructs, only those surrogate ligands that trigger clathrin dependent endocytosis, analogous to the mechanism of entry of endogenous DT, are functional. There are currently more than 20 different fusion protein toxins under clinical development. Since DAB_{389}IL-2 binds with greater affinity to its receptor compared to native DT, this fusion protein toxin has proven to be an effective and novel probe for studying internalization of the C-domain by target cells.

3. Endocytosis

Receptor bound DT is concentrated in clathrin coated pits and internalized into clathrin coated vesicles (CCVs), which are then converted into early endosomes (Moya et al. 1985). Assembly of the clathrin coat is inhibited by depletion of intercellular potassium, and cells are protected against DT under such conditions (Moya et al., 1985; Sandvig et al., 1985). Sequestration of the coated pit from the plasma membrane requires additional proteins, including the GTPase dynamin (Simpson et al., 1998). Simpson et al. (1998) demonstrated that over expression of dominant negative dynamin blocks clathrin dependent endocytosis and protects cells against DT. Successful detachment of the coated pit results in CCVs which are subsequently released into the cytoplasm. After entering the cytoplasm, the CCVs are uncoated in an ATPase dependent manner and the subsequent homotypic fusion of uncoated vesicles results in the formation of early endosomes (Luzio et al., 2001). The clathrin triskelon is replaced with a new set of protein components on the vesicle membrane that includes Arf-1, COPI complex, Rab-5, early endosomal antigen (EEA1), and vesicular (v)-ATPase. Although the precise mechanism is unclear, the dynamic docking and release of these factors activates the process of membrane fusion through the formation of a fusion pore and activation of v-ATPase (Luzio et al, 2001).

The characteristic feature of endosomes is acidification of the lumen by v-ATPase. Acidification promotes protein sorting by dissociating ligand-receptor complexes and allowing some receptors to be recycled back to the plasma membrane. Acidification is also required for the formation of endosomal carrier vesicles (ECVs), which carry ligands and non-dissociated ligand-receptor complexes from early to late endosomes. Bafilomycin A1, a specific inhibitor of v-ATPase, blocks acidification and prevents the formation of ECVs, resulting in the accumulation of early endosomes (Bowman, et al.,1988). The formation of ECVs requires the binding of both β'COP (Sec 27) and ADP-ribosylation factor 1 (ARF1) to the cytoplasmic surface of the endosomal membrane, and binding of both factors is dependent upon a low pH within the endosomal lumen (Aniento et al., 1996). Inward invaginations of the endosomal membrane also occurs during ECV formation, resulting in the production of multi-vesicular bodies (Futter et al., 1996).

Several studies have confirmed the early endosomal compartment as the site fragment A translocation. Merion et al. (1983) showed that endosomes isolated from DT resistant mutants of chinese hamster ovary (CHO)-K1 cells were defective in acidification. In contrast, lysosomes isolated from the same mutants were not defective in acidification, suggesting that the endosomal compartment was the site of fragment A translocation (Merion et al., 1983). Umata et al. (1990) demonstrated that Bafilomycin A1, which prevents acidification of the endosomal lumen, protected cells against DT intoxication.

Cell fractionation experiments provided the best evidence that DT translocation occurs from early endosomes (Papini et al., 1993a; Papini et al. 1993b; Lemichez et al., 1997). While the DT C domain is most efficiently translocated from early endosomes, the majority of the toxin is actually sorted into ECVs and late endosomes where translocation of the C domain into the cytosol is marginal (Lemichez et al., 1997). Toxin trapped within ECVs and late endosomes is ultimately targeted for lysosomes and degraded. Lemichez et al. (1997) provided two possible explanations for why toxin failed to translocate from ECVs or late endosomes: First, there might be cytosolic factors specific to early endosomes required for translocation. Second, translocation events might actually be occurring in the ECVs, but such events within the multi-vesicular body would result in the vectorial transfer of the DT C domain into the lumen of another intra-vaculolar vesicle rather than the cytosol.

4. Role for acidification

Ammonium salts (e.g., NH_4Cl), glutamine and other amines, and choloroquine were the first compounds found to inhibit the cytosolic entry of the DT (Kim et al., 1965; Sandvig et al., 1980). Although these compounds had no effect upon neither enzymatic activity nor receptor binding, these reagents did protect sensitive cells against DT intoxication. Choloroquine and ammonium salts are ionophores, and they raise the luminal pH of endosomes and lysosomes. These results led to the hypothesis that passage of DT through a low pH compartment was a required step for intoxication. Umata et al. (1990) confirmed this hypothesis by demonstrating that acidification of the endosomal lumen by membrane associated vesicular (v)-ATPase was a required step in DT intoxication.

In contrast to the endosomal route, low pH (5.5) exposure of toxin bound to the surface of cells results in decreased protein synthesis even in the presence of choloroquine and ammonium ions (Sandvig et al., 1980). This same study demonstrated that the entry of pre-nicked diphtheria toxin through the cell membrane in the low pH environment was time and temperature dependent. Using the same system, Sandvig and Olsnses (1981) also demonstrated that the cytosolic entry of the DT C domain could be blocked by the metabolic inhibitors 2-deoxyglucose and sodium azide, implying that a cellular ATPase was required for the membrane translocation of the DT C domain (Sandvig et al., 1981).

Pronase protection assays were used to examine which portions of DT inserted into the plasma membrane when toxin bound cells were exposed to low pH (Moskaug et al., 1991). Moskaug et al. (1991) found a translocated fragment A (20 kD) in the cytosol and a plasma membrane associated 25 kDa peptide derived from fragment B. Furthermore, an inwardly directed proton gradient was required for the translocation of fragment A, but not for membrane insertion of fragment B (Sandvig et al., 1988). Analogously, it has also been shown that translocation of fragment A requires a lower pH as compared to the membrane insertion of fragment B (Falnes et al., 1992).

5. Pore formation

Exposure of DT transmembrane (T) domain to artificial lipid bilayers at low pH results in spontaneous membrane insertion and the formation of voltage dependent and cation selective channels (Boquet et al., 1976; Donovan et al., 1981). Kagan et al. (1981) observed a channel diameter of approximately 18-22 Å, which is theoretically large enough to accommodate the passage of a fully denatured fragment A. The crystal structure of DT shows that the T domain is composed of nine α-helices (TH1-9) and their connecting loops, and that the helices are arranged in three layers (Figure 1, Choe et al., 1992). The first three helices (TH1-3) comprise the first layer and are amphipathic in nature. Helices TH5, 6, and 7 compose a second hydrophobic layer. The third, central core layer is composed of the hydrophobic helices TH8 and 9, connected by transmembrane loop 5 (TL5).

Insertion of this third α-helical layer (Th8-9) is required for pore formation, which is then stabilized by the second α-helical layer (TH5, 6, and 7). Assays used to measure the formation and conductance of membrane pores, such as patch clamp experiments, molecular marker exclusion studies, and pH sensitive dyes have been used in conjunction with diphtheria toxin mutants to demonstrate the importance of specific residues in pore formation and support this model of helix insertion (Figure 3). Upon acidifcation of the endosomal lumen, residues Glu 349 and Asp 352 located at the tip of loop (TL5) connecting TH8 and TH9 are protonated, and the third helical layer spontaneously inserts into the membrane and forms a cation selective channel (O'Keefe et al., 1992; Mindell et al., 1994). Deletion or disruption of these helices by introducing proline residues ablates channel formation and results in non-cytotoxic mutants (vanderSpek et al., 1994a; Hu et al., 1998), suggesting that the full length helices arranged in a specific conformation is required for channel formation. While helices TH8 and 9 alone can create pores (Silverman et al., 1994), pore formation by TH8 and 9 alone is not sufficient for effective delivery of the C domain (vanderSpek et al., 1994a).

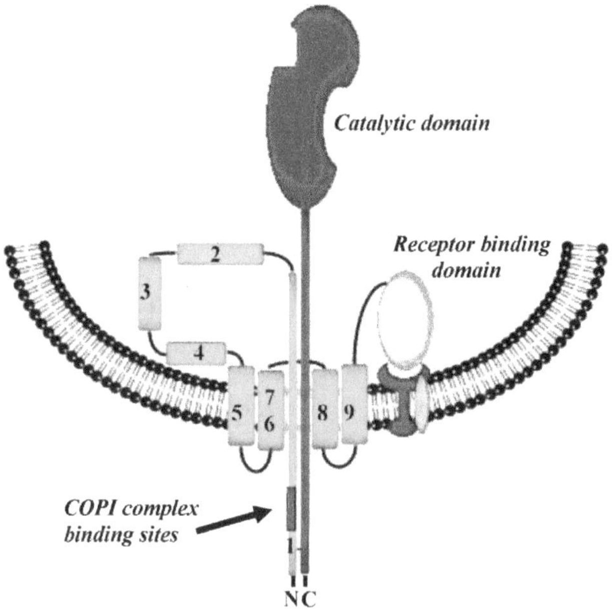

Fig. 3. Schematic of DT transmembrane (T) domain membrane insertion and pore formation. Following furin mediated nicking at Arg194 and denaturation of the catalytic (C) domain, the *N*-terminal portion of the T domain with the disulfide bond linked C-terminal end of the C domain is threaded into the pore. Emergence of one or more of the KXKXX motifs in first alpha helix (TH1) of the T domain on the cytosolic side of the vesicle membrane allows for binding of the COPI complex required for translocation of the catalytic domain. Reproduced from Murphy (2011).

The role that the Pro 345 residue, located at the end of TH8, plays in channel formation remains unclear. Mutation of Pro 345 to either a Glu residue, an α-helix former, or to a Gln residue, an α-helix breaker, resulted in a marked decrease in DT toxicity (Johnson et al., 1993). The *cis-trans* isomerization of proline by membrane associated peptidylprolyl *cis-trans* isomerases (PPIases), or cyclophilins, is important in the gating mechanisms of other cation selective channels, and a role for PPIases in DT channel formation or translocation of the DT C domain have been proposed (Johnson et al., 1993).

Following membrane insertion of the third helical layer, the second helical layer is subsequently inserted next and is thought to stabilize the channel formed by helices TH8 and 9 (Cabiaux et al., 1993; Cabiaux et al. 1994). Insertion of proline residues into the second helical layer of $DAB_{389}IL$-2 resulted in non-cytotoxic mutants with abnormal channel formation (Hu et al., 1998). Although this layer is not required for channel formation, it appears that the second helical layer is required for the formation of productive channels capable of supporting C domain translocation across the early endosomal membrane.

Deletion of the first three helices of $DAB_{389}IL$-2 resulted in a non-cytotoxic mutant that still formed characteristic channels and retained enzymatic activity (vanderSpek et al., 1993). The amino terminal residues of TH1 are translocated across the membrane and presented to the cytosol (Madshus et al., 1994a). Replacement of the charged residues in TH1 with uncharged residues strongly inhibits translocation of TH1 (Madshus et al., 1994a, vanderSpek et al., 1994b). The insertion of proline residues into the first helical layer also resulted in non-cytotoxic mutants that formed characteristic channels and retained enzymatic activity (Hu et al., 1998).

Taken together, these results suggested that the first helical layer facilitates the orientation and insertion of the C domain through the nascent channel formed by the T domain. Assuming that the disulfide bond connecting fragments A and fragment B remains intact, translocation of amino terminal residues of TH1 across the endosomal membrane would be anticipated to effectively thread the carboxy terminal residues of the C domain through the nascent channel and present them to the cytosol (vanderSpek et al., 1994b), and this work implied possible interactions with an unidentified translocation apparatus. These early findings were prescient of the recent identification of the T1 motif in TH1 by Ratts et al (2005) and role of the di-lysine motif KXKXX in recruiting components COPI complex required for toxin entry that is discussed below (Trujillo et al., 2010).

6. Unfolding of the catalytic domain

Unfolding of the DT C domain occurs *in vitro* in acidic conditions similar to those found inside the lumen of the endosome, and unfolding is required for delivery. Given the limited size of the pore, unfolding of the DT C domain was postulated as a pre-requisite for translocation (Donovan et al., 1981; Kagan et al., 1981). The necessity for complete denaturation of the DT C domain prior to translocation was then indirectly demonstrated by (Wiedlocha et al., 1992) and by (Falnes et al., 1994). Wiedlocha et al. (1992) fused acidic fibroblast growth factor (aFGF) to the amino terminus of fragment A. This aFGF-DT fusion protein construct was cytotoxic, confirming the observation that polypeptides fused to fragment A are delivered into the cytosol of targeted cells (Stenmark et al., 1991). In the presence of heparin, however, aFGF retains a rigid tertiary structure and the aFGF-DT fusion protein was no longer cytotoxic, implying that unfolding is a requirement for delivery through the nascent channel formed by the T domain. Falsnes et al. (1994) also created a double cysteine mutant which formed a disulfide bond within fragment A. With the disulfide bond intact, unfolding of fragment A does not occur. This mutant retained ADP-ribosyltransferase activity, but it was not cytotoxic. Taken together, these studies indicated that the cytosolic delivery of the C domain occurs in at least a partially unfolded state and that once delivered into the cytosol, the C domain must be refolded into an active conformation.

7. Reduction of the interchain disulfide bond

The C domain is separated from the T and R domains by a protease sensitive loop that is sub-tended by the disulfide bond between residues Cys 186 and Cys 201. Upon binding and internalization of the toxin-receptor complex, this loop is nicked by the enzyme furin (Tsuneoka et al., 1993). Retention of the interchain disulfide bond following nicking is a pre-requisite for intoxication (Falsnes et al., 1992), and it presumably mediates threading the DT C domain through the channel formed by the T domain. The pivotal role of reducing the inter-chain disulfide bond is underscored by the observation that reduction and release of the C domain appears to be the rate limiting step for the entire intoxication process (Papini et al., 1993b).

The precise location where reduction of the DT inter-chain dilsulfide bond occurs remains somewhat controversial. Moskaug et al. (1987) showed that only membrane permeate sulfhydryl blockers were able to prevent the release of the C-domain into cytosol. Papini et al. (1993b) reported that reduction of the DT interchain disulfide bond occurs after the low pH induced membrane insertion of the T domain within the early endosome. Since unreduced DT C domain and membrane inserted DT fragment B are both targeted for proteolytic degradation (Madshus et al. 1994b), these results suggested that reduction of the interchain disulfide bond occurs during or post-translocation. In contrast, Ryser et al. (1991) found that membrane impermeate sulfhydryl blockers prevented DT intoxication, and proposed that reduction occurs prior to translocation, presumably on the cell surface or within the endosomal lumen. *In vitro* studies have shown that thioredoxin 1 (Trx-1) (12 kDa) reduces the DT inter-chain disulfide bond under acidic conditions (Moskaug et al., 1987). This result is consistent with observations that exposure of the DT interchain disulfide bond on the protein surface occurs upon denaturation (Blewitt et al., 1985). Trx-1 is predominately cytosolic, but a shorter form (10 kDa) is actively secreted by a non-classical ER-Golgi independent pathway and is present on the luminal side of the endosomal membrane (Rosen et al., 1995). It is not known whether or not Trx-1 interacts directly with DT *in vivo*.

8. Model for autonomous delivery

Initial studies of T domain insertion and pore formation in artificial lipid bilayers in the presence of a pH gradient led to the hypothesis of autonomous delivery of the C domain, and Deleers et al (1983) first suggested that a pH gradient was required to facilitate C-domain delivery. Shiver and Donovan (1987), using asolectin vesicles, demonstrated that diphtheria toxin could deliver its own C-domain across the artificial bilayer in a pH dependent fashion, independent of added proteins or factors. These studies demonstrated a requirement for a pH gradient, in which the endocytic vesicle luminal pH is optimally between 4.7 and 5.5 and the cytosolic pH is at or near 7.4. The topography of DT inserted into both cell plasma membranes and artificial bilayers has been studied using protease digestion and analyzing the enzymatic cleavage products (Moskaug et al, 1991, Cabiaux et al, 1994). Although insertion of transmembrane helices 8 and 9 is a common finding of these studies, discrepancies arise in interpreting cleavage products that include the C-domain and whether or not they represent translocation intermediates (Madhus, 1994). Taken together, the apparent ability of DT to transfer its C-domain across synthetic lipid bilayers, in the absence of other proteins, led to a model of autonomous C-domain delivery.

The model of autonomous C-domain delivery was advanced by Oh et al. (1999) using planar lipid membranes and DT labeled with an *N*-terminal histidine tag (6× His). Since addition of Ni2+ to the *trans* compartment prevented the rapid closure of pores, these investigators concluded that the N- terminal end of the C-domain containing the His tag was translocated from the *cis* to the *trans* side of the lipid bilayer upon channel formation by the T-domain. These investigators also used biotin to label cysteine site-directed mutants at either position 58 or 148. The addition of streptavidin to the *trans* side of the planar lipid membrane also interfered with the channel closure. Again, these results suggested that Cys_{58} and Cys_{148} were on the *trans* side of the membrane following channel formation.

Also using artificial lipid bilayers, Ren et al. (1999) demonstrated that in a low pH environment, the presence of proteins in a partly unfolded molten globule-like conformation (e.g. unfolded C-domain) were able to convert the T domain from a shallow membrane inserted form to a fully *trans*- membrane inserted form. Hammond et al (2002) confirmed that the DT T-domain has chaperonin-like properties, but also observed that the T domain had a significantly greater affinity for other molten globule-like polypeptides compared to its own C-domain. The chaperonin-like property of membrane inserted T domain towards unfolded substrates under acidic conditions has been confirmed (Hayashibara *et al*, 2005; Chassaing *et al.*, 2011).

In the autonomous translocation model, delivery of the C-domain is thought to be achieved through the chaperonin-like activity of the T-domain. Although these studies clearly demonstrate ability for DT to utilize a pH gradient, in conjunction with a relatively high membrane potential, to mediate autonomous translocation *in vitro*, it is not at all clear that these conditions occur *in vivo*. Many proteins are imbedded in the endosomal membrane and decorate both the luminal and cytosolic face of endocytic vesicles, and the impact these proteins may have on toxin delivery across the endosomal membrane are not included in artificial membrane bilayer systems. Since protease digestion patterns of DT inserted into planar lipid bilayers differ from those of DT inserted into the plasma membrane (Moskaug et al., 1991; Cabiaux et al., 1994), it seems likely that interaction(s) between the toxin and proteins associated with the endosomal membrane influence the orientation and/or stoichiometry of T-domain membrane insertion and translocation of the C-domain.

9. Model for facilitated delivery

A role for cellular factors in facilitating DT membrane translocation was first suggested by Sandvig and Olsnses (1981) with their observation that the successful delivery of toxin artificially inserted into the plasma membrane under acidic conditions required the function of a cellular ATPase. This hypothesis was expanded by Kaneda et al (1984), who established hybrid cell lines resistant to DT and demonstrated that the resistance of these cell lines appeared to be independent of receptor binding, receptor trafficking, and susceptibility of EF2 to ADP-ribosylation. They concluded that the resistance of these hybrid lines was due to cellular factors required for toxin entry.

The rationale for cellular factors facilitating the delivery of the DT C-domain across the endosomal membrane is congruent with other known and similar mechanisms of protein translocation across membranes within eukaryotic cells such as mitochondrial import, ER synthesis, and the retrograde translocation of toxins from the ER. During mitochondrial import, an electrochemical membrane potential is initially required for insertion of the proteins synthesized in the cytosol into the translocation complex and its subsequent transfer to the translocation complex present on the mitochondrial inner membrane (Bauer et al., 2000). The inward movement of the protein, however, requires unfolding and its translocation into the mitochondrial matrix is mediated by an ATP dependent import motor consisting of at least three components, including mitochondrial heat shock protein 70 (Hsp 70) (Bauer et al., 2000). The translocation of newly synthesized proteins into the ER occurs co-translationally through channels formed by the Sec 61 translocon complex (Tsai et al., 2002). Bip, an ER luminal resident homologue of Hsp 70, functions analogously to mitochondrial Hsp 70 in mediating protein translocation into the ER lumen (Baker et al., 1996). In contrast, the ERAD pathway involves the retro-translocation of misfolded proteins, as well as several toxins (*e.g.* cholera, pseudomonas exotoxin A, ricin), from the ER lumen into the cytosol through the same Sec 61 channel (Tsai et al., 2002). In ERAD, as reviewed by Tsai et al (2002), misfolded luminal proteins are recognized and unfolded by chaperones prior to retro-translocation through the Sec 61 channel. Cellular factors that are conserved from yeast to humans, are then required for the extraction of from the ER membrane and their subsequent release into the cytosol. In all of these systems, translocation is facilitated by the sequential binding and refolding of denatured proteins by chaperonins as they emerge through the membrane.

Lemichez et al (1997) provided the first direct evidence supporting the hypothesis that delivery of the C-domain across the endosomal membrane requires both ATP and cytosolic factors. This pivotal study demonstrated that DT translocation occurs from within early endosomes, and that Bafilomycin A1 resulted in the accumulation of DT within the lumen of arrested early endosomes. These investigators established an *in vitro* translocation assay system using purified early endosomes pre-loaded with DT from cells treated with bafilomycin A1. The *in vitro* translocation of the C-domain across the endosomal membrane required the addition of both ATP and cytosolic factors. Lemichez et al (1997) also observed that DT co-localizes with β'COP in tubular structures, and that antibodies to β'COP inhibited the *in vitro* translocation of the DT C domain across the endosomal membrane.

10. Defining the DT Cytosolic Translocation Factor (CTF) complex

Using the *in vitro* translocation assay developed by Lemichez *et al.* (1997) as a purification assay, Ratts *et al.* (2003) confirmed and extended the observations that cytosolic translocation factors (CTFs) are essential for the translocation and release of the DT C-domain from the lumen of early endosomes pre-loaded with the fusion protein toxin DAB_{389}IL-2. Control endosomes loaded with horse radish peroxidase and a pH sensitive dye

(OG514) demonstrated that endosomal lysis did not occur and that the cytosolic factors were not required for endosomal acidification, respectively, under assay conditions. Protein complexes mediating toxin translocation were then partially purified from both human and yeast cytosolic extracts, and individual proteins were identified using mass spectrometry sequencing. The potential role of individual proteins as putative CTFs were then examined using specific inhibitors and/or neutralizing antibodies. Ratts et al (2003) showed that both heat shock protein 90 (Hsp 90) and thioredoxin reductase 1 (TrR-1), and their yeast homologues Hsp 82 and TrR, respectively, are components of the CTF complex required for DT entry. Importantly, CTF activity was limited to the translocation step and neither factor inhibited the enzymatic ADP-ribosylation of EF2 by the DT C-domain. Finally, a physiologic role for Hsp 90 and TrR-1 was confirmed using specific inhibitors in cytotoxicity assays to protect cells against toxin. Although Hsp 90, TrR-1, β-COP have all been confirmed as CTFs for the entry of diphtheria toxin, these factors alone are not sufficient for translocation (Ratts et al., 2003; Ratts et al 2005). The additional required components of the CTF remain to be identified. The *in vitro* translocation assay utilized by Lemichez et al (1997) and Ratts et al (2003) cannot distinguish between direct translocation of the DT C domain across the endosomal membrane and the release of the DT C domain from the cytosolic surface of the endosomal membrane. In either scenario, the assay system does accurately assess the physiological delivery of C-domain from lumen of early endosomes into the cytosol and the *in vitro* translocation assay has rapidly become the gold standard for studying toxin translocation across the endosomal membrane.

Protein complexes of similar composition to the diphtheria toxin CTF complex have been described in the protein-trapping proteomic analysis of yeast by Ho et al. (2002). Cyclophilin (Cpr6) trapped complexes from yeast contain Hsp 82, TrR-1 and Sec 27 (β-COP) (Ho et al, 2002). There are two considerations for interpreting the data obtained from protein-trapping proteomic analysis: First, the protein complexes are most likely of heterologous nature. Second, only the proteins that were readily detectable are included. Cyclophilin is functionally active in Hsp 90 chaperonin complexes, and a role for cyclophilin as a putative CTF will be discussed below. Surprisingly, EF-2 is present in several yeast complexes containing the diphtheria toxin CTFs (Ho et al., 2002), and Hsp 90 has previously been shown to directly interact with elongation factor-2 kinase (Palmquist et al., 1994). Recently, Bektas et al. (2011) provided evidence that EF-2 itself may augment the *in vitro* translocation of the DT C domain across endosomal membranes in the presence of actin filaments .

10.1 Hsp 90 functions as a CTF

Hsp 90 is ubiquitously expressed and comprises the core of several multi-molecular chaperonin complexes that are highly conserved in eukaryotes (Schulte et al., 1998). These complexes also contain additional chaperones, co-chaperones, and adapter proteins. Interaction of these proteins with Hsp 90 is mediated through a tetracopeptide repeat acceptor site (TPR domain) found in Hsp 90, and the formation of discrete subcomplexes with distinct co-chaperones mediates Hsp 90 substrate recognition (Caplan, 1999). Although Hsp 90 does not usually directly bind nor refold nascent polypeptides, it is known to refold a growing list of proteins including membrane associated protein kinases (Bijlmakers et al., 2000). In addition to its refolding activity, Hsp 90 complexes are also known to regulate the trafficking of membrane associated proteins through interactions with cytoskeletal motors (Pratt et al., 1999).

Ratts et al (2003) established a functional role for human Hsp 90, and the yeast homologue Hsp 82, as a component of the CTF complex by immunoprecipitation and the use of specific inhibitors in both the *in vitro* translocation assay and cytotoxicity assays. Using the Hsp 90 specific inhibitors geldanamycin and radicicol, Ratts et al (2003) demonstrated that Hsp 90 ATPase activity is capable of refolding *in vitro* denatured DT C domain into a biologically active conformation. Geldanamycin binds to the Hsp 90 active site, blocks the binding of ATP, and consequently inhibits substrate dissociation from the Hsp 90 refolding complex (Grenert et al., 1997). Radicicol, different in structure from geldanamycin, binds to a different location within the ATP binding pocket of Hsp 90 but also blocks the binding of ATP, and consequently inhibits substrate dissociation from the Hsp 90 refolding complex (Schulte et al., 1998).

Surprisingly, neither the addition of geldanamycin nor radicicol alone inhibited the *in vitro* translocation of the DT C-domain (Ratts et al., 2003). There are several reports demonstrating the synergistic inhibitory effects of geldanamycin and radicicol on Hsp 90, and inhibition is thought to result from either the disruption of substrate binding or the interaction with co-chaperonins (Schulte et al., 1998). When both inhibitors were used together, the *in vitro* translocation of the DT C-domain was inhibited (Ratts et al., 2003). The synergistic inhibition of C domain translocation was specific to Hsp 90, and protected cells against toxin. These results indicated that refolding of the denatured C-domain into an active conformation and translocation of the C domain across the early endosomal membrane were mutually exclusive events, and that redundant mechanisms exist for refolding any unfolded DT C domain following translocation. Dmochewitz et al (2011) confirmed and extended the observations made by Ratts et al (2003) using the anthrax pore to deliver the DT C domain across endosomal membranes *in vitro*. In this system, the *in vitro* translocation of the DT C domain across endosomal membranes was dependent on Hsp 90 ATPase activity. This study also demonstrated that the *in vitro* translocation of the DT C domain through the anthrax pore required the activity of cyclophilin, a known Hsp-90 co-chaperone. Dmochewitz et al. (2011) also provided the first evidence for interaction between the DT C domain and Hsp 90, either directly or in the presence of an adaptor protein.

Hsp 90 mediates the entry of other bacterial toxins from the lumen of endosomes including the *C. botulinum* C2 toxins (Haug et al., 2003), iota toxin (Haug et al., 2004), and *C. perfingens* toxin (Haug et al. 2004). Like diphtheria toxin, passage through a low pH compartment and unfolding of the *C. botulinum* C2 toxin catalytic domain are pre-requisites for entry (Barth et al., 2011). In the case of the *C. botulinum* C2 toxins, Haug et al (2003) clearly demonstrated that Hsp 90 ATPase activity was not acting as an allosteric regulator of v-ATPase, and ruled out the possibility that Hsp 90 inhibition resulted in the enhanced proteosomal degradation of toxin. In addition to bacterial protein toxins, Hsp 90 has also been show to to mediate the endosomal membrane translocation of the HIV viral TAT protein (Vendeville et al, 2004), the endogenous protein fibroblast growth factor (Wesche, et al. 2006). Hsp 90 mediated translocation is not limited to the endosomal membrane, and Hsp 90 function is also required cytosolic entry of cholera toxin, another ADP-ribosylating toxin, from the ER via the ERAD pathway (Taylor et al, 2010).

Subtle differences between these toxins and their interaction with CTFs may reveal insight into the precise molecular role of Hsp 90 within the CTF complex. All of the bacterial protein toxins requiring Hsp 90 for cytosolic entry that have been identified to date are ADP-ribosyltransferases, and Barth (2011) has hypothesized that there is some conserved component of the ADP-ribosyltransferase domain that mediates interaction with Hsp 90, either directly or indirectly through an adaptor protein or co-chaperone.

10.2 TrR-1 functions as a CTF

TrR-1 is an ubiquitously expressed homodimeric NADPH-dependent flavin adenine dinucleotide containing reductase, and is the only protein known to date to reduce thioredoxin (Trx-1) (Mustacich et al., 2000). Trx-1 reduces *in vitro* the DT inter-chain disulfide bond under acidic conditions (Moskaug et al., 1987), and reduced Trx-1 has also been shown to bind a variety of misfolded cytosolic proteins and directly facilitate refolding (Hawkins et al., 1991). Ratts et al (2003) established a functional role for TrR-1 and the yeast homologue as a component of the CTF complex by both immunoprecipitation, affinity depletion, and the use of the TrR-1 specific inhibitor *cis*-13-retinoic acid in both *in vitro* translocation assays and cytotoxicity assays. Under reducing conditions, TrR-1 was an essential component of the CTF complex indicating that it is structurally present or directly interacting with other CTFs that are required for DT C domain translocation, and this role is independent of its enzymatic activity. Ratts et al. (2003) demonstrated that TrR-1 function *in vitro* is required for translocation and/or release of the C-domain from early endosome under non-reducing conditions.

TrR-1 may be important for the entry of other bacterial protein toxins. TrR-1 reduces *in vitro* the inter-chain disulfide bond in both the botulinum neurotoxins and tetanus neurotoxins (Kistner et al., 1992; Kistner et al., 1993). These toxins are organized in a similar fashion to DT, and their mechanism across endosomal membranes parallels that of DT (Montecucco et al., 1996). An *in vivo* role for TrR-1 in mediating the entry of these neurotoxins, however, has not been shown. A role for TrR-1 in the intoxication of ricin has recently been reported by Bellisola et al. (2004), who showed that Trx and PDI mediated *in vitro* reduction of the ricin inter-chain disulfide bond depends upon TrR-1 activity under non-reducing conditions. When cytosolic extracts were depleted of TrR-1, effective reduction of ricin into two fragments still occurred, but protein(s) or protein fragment(s) of 15 kDa were associated with the ricin catalytic domain. Bellisola et al. (2004) hypothesized that this factor(s) associated with the ricin catalytic domain were chaperones required for toxin entry.

10.3 Cyclophilin may function as a CTF

Cyclophilin is a peptidylprolyl *cis-trans* isomerase and co-chaperone of Hsp 90, and mammalian cyclophilin - Hsp 90 complexes are conserved in yeast (Dolinski et al., 1998). A potential role for proyl isomerases in DT T domain membrane insertion and channel formation has been proposed (See Pore Formation above). Cyclophilin does facilitate the cytosolic entry of the *C. botulinum* C2 toxin, *C. perfingens* toxin, and the *C difficile* actin-ADP ribosylating CDT toxin (Kaiser et al., 2011). Dmochewitz et al (2011) demonstrated that *in vitro* translocation of the DT C domain across endosomal membranes using the anthrax pore was inhibited by cyclosporin, a specific inhibitor of cyclophilin. It has not yet been demonstrated, however, if translocation of the DT C domain using the DT T domain requires cyclophilin. Cyclophilin has not yet been identified in the purified diphtheria CTF complex, but cyclophilin trapped complexes from yeast do contain the other known CTFs required for diphtheria toxin entry. Although additional analysis is required to confirm that cyclophilin plays a role in the diphtheria toxin CTF complex, cyclophilin does play a role in the entry of other toxins.

11. Identification of the T1 motif

Since a highly conserved CTF complex is required for DT entry, we reasoned that a sequence specific binding site mediating interaction between toxin and the CTF complex exists. Given the common route of entry of diphtheria toxin, the anthrax lethal and edema factors, and the botulinum neurotoxins across endosomal membranes, we performed *in silico* sequence analysis of these toxins. Initial analysis was limited to portions of the DT C domain (residues 140-193) and T domain (residues 194-272) which were hypothesized to be the first portions of the toxin threaded through the nascent pore and presented to cytosol, using position-specific-iterated (PSI)-BLAST (Basic Local Alignment Search Tool) analysis (Karlin and Altschul, 1990). This initial analysis elucidated a 12 amino acid motif corresponding to DT residues 212-223 in transmembrane helix 1, and was therefore named the T1 motif (Figure 4) (Ratts dissertation 2004). Next, *in silico* analysis of the entire primary amino acid sequence of DT that employed PSI-BLAST, Clustal W Alignment (Thompson et al, 1994), and MEME (Multiple Expectation maximization for Motif Elucidation) (Bailey et al, 1994) using overlapping 12 amino acid sequences from DT to probe the data base revealed a conserved 10 amino acid motif corresponding to the same region within diphtheria toxin, anthrax lethal factor, anthrax edema factor and botulinum neurotoxins serotype A, C, and D (Figure 4) (Ratts et al., 2005). Although these two methods essentially defined the same motif, the two algorithm derived consensus sequences contain subtle differences highlighting the import of functional analysis to confirm any physiological relevance such motifs may have in mediating protein-protein interactions.

Anthrax			p-value
Edema Factor	50-65	EKNKTEKEKFKDSINN	2.4 x 10-7
	404-420	KLDHLRIEELKENGII	1.8 x 10-6
Lethal Factor	27- 42	ERNKTQEEHLKEIMKH	5.5 x 10-8
Botulinum neurotoxin			
Serotype A	719-734	AKVNTQIDLIRKKMKE	5.4 x 10-6
	828-843	GTLIGQVDRLKDKVNN	2.1 x 10-7
Serotype C1	755-770	ENIKSQVENLKNSLDV	2.4 x 10-9
Serotype D	751-766	ENIKSQVENLKNSLDV	2.4 x 10-9
Diphtheria toxin			
	212-227	DKTKTKIESLKEHGPI	9.0 x 10-8
MEME Consensus		TQIENLKEKGX	
Blast Consensus		EKXKTXXEXLKE	

DT 198-SSLSCINLDWDVIRDKTKTKIESLKEHGPIKNKMSESPNKTVSEEKAKQYLEE-250
LF 10-KEKEKNKDENKRDEERNKTQEEHLKEIMKHIVKIEKGEEAVKKEAAEKLLEKV-65

Fig. 4. BLAST and MEME analysis of anthrax edema and lethal factor (LF), botulinum neurotoxins, and diphtheria toxin (DT). P-values are for toxins compared to MEME consensus sequence. Longer sequence for LF and DT are shown indicating the flanking di-lysine motifs as underlined and described in the text.

For each toxin, the T1 motif is positioned on the surface of the protein within an amphipathic alpha helix that is located in a region of the toxin consistent with potential function in the translocation process. For diphtheria, the T1 motif is present within the first amphipathic helix of the DT T domain - TH1 – which is responsible for threading the DT C domain into the nascent pore formed by the remainder of the T domain. Deletion of TH1, proline disruption of TH1, or change in the charge distribution within this region all result in the loss of toxicity (vanderSpek et al., 1993; vanderSpek et al., 1994b). Furthermore, these mutations had no effect upon receptor binding, channel conductance in artificial lipid bilayers, nor the ADP-ribosyltransferase activity of the C domain.

The proposed 'entry' motif is also consistent with the known mechanism of entry for anthrax lethal factor. Anthrax toxin is a binary complex assembled from three distinct protein chains: protective antigen (PA), lethal factor (LF), and edema factor (EF) (for review see Mourez et al., 2002). Protective antigen (PA83) binds to a universal cell surface receptor and a 20 kDa fragment is removed by furin digestion (Molloy et al., 1992). The remaining 63 kDa fragment (PA63) remains on the cell surface and spontaneously oligomerizes into a heptamer. The heptameric complex is then capable of binding either LF or EF (Pimental et al., 2004). The overall route of entry closely follows that of diphtheria. PA bound with either LF or EF, is internalized into an endosomal compartment, where acidification induces a conformational change in PA, driving membrane insertion and formation of a cation selective channel (Abrami et al 2003; Blaustein et al., 1989). Wesche et al. (1998) showed that the acid-induced translocation of LF, like diphtheria, must undergo complete unfolding for passage through the channel formed by PA, and is then refolded into an active conformation in the cytosol (Wesche et al., 1998). In contrast, EF remains associated with the vesicle compartment (Guidi-Rontani et al., 2000). In the case of anthrax LF, the putative entry motif is located between amino acid residues 27 - 39 in the mature protein, a region N-terminal to the PA binding domain. Analysis of anthrax LF N-terminal deletion mutagenesis (Arora and Leppla, 1993) demonstrated that the deletion of amino acids 1 - 40 in lethal factor results in a complete loss of toxicity for macrophages. More recently, Lacy et al. (2002) confirmed these results, and also showed that deletion of the N-terminal 27 amino acids had no effect. Although results by Lacy et al. (2002) suggested that the deletion of amino acid residues 1-40 may abrogate LF binding to PA, it is clear that the region is required for toxicity.

12. β COP Functions as a CTF

To demonstrate that the T1 motif mediates physiologically relevant interaction with CTFs, Ratts et al. (2005) engineered toxin resistant cells by transfecting a mini-gene encoding the T1 motif (amino acids 210-229 of DT). Cells expressing the T1 peptide were resistant to both DAB_{389}IL-2 and wild type DT, but were not protected against pseudomonas exotoxin A which enters cells through the ER and once delivered to the cytosol inhibits protein synthesis via an identical NAD+ dependent ribosylation of EF2. These results suggested that the T1 motif was not interfering with receptor binding, receptor trafficking, nor inhibiting the ability of toxin to ADP-ribosylate EF-2. Ratts et al (2005) then showed that knockdown of the T1 motif mini-gene using siRNA restored sensitivity to toxin, and we reasoned the T1 peptide was inhibiting an essential protein-protein interaction with CTFs.

In order to confirm such an interaction, a fusion protein was constructed between GST and DT amino residues 140-271 (Ratts et al., 2005). Because other regions outside the T1 motif might also be important in the entry process we used a longer segment of DT, corresponding to regions of T domain and C domain that are first threaded through the pore and presented to the cytosol. While the T1 motif alone might be sufficient in blocking protein-protein interactions, additional regions of the toxin may be required for actually binding CTFs. In pull down experiments, Ratts et al (2005) affinity purified several proteins that specifically bound to DT140-271, and identified them by mass spectrometry sequencing. One of these identified proteins was β-COP. Using labeled [35S]-β-COP that was synthesized *in vitro* using a rabbit reticulocyte transcription and translation reaction mixture, we found that GST-DT140-271 specifically bound β-COP and that bind was inhibited by synthetic T1-motif peptide. Confirming and extending Lemichez et al. (1997), there results suggested direct interaction between toxin and β-COP via the T1 motif.

A role for the DT T1 Motif in mediating the cytosolic entry of anthrax lethal factor (LF) was demonstrated by Tamayo et al. (2008) using an *in vitro* translocation assay consisting of early endosomes pre-loaded with anthrax protective antigen (PA) and the anthrax LFn-DTa fusion protein construct. The LFn-DTa is a fusion protein consisting of the LF binding domain for PA and the C domain of diphtheria. Tamayo et al. (2008) clearly demonstrated that the anthrax LFn-DTa fusion protein construct was translocated across the endosomal membrane in an ATP and cytosol dependent fashion, and this observation was confirmed by Dmochewitz et al (2011). Tamayo et al. (2008) also demonstrated using GST-LFn pull downs that the T1 motif in anthrax lethal factor directly binds β-COP, as well as zeta (ζ)-COP, and that a synthetic peptide containing the DT T1 motif blocked this interaction.

13. Lysines adjacent to the T1 motif region bind COPI

COPI is a heptameric structure that is composed of α-, β-, β'-, γ-, ε-, δ-, δ-subunits, and this complex functions to facilitate endosomal vesicular trafficking, the retrograde transport of vesicles between Golgi compartments, and between the Golgi apparatus and the endoplasmic reticulum (Serafini et al, 1991; Waters et al., 1991; Whitney et al., 1995). As previously mentioned, both β'COP (Sec 27) and ADP-ribosylation factor 1 (ARF1) bind to the cytoplasmic surface of the endosomal membrane to promote ECV formation, and the binding of both factors is dependent upon a low endosomal lumen pH (Aniento et al., 1996). COPI complexes have also been shown to be recruited to the cytosolic surface of vesicle membranes *en bloc* by Arf-GTP (Donaldson et al, 1992; Palmer et al., 1993). The recognition of di-lysine motifs (KXKXX, KKXX) by coatomer in the cytoplasmic tails of cargo proteins is well established (Cosson et al., 1994; Eugster et al., 2004). Interactions between COPI and the p23/24 adaptor is also mediated by a di-lysine motif, and is thought stabilize coatomer binding to the membrane surface (Harter et al., 1998).

Trujillo et al (2010) hypothesized that the multiple di-lysine motifs adjacent to the T1 motif in DT are the specific amino acid residues that interact with coatomer. This hypothesis was then confirmed by site-directed mutagenesis of the specific lysine residues K213, K215, K217, and K222 demonstrating that at least three of the four lysine residues in the region of the T1 motif are required for both COPI binding and for the cytotoxic activity of DAB389IL-2 (Trujillo et al., 2010). Using a similar *in vitro* COPI precipitation assay as described by Hudson and Draper (1997), Trujillo et al (2010) demonstrated that synthetic peptides of the DT T domain transmembrane helix 1 would cross-link and induce precipitation of COPI complexes *in vitro*. Synthetic peptides containing lysine to alanine mutations at either the N-terminal or C-terminal end of the peptide, or all five positions failed to precipitate COPI *in vitro*. The addition of monoamine 1,3-cyclohexanebis (methylamine), CBM, to the reaction mixture also blocked peptide binding to COPI complex. Trujillo et al. (2010) also demonstrated that DT directly interacts with only the β-COP and γ_1-COP components.

These observations suggested that the ε-amino moieties of the lysine residues immediately adjacent to the T1 motif specifically bind to COPI, and Trujillo et al (2010) reasoned that this region within DT was functioning as a mimetic of the cytoplasmic tail regions of either the cargo or p23/24 adaptor proteins that are normally recognized by COPI. This theory was validated by domain swapping the 13 amino acid COPI binding sequence from the cytoplasmic tail region of the p23 adaptor protein with native T1 motif and adjacent upstream lysine residues in DAB_{389}IL-2. The COPI domain swap fusion toxin mutant $DAB_{(212p23)389}$IL-2 retained full cytotoxic potency relative to the wild type-fusion protein toxin (Trujillo et al., 2010). Regardless of sequence, a major role for the DT transmembrane helix 1 is COPI complex binding and this interaction is essential for toxin entry.

14. A new model for translocation

The autonomous model for entry explains the initial steps in toxin translocation across the endosomal membrane, while the completion of translocation and release of the DT C domain into cytosol requires cytosolic factors. Acidification within the endosomal lumen promotes unfolding of the C domain and membrane insertion of the T domain in a mutually augmented process. It is not known if any host cell proteins help facilitate unfolding. The chaperonin-like qualities of the T domain then appear to thread the C-terminal end of the C domain, connected by its disulfide bond to the *N*-terminal end of the T domain, into the nascent pore. Presentation of the di-lysine motifs (KXKXX) in the N-terminal end of the T domain to the cytosolic side of the endosomal membrane then allows for targeting of the toxin by the COPI complex. Coatomer recognition of the toxin as cargo or a p23 mimetic essentially designates the N-terminal end of the T domain for "retrieval" into endogenous membrane sorting pathways. The effect of coatomer is to normally retrieve, or pull, membrane bound proteins into carrier vesicles. The effect of retrieving, or pulling, the mobile region of the N-terminal T domain actually results in the "retrieval" of the disulfide linked C domain through the pore and facilitating its complete translocation.

During this translocation process, Hsp 90 and TrR-1 perform critical steps that are required for toxin entry. Coatomer binding is a dynamic process consisting of many factors, and whether or not Hsp 90 and TrR-1 directly interact with the toxin or are rather involved in regulating or stabilizing coatomer remains to be elucidated. It is interesting that coatomer stabilization and release from the membrane is regulated by an endogenous ADP-ribosylation factor, and that the role of Hsp 90 in mediating toxin entry appears to be limited to toxins whose catalytic domains, like diphtheria, are ADP-ribosyltransferases. Likewise, the potential role for cyclophilin within the CTF complex also needs clarification.

Potential models for Hsp 90 function in the CTF complex include (but are not limited to): power stoke, regulation of other CTFs, Brownian ratchet, or architectural adaptor. The power stroke model implies that the Hsp 90 ATPase functions as a motor that directly drives the translocation, and is unlikely to apply to diphtheria entry since Ratts et al. (2003) demonstrated that translocation of the DT C domain across the endosomal membrane did not require processive cycles of Hsp 90 ATPase function. Dmochewitz (et al. 2011) has demonstrated interaction between the C domain and Hsp 90, implying that Hsp 90's role is direct rather than indirect, i.e. regulatory, within the CTF complex. In the Brownian ratchet model, Hsp 90 would bind to progressive nascent regions of translocating C domain, preventing retrograde translocation back into the endosome. In other words, Hsp 90 binding and stabilization of exposed hydrophobic residues in the DT C domain as they emerge from the endosome effectively facilitates translocation. The Brownian ratchet model would be consistent with the observed synergistic inhibition by geldanamycin and radical - only when both inhibitors are used concomitantly, the emerging diphtheria toxin residues are no longer recognized by Hsp 90 and translocation is inhibited. Alternatively, Hsp 90 may function merely as an architectural adaptor, i.e. scaffold, within the CTF complex mediating a purely structural interaction between the toxin C domain and other CTFs.

Whether or not TrR-1 directly reduces the DT inter-chain disulfide bond *in vivo* remains unknown. It is possible that TrR-1 first reduces another reductase, which then directly reduces the DT inter-chain disulfide bond. Potential candidates include (Trx-1), presumably present on the endosomal membrane. Thioredoxin peroxidases, such as the alkyl hydroperoxide reductase-1 (Ahp1) identified in the yeast partially purified CTF complex; or a hitherto unidentified reductase, such as the novel protein YOR011C identified in the yeast partially purified CTF complex that bears homology to known NADPH oxidoreductases (Ratts et al. 2003). Conversely, another reductase might first reduces the DT inter-chain disulfide bond, and TrR-1 then subsequently mediates the release of the DT C domain by reducing the newly formed intermediate disulfide bond. A third possibility is that TrR-1 plays no role in reduction of the DT inter-chain disulfide bond during intoxication. Rather, TrR-1 may be responsible for the reduction of a key component of the CTF machinery required for translocation. For example, the reactivity of the free cysteines in Hsp 90 have been implicated in mediating chaperonin activity (Nardai et al., 2000).

As we learn more about toxin entry, our models will continue to need refinement. In the case of anthrax lethal factor, for example, Tamayo et al. (2011) recently reported that the chaperone Grp78 is required for intoxication and it unfolds the LF catalytic domain within the endosomal lumen. This finding appears to contradict long held beliefs that unfolding of the anthrax LF catalytic domain naturally occurs solely under acidic conditions *in vitro* and that the pore formed by protective antigen has chaperonin-like properties that facilitates autonomous delivery - both of which parallel and are analogous to models of diphtheria toxin entry. The report by Tamayo et al. (2011) reiterates the importance of studying toxin entry in biologically relevant systems containing the heterogeneous population of proteins naturally encountered by the toxin during intoxication. While the chaperones facilitating translocation of anthrax LF and DT have so far been found on opposite sides of the endosomal membrane, the entry of both toxins requires COPI binding in the cytosol. The identification of any other additional CTFs will further refine our models of toxin entry.

15. Conclusion

Diphtheria was the first investigated bacterial protein toxin, and more than a century later remains a paradigm for toxin entry. While there is no longer any question that cytosolic translocation factors (CTFs) facilitate the entry of diphtheria toxin, much work remains. The remaining components of the CTF complex required for the cytosolic entry of diphtheria toxin need to be identified, and the precise role each cellular factor performs during translocation requires definition. Current methods for the purification of CTF complexes remain limited, and novel techniques that are more cost effective and readily available are desperately needed.

It is now apparent that a divergent group of toxins have convergently evolved to exploit similar mechanisms of entry to that of diphtheria toxin, and comparing and contrasting the differences in the CTF complexes for each toxin will serve as a valuable probe into the endogenous functions of coatomer assembly, cyclophilin and Hsp 90 function, thioredoxin redox pathways, and any other yet unidentified factors. Defining the precise molecular interaction between toxins and the CTF complex will allow for the design of novel therapeutics targeted towards virulence factors. Indeed, geldanamycin has already been shown to protect rat ileal gut from cholera toxin (Taylor et al., 2010) and clinical trials will likely soon follow. In light of the apparent evolutionary pressures, it is tempting to hypothesize that the CTF complex described for diphtheria toxin entry endogenously participates in discrete inter-intracellular signaling mechanisms that are highly conserved in eukaryotes.

16. Acknowledgements

Ryan Ratts is supported by a Hitchcock Foundation Pilot Research Grant. John Murphy is supported by Public Health Service grant AI-021628 and by grant AI-057159 from the New England Regional Center of Excellence in Emerging Infectious Diseases and Biodefense.

17. References

Abrami, L, Liu, S, Cosson, P., Leppla, S.H., and van der Goot, F.G. Anthrax toxin triggers endocytosis of its receptor via a lipid raft-mediated clathrin-dependent process. *J Cell Biol* 2003 160: 321-328.

Aniento, F, Emans, S, Griffiths, G, & Gruenberg, J. An endosomal bCOP is involved in the pH-dependent formation of transport vesicles destined for late endosomes. *J Cell Biol*, 1993; 133: 29-41.

Ariansen, S, Afanasiev, BN, Moskaug, JO, Stenmark, H, Madhaus, IH, & Olsnes, S. Membrane translocation of diphtheria toxin A-fragment: role of carboxy-terminal region. *Biochemistry*, 1993; 32: 83-90.

Arora, N. and Leppla, S.H. Residues 1-254 of anthrax lethal factor are sufficient to cause cellular uptake of fused polypeptides. *J Biol chem.* 268: 3334-41

Bacha, P, Waters, C, Williams, J, Murphy, JR, & Strom, TB. Interleukin-2 targeted cytotoxicity: Selective action of a diphtheria toxin-related interleukin-2 fusion protein. *J Exp Med*, 1988; 167: 612-622.

Bailey, T.L.; Elkan, C. Fitting a mixture model by expectation maximization to discover motifs in biopolymers. *Proc. Int. Conf. Intell. Syst. Mol. Biol.* 1994, 2, 28–36.

Baker, A, Kaplan CP, & Pool, MR. Protein targeting and translocation, a comparative review. *Biol Rev Camb Philos Soc* 1996, 71(4):637-702.

Bauer, M. F., S. Hofmann, W. Neupert and M. Brunner. Protein translocation into mitochondria: the role of TIM complexes. *Trends Cell Biol* 2000, 10(1): 25-31.

Barth, H. Exploring the role of host cell chaperones/PPIases during cellular up-take of bacterial ADP-ribosylating toxins as basis for novel pharmacological strategies to protect mammalian cells against these virulence foactors. *Naunyn. Schmiedebergs Arch. Pharmacol.* 2011, *383*, 237–245.

Bektaş M, Hacıosmanoğlu E, Ozerman B, Varol B, Nurten R, Bermek E. On diphtheria toxin fragment A release into the cytosol-Cytochalasin D effect and involvement of actin filaments and eukaryotic elongation factor 2. Int J Biochem Cell Biol. 2011 Jun 12.

Bellisola, G., G. Fracasso, R. Ippoliti, G. Menestrina, A. Rosen, S. Solda, S. Udali, R. Tomazzolli, G. Tridente and M. Colombatti. Reductive activation of ricin and ricin A-chain immunotoxins by protein disulfide isomerase and thioredoxin reductase. Biochem Pharmacol 2004, 67(9): 1721-31.

Bijlmakers, M. J. and M. Marsh. Hsp90 is essential for the synthesis and subsequent membrane association, but not the maintenance, of the Src-kinase p56(lck). Mol Biol Cell 2000, 11(5): 1585-95.

Blaustein, RO, Koehler, TM, Collier, RJ, & Finkelstein, A. Anthrax toxin: channel forming activity of PA in planar phospholipid bilayers. *Proc Natl Acad Sci, USA*, 1989; 86: 2209-2213.

Blewitt, M. G., L. A. Chung and E. London. Effect of pH on the conformation of diphtheria toxin and its implications for membrane penetration. Biochemistry 1985, 24(20): 5458-64.

Bowman, E.J.; Siebers, A.; Altendorf, K. Bafilomycins: A class of inhibitors of membrane ATPases from microorganisms, animal cells, and plant cells. *Proc. Natl. Acad. Sci. USA* 1988, *85*, 7972–7976.

Boquet, P, Silverman MS, Pappenheimer, AM, Jr, & Vernon WB. Binding of Triton X-100 to diphtheria toxin, cross reacting material 45, and their fragments. *Proc Natl Acad Sci, USA*, 1976; 73: 4449-4453.

Brown, JG, Almond, BD, Naglich, JG, & Eidels L. Hypersensitivity to DT by mouse cells expressing both DT receptor and CD9 antigen. *Proc Natl Acad Sci, USA*, 1993; 90: 8184-8188.

Cabiaux, V.; Quertenmont, P.; Conrath, K.; Brasseur, R.; Capiau, C.; Ruysschaert, J.M. Topology of diphtheria toxin B fragment inserted in lipid vesicles. *Mol. Microbiol.* 1994, *11*, 43–50.

Caplan, A. J. Hsp90's secrets unfold: new insights from structural and functional studies. *Trends Cell Biol* 1999, 9(7): 262-8.

Chassaing, A, Prichard, S. Araye-Guet, A, Barbier, J, Forge V., & Gillet D. Solution and membrane-bound chaperone activity of DT T domain towards the C domain. *FEBS* 2011, Epub Feb 18.

Choe et al., S Choe, M J Bennett, G Fujii, P M Curmi, K A Kantardjieff, R J Collier and D Eisenberg The crystal structure of diphtheria toxin. *Nature* 1992 357(6375): 216-22.

Collier, R. J. and H. A. Cole. Diphtheria toxin subunit active in vitro. *Science* 1969 164 (884): 1179-81.

Collier, R.J.; Kandel, J. Structure and activity of diphtheria toxin. I. Thiol-dependent dissociation of a fraction of toxin into enzymically active and inactive fragments. *J. Biol. Chem.* 1971, *246*, 1496–1503.

Cosson, P.; Letourneur, F. Coatomer interaction with di-lysine endoplasmic retention motifs. *Science* 1994, *263*, 1629–1631.

Deleers, M.; Beugnier, N.; Falgmagne, P.; Cabiaux, V.; Ruysschaert, J.M. Localization in diphtheria toxin fragemnt B of a region that induces pore formation in planar lipid bilayers at low pH. *FEBS Lett.* 1983, *160*, 82–86.

Dmochewitz L, Lillich M, Kaiser E, Jennings LD, Lang AE, Buchner J, Fischer G, Aktories K, Collier RJ, Barth H Role of CypA and Hsp90 in membrane translocation mediated by anthrax protective antigen. *Cell Microbiol.* 2010 Oct 14

Donaldson, J.G.; Cassel, D.; Kahn, R.A.; Klausner, R.D. ADP-ribosylation factor, a small GTP-binding protein, is required for binding of coatomer protein beta-COP to membranes. *Proc. Natl. Acad. Sci. USA* 1992, *89*, 6408–6412.

Dolinski, K. J., M. E. Cardenas and J. Heitman (1998). CNS1 encodes an essential p60/Sti1 homolog in Saccharomyces cerevisiae that suppresses cyclophilin 40 mutations and interacts with Hsp90. Mol Cell Biol 1998, 18(12): 7344-52.

Donovan, Jj, Simon, MI, Draper RK, & Montal, M. Diphtheria toxin forms transmembrane channels in planar lipid bilayers. *Proc Natl Acad Sci, USA*, 1981; *78:* 172-176.

Drazin, R, Kandel, J, & Collier, RJ. Structure and activity of DT II. Attack by trypsin at a specific site within the intact molecule. *J Biol Chem*, 1971; 246: 1504-1510.

Duprez, V, Smoljanovic, M, Lieb, M, & Dautry-Varsat, A. Trafficking of interleukin 2 and transferring in endosomal fraction of T cells. J cell Sci, 1994; 107: 1289-1295.

Eugster, A.; Frigerio, G.; Dale, M.; Duden, R. The alpha- and beta'-COP WD40 domains mediate cargo-selective interactions with distinct di-lysine motifs. *Mol. Biol. Cell* 2004, *15*, 1011–1023.

Falnes, PO, Madshus, IH, Sandvig, K, & Olsnes, S. Replacement of negative by positive charges in the presumed membrane-inserted part of diphtheria toxin B fragment. Effect on membrane translocation and on formation of cation channels. *J Biol Chem*, 1992; 267: 12284-12290.

Falnes, P. O., S. Choe, I. H. Madshus, B. A. Wilson and S. Olsnes Inhibition of membrane translocation of diphtheria toxin A-fragment by internal disulfide bridges *J Biol Chem* 1994 269(11): 8402-7.

Futter, C. E., A. Pearse, L. J. Hewlett and C. R. Hopkins. Multivesicular endosomes containing internalized EGF-EGF receptor complexes mature and then fuse directly with lysosomes. J Cell Biol 1996. 132(6): 1011-23.

Gill, DM, & Pappenheimer, AM, Jr. Structure activity relationships in diphtheria toxin. *J Biol Chem*, 1971; 246: 1485-1491.

Greenfield L, Bjorn MJ, Horn G, Fong D, Buck GA, Collier RJ, & Kaplan D. Nucleotide sequence of the structural gene for diphtheria toxin carried by corynebacteriophage *Proc Natl Acad Sci, USA*, 1983; 80: 6853-6857.

Grenert, J. P., W. P. Sullivan, P. Fadden, T. A. Haystead, J. Clark, E. Mimnaugh, H. Krutzsch, H. J. Ochel, T. W. Schulte, E. Sausville, et al.. The amino-terminal domain of heat shock protein 90 (hsp90) that binds geldanamycin is an ATP/ADP switch domain that regulates hsp90 conformation. J Biol Chem 1997, 272: 23843-50.

Guidi-Rontani, C, Weber-Levy, M, Mock, M, & Cabiaux, V. Translocation of Bacillus anthracis lethal and oedema factors across endosome membranes. *Cell Microbiol*, 2000; 2: 259-264.

Hammond, K., G. A. Caputo and E. London Interaction of the membrane-inserted diphtheria toxin T domain with peptides and its possible implications for chaperone-like T domain behavior. Biochemistry 2002, 41: 3243-53.

Haug G, Aktories K, Barth H. The host cell chaperone Hsp90 is necessary for cytotoxic action of the binary iota-like toxins. *Infect Immun.* 2004 May;72(5):3066-8

Haug G, Leemhuis J, Tiemann D, Meyer DK, Aktories K, Barth H The host cell chaperone Hsp90 is essential for translocation of the binary Clostridium botulinum C2 toxin into the cytosol. *J Biol Chem.* 2003 Aug 22;278(34):32266-74.

Hawkins, H. C., E. C. Blackburn and R. B. Freedman (1991a). Comparison of the activities of protein disulphide-isomerase and thioredoxin in catalysing disulphide isomerization in a protein substrate. Biochem J 1991, 275: 349-53.

Hayashibara, M.; London, E. Topography of diphtheria toxin A chain inserted into lipid vesicles. *Biochemistry* 2005, *44*, 2183–2196.

Harter, C.; Weiland, F.T. A single binding site for dilysine retrieval motifs and p23 with the gamma subunit of coatomer. *Proc. Natl. Acad. Sci. USA* 1998, *95*, 11649–11654.

Hudson, R.T.; Draper, R.K. Interaction of coatomer with aminoglycoside antibiotics: evidence that coatomer has at least two dilysine binding sites. *Mol. Biol. Cell* 1997, *8*, 1901–1910.

Ho, Y., A. Gruhler, A. Heilbut, G. D. Bader, L. Moore, S. L. Adams, A. Millar, P. Taylor, K. Bennett, K. Boutilier, et al. Systematic identification of protein complexes in Saccharomyces cerevisiae by mass spectrometry. *Nature* 2002 415(6868): 180-3.

Hu, H-Y, Hunth PD, Murphy, JR, & vanderSpek, JC. The effects of helix breaking mutations in the diphtheria toxin transmembrane domain helix layers of the fusion toxin DAB_{389}IL-2. *Protein engn*, 1998; 11: 101-107.

Iwamoto, R.; Higashiyama, S.; Mitamura, T.; Taniguchi, N.; Klagsbrun, M.; Mekada, E. Heparin-binding EGF-like growth factor, which acts as the DT receptor, forms a complex with membrane protein DRAP27/CD9, which up-regulates functional receptors and DT sensitivity. *EMBO J.* 1994, *13*, 2322–2330.

Johnson, V. G., P. J. Nicholls, W. H. Habig and R. J. Youle. The role of proline 345 in diphtheria toxin translocation. *J Biol Chem* 1993, 268(5): 3514-9.

Kaczorek M, Delpeyroux F, Chenciner N, Streek RE, Murphy JR, Boquet P, & Tiollais P. Nucleotide sequence and expression of the diphtheria *tox*228 gene in *Escherichia coli*. *Science*, 1983; Science, 221: 855-858.

Kagan, BL, Finkelstein, A, & Colombini, M. Diphtheria toxin fragment forms large pores in phospholipids bilayer membranes. *Proc Natl Acad Sci, USA*, 1981; 78: 4950-4954.

Kaiser, E., Kroll, C., Ernst, K., Schwan, C, Popoff, M, Fischer, G, Buchner, J, Aktories, K, Barth, H. Membrane translocation of binary ADP-ribosylating toxins from C. difficile and C. perfingines is facilitated by cyclophilin and Hsp 90. Infect Immun, 2011 Epub Jul 18.

Kaneda, Y., Uchida, T., Mekada, E.; Nakanishi, M.; Okada, Y. Entry of diphtheria toxin into cells: possible existence of cellular factor(s) for entry of diphtheria toxin into cells was studied in somatic cell hybrids and hybrid toxins. *J. Cell Biol.* 1984, *98*, 466–472.

Karlin, S and Altschul, SF. Methods for assessing the statistical significance of molecular sequence features by using general scoring themes. *Proc Natl Acad Sci USA* 1990, 87(6)2264-8.

Kim, K.; Groman, N.B. *In vitro* inhibition of diphtheria toxin action by ammonium salts and amines. *J. Bacteriol.* 1965, *90*, 1552–1556.

Kistner, A. and E. Habermann. Reductive cleavage of tetanus toxin and botulinum neurotoxin A by the thioredoxin system from brain. Evidence for two redox isomers of tetanus toxin. *Naunyn Schmiedebergs Arch Pharmacol* 1992, 345(2): 227-34.

Kistner, A., D. Sanders and E. Habermann. Disulfide formation in reduced tetanus toxin by thioredoxin: the pharmacological role of interchain covalent and noncovalent bonds. *Toxicon* 1993, 31(11): 1423-34.

Lacy, D. B. and R. J. Collier, Structure and function of anthrax toxin. *Curr Top Microbiol Immunol* 2002, 271: 61-85.

Lemichez, E, Bomsel, M, Devilliers, G, vanderSpek, J, Murphy, JR, Lukianov, EV, Olsnes, S, & Boquet, P. Membrane translocation of diphtheria toxin fragment A exploits early to late endosome trafficking machinery. *Molec Microbiol*, 1997; 23: 445-457.

Love, J.F. and Murphy, J.R. Design and development of a novel genetic probe for the analysis of repressor-operator interactions. *J Microbiol Methods* 2002, 51(1):63-72.

Luzio, J. P., B. M. Mullock, P. R. Pryor, M. R. Lindsay, D. E. James and R. C. Piper, Relationship between endosomes and lysosomes. *Biochem Soc Trans 2001*, 29: 476-80.

Madshus, I.H. The *N*-terminal alpha-helix of fragment B of diphtheria toxin promotes translocation of fragment A into the cytoplasm of eukaryotic cells. *J. Biol. Chem.* 1994, *269*, 17723–17729.

Madshus, I.H.; Wiedlocha, A.; Sandvig, K. Intermediates in translocation of diphtheria toxin across the plasma membrane. *J. Biol. Chem.* 1994, *269*, 4648–4652.

Merion, M., P. Schlesinger, R. M. Brooks, J. M. Moehring, T. J. Moehring and W. S. Sly. Defective acidification of endosomes in Chinese hamster ovary cell mutants "cross-resistant" to toxins and viruses. *Proc Natl Acad Sci U S A* 1983, 80(17): 5315-9.

Mindell, J.A.; Silverman, J.A.; Collier, R.J.; Finkelstein, A. Structure function relationships in diphtheria toxin channels: II. A residue responsible for the channel's dependence on *trans* pH. *J. Memb. Biol.* 1994, *137*, 29–44.

Mitamura, T, Iwamoto, R, Umata, T, Yomo, T, Urabe, M, Tsuneoka, M, & Mekada, E. The 27-kD DT receptor-associated protein (DTRAP27) from Vero cells is the monkey homolog of human CD9 antigen: expression of DRAP27 elevates the number of DT receptors on toxin sensitive cells. J Cell Biol, 1992; 118: 1389-1399.

Molloy, SS, Bresnahan, PA, Leppla, SH, Klimpel, KR, & Thomas, G. Human furin is a calcium-dependent serine endoprotease that recognizes the sequence Arg-X-X-Arg and efficiently cleaves anthrax toxin protective antigen. *J Biol Chem*, 1992; 267: 16396-16402.

Montecucco, C., E. Papini and G. Schiavo. Bacterial protein toxins and cell vesicle trafficking. *Experientia* 1996, 52(12): 1026-32.

Moskaug, J. O., K. Sandvig and S. Olsnes. Cell-mediated reduction of the interfragment disulfide in nicked DT. A new system to study toxin entry at low pH." *J Biol Chem* 1987, 262(21): 10339-45.

Moskaug, JO, Stenmark, H, & Olsnes, S. Insertion of diphtheria toxin B-fragment into the plasma membrane at low pH. Characterization and topology of inserted regions. *J Biol Chem*, 1991; 266: 2652-2659.

Mourez, M, Lacy, DB, Cunningham, K, Legmann, R, Sellman, BR, Mogridge, J, & Collier RJ. 2001: a year of major advances in anthrax toxin research. *Trends in Microbiology*, 2002; 10: 287-293.

Moya, M.; Dautry-Varsat, A.; Goud, B.; Louvard, D.; Boquet, P. Inhibition of coated pit formation in Hep2 cells blocks the cytotoxicity of diphtheria toxin but not that of ricin toxin. *J. Cell Biol.* 1985, *101*, 548–559.

Murphy, JR. Mechanism of DT C domain delivery to eukaryotic cell cytosol and the cellular factors that directly participate in the process. *Toxins*, 2011, 3(3):294-308.

Murphy, J.R.; Bishai, W.; Borowski, M.; Miyanohara, A.; Boyd, J.; Nagle, S. Genetic construction, expression, and melanoma-selective cytotoxicity of a diphtheria toxin-related alpha-melanocyte-stimulating hormone fusion protein. *Proc. Natl. Acad. Sci. USA* 1986, *83*, 8258–8262.

Mustacich, D. and G. Powis. Thioredoxin reductase. *Biochem J* 2000, 346 Pt 1: 1-8.

Naglich, JG, Matherall, JE, Russell, DW, & Eidels L. Expression cloning of a diphtheria toxin receptor: identity with a heparin-binding EGF-like growth factor precursor. *Cell*, 1992; 69: 1051-1061.

Nardai, G., B. Sass, J. Eber, G. Orosz and P. Csermely. Reactive cysteines of the 90-kDa heat shock protein, Hsp90. *Arch Biochem Biophys* 2000, 384(1): 59-67.

Oh, JO, Senzel, L, Collier, RJ, & Finkelstein, A. Translocation of the catalytic domain of diphtheria toxin across planar phospholipids bilayers by its own T-domain. Proc *Natl Acad Sci, USA*, 1999; 96: 8467-8470.

O'Keefe, DO, Cabiaux, V, Choe, S, Eisenberg, D, & Collier, RJ. pH-dependent insertion of proteins into membranes: B-chain mutation of diphtheria toxin that inhibits membrane translocation, Glu-349-Lys. *Proc Natl Acad Sci, USA*, 1992; 89: 6202-6206.

Palmer, D.J.; Helms, J.B.; Beckers, C.J.; Orci, L.; Rothman, J.E. Binding of coatomer to Golgi membranes requires ADP-ribosylation factor. *J. Biol. Chem.* 1993, *268*, 12083–12089.

Palmquist, K., B. Riis, A. Nilsson and O. Nygard.. Interaction of the calcium and calmodulin regulated eEF-2 kinase with heat shock protein 90. *FEBS Lett* 1994, 349(2): 239-42.

Papini, E., R. Rappuoli, M. Murgia and C. Montecucco. Cell penetration of diphtheria toxin. Reduction of the interchain disulfide bridge is the rate-limiting step of translocation in the cytosol. *J Biol Chem* 1993, 268(3): 1567-74.

Pappenheimer, AM, Jr. Diphtheria toxin. *Annu. Rev. Biochem.*, 1977; 46: 69-94.

Pimental, R.A., Christensen, K.A., Krantz, B.A., and Collier, R.J. (2004) Anthrax toxin complexes: heptameric protective antigen can bind lethal factor and edema factor simultaneously. *Biochem Biophys Res Commun* 322: 258-262

Pratt, W. B., A. M. Silverstein and M. D. Galigniana. A model for the cytoplasmic trafficking of signalling proteins involving the hsp90-binding immunophilins and p50cdc37. *Cell Signal* 1999, 11(12): 839-51.

Ratts, R. Purification, Identification and Characterization of the DT CTF complex. PhD Thesis. Copyright 2004. Boston University

Ratts R, Trujillo C, Bharti A, vanderSpek J, Harrison R, Murphy JR A conserved motif in transmembrane helix 1 of DT mediates catalytic domain delivery to the cytosol. Proc Natl Acad Sci U S A. 2005 Oct 25;102(43):15635-40. Epub 2005 Oct 17.

Ratts, R and vanderSpek, JC. DT: structure function and its clinical applications. In, *Chimeric Toxins*. H. Lorberboum-Galski and P. Lazarovici (Eds). Taylor and Francis, London 2002, 14-36

Ratts, R, Zeng, H, Berg EA, Blue, C, McComb, ME, Costello, CE, vanderSpek, JC, & Murphy, R. The cytosolic entry of diphtheria toxin catalytic domain requires a host cell cytosolic translocation factor complex. *J Cell Biol*, 2003 Mar 31;160(7):1139-50

Ren, J, Kachel, K, Kim, H, Malenbaum, S, Collier, RJ, & London, E. Interaction of diphtheria toxin T domain with molten globule-like proteins and its implicatios for translocation. *Science*, 1999; 248: 955-957.

Rosen, A., P. Lundman, M. Carlsson, K. Bhavani, B. R. Srinivasa, G. Kjellstrom, K. Nilsson and A. Holmgren. A CD4+ T cell line-secreted factor, growth promoting for normal and leukemic B cells, identified as thioredoxin. *Int Immunol* 1995, 7(4): 625-33.

Ryser, H-J, Mandel, R, & Ghani, F. Cell surface sulfhydryls are required for the cytotoxicity of DT but not ricin toxin in Chinese hamster ovary cells. *J Biol Chem*, 1991; 266: 18439-18442.

Sandvig, K. and S. Olsnes. Diphtheria toxin entry into cells is facilitated by low pH. *J Cell Biol* 1980, 87(3 Pt 1): 828-32.

Sandvig, K. and S. Olsnes. Rapid entry of nicked diphtheria toxin into cells at low pH. Characterization of the entry process and effects of low pH on the toxin molecule. *J Biol Chem* 1981, 256(17): 9068-76.

Sandvig, K. and S. Olsnes. Diphtheria toxin-induced channels in Vero cells selective for monovalent cations. *J Biol Chem* 1988, 263(25): 12352-9.

Sandvig, K., A. Sundan and S. Olsnes. Effect of potassium depletion of cells on their sensitivity to diphtheria toxin and pseudomonas toxin. *J Cell Physiol* 1985, 124(1): 54-60.

Serafini, T.; Stenbeck, G.; Brecht, A.; Lottspiech, F.; Orci, L.; Rothman, J.E.; Wieland, F.T. A coat subunit of Golgi-derived nonclathrin—coated vesicles with homology to the clathrin-coated vesicle protein beta-adaptin. *Nature* 1991, *349*, 215–220.

Schulte, T. W., S. Akinaga, S. Soga, W. Sullivan, B. Stensgard, D. Toft and L. M. Neckers. Antibiotic radicicol binds to the N-terminal domain of Hsp90 and shares important biologic activities with geldanamycin. *Cell Stress Chaperones* 1998, 3(2): 100-8.

Shiver, J.W.; Donovan, J.J. Interactions of diphtheria toxin with lipid vesicles: Determinants of ion channel formation. *Biochim. Biophys. Acta* 1987, *903*, 48–55.

Silverman, J.A.; Mindell, J.A.; Collier, R.J.; Finkelstein, A. Structure-function relationships in diphtheria toxin channels: I. Determining a minimal channel-forming domain. *J. Membr. Biol.* 1994, *137*, 17–28.

Simpson, J.C.; Smith, D.C.; Roberts, L.M.; Lord, J.M. Expression of mutant dynamin protects cells against diphtheria toxin but not against ricin. *Exp. Cell Res.* 1998, *239*, 293–300.

Smith, WP, Tai, PC, Murphy, JR, & Davis BD. A precursor in the cotranslational secretion of diphtheria toxin. *J Bacteriol*, 1980; 141: 184-189.

Stenmark, H., S. Olsnes and I. H. Madshus. Elimination of the disulphide bridge in fragment B of diphtheria toxin: effect on membrane insertion, channel formation, and ATP binding. *Mol Microbiol* 1991, 5(3): 595-606.

Tamayo AG, Bharti A, Trujillo C, Harrison R, Murphy JR. COPI coatomer complex proteins facilitate the translocation of anthrax lethal factor across vesicular membranes in vitro. *Proc Natl Acad Sci* U S A. 2008 Apr 1;105(13):5254-9.

Tamayo AG., Slater, L, Taylor-Parker, J, Bharti, A., Harrison, R., Hung, D, Murphy, JR. GRP78(BiP) facilitates the cytosolic delivery of anthrax lethal factor (LF) in vivo and functions as an unfoldase in vitro. Mol Microbiol 2011, 81(5): 1390-401.

Taylor M, Navarro-Garcia F, Huerta J, Burress H, Massey S, Ireton K, Teter K. Hsp90 is required for transfer of the cholera toxin A1 subunit from the endoplasmic reticulum to the cytosol. *J Biol Chem*. 2010 Oct 8;285(41):31261-7. Epub 2010 Jul 28.

Thompson, J.D.; Higgins, D.G.; Gibson, T.J. CLUSTAL W: Improving the sensitivity of progressive multiple sequence alignment through sequence weighting, position-specific gap penalties, weight matrix choice. *Nucleic Acids Res.* 1994, *22*, 4673–4680.

Trujillo C, Taylor-Parker J, Harrison R, Murphy JR Essential lysine residues within transmembrane helix 1 of diphtheria toxin facilitate COPI binding and catalytic domain entry. *Mol Microbiol.* 2010 May;76(4):1010-9. Epub 2010 Apr 14.

Tsai, B., Y. Ye and T. A. Rapoport. Retro-translocation of proteins from the endoplasmic reticulum into the cytosol. *Nat Rev Mol Cell Biol* 2002, 3(4): 246-55.

Tsuneoka, M, Nakayama, K, Hatsuzawa, K, Komada, M, Kitamura, N, & Mekada E. Evidence for the involvement of furin in cleavage and activation of diphtheria toxin. *J Biol Chem*, 1993; 268: 26461-26465.

Uchida, T, Gill, DM, & Pappenheimer, AM, Jr. Mutation in the structural gene for diphtheria toxin carried by temperate phage . *Nature*, 1971; 233: 8-11.

Umata, T.; Moriyama, Y.; Futai, M.; Mekada, E. The cytotoxic action of diphtheria toxin and its degradation in intact Vero cells are inhibited by bafilomycin A1, a specific inhibitor of vacuolar-type H(+)-ATPase. *J. Biol. Chem.* 1990, *265*, 21940–21945.

Waters, CA, Schimke, P, Snider, CE, Itoh, K, Smith, KA, Nichols, JC, Strom, TB, & Murphy, JR. Interleukin-2 receptor targeted cytotoxicity: Receptor requirements for entry of IL-2-toxin into cells. *Eur J Immunol*, 1990; 20: 785-791.

Waters, M.G.; Serafini, T.; Rothman, J.E. Coatomer a cytosolic protein complex containing subunits of non-clathrin-coated Golgi transport vesicles. *Nature* 1991, *349*, 248–251.

Wesche, J, Malecki, J, Wiedlocha A, Skjerpen, CS and Olsnes, S. FGF-1 and FGF-2 require the cytosolic chaperone Hsp 90 for translocation into the cytosol and nucleus. *J Cell Sci* 2006, 119:4332-41

Wesche, J, Elliott, JL, Falnes, PO, Olsnes, S, Z& Collier, RJ. Characterization of membrane translocation by anthrax protective antigen. *Biochemistry*, 1998; 37: 15737-15746.

Whitney, J.A.; Gomez, M.; Sheff, D.; Kries, T.E.; Mellman, I. Cytoplasmic coat proteins involved in endosome function. *Cell* 1995, *83*, 703–713.

Wiedlocha, A., I. H. Madshus, H. Mach, C. R. Middaugh and S. Olsnes. Tight folding of acidic fibroblast growth factor prevents its translocation to the cytosol with diphtheria toxin as vector. 1992 *Embo J* 11(13): 4835-42.

Williams, D, Parker, K, Bishai, W, Borowski, M, Genbauffe, F, Strom, TB, & Murphy, JR. DT receptor binding domain substitution with IL-2: genetic construction and properties of the DT-related IL-2 fusion protein. *Protein Engn*, 1987; 1: 493-498.

Williams, DP, Snider, CE, Strom TB, & Murphy JR. Structure function analysis of IL-2-toxin (DAB_{486}IL-2): Fragment B sequences required for the delivery of fragment A to the cytosol of target cells. *J Biol Chem*, 1990; 265: 11885-11889.

VanderSpek, C, Cassidy, D, Genbauffe, F, Huynh, PD, & Murphy, JR. An intact transmembrane helix 9 is essential for the efficient delivery of the diphtheria toxin catalytic domain to the cytosol of target cells. *J Biol Chem*, 1994; 269: 21455-21459.

VanderSpek, C, Howland, K, Friedman, T, & Murphy, JR. Maintenance of the hydrophobic face of the diphtheria toxin amphipathic transmembrane helix 1 is essential for the efficient delivery of the catalytic domain to the cytosol of target cells. *Protein Engn*, 1994; 7: 985-989.

vanderSpek JC, Mindel J, Finkelstein A, & Murphy JR. Structure function analysis of the transmembrane domain of the interleukin-2 receptor targeted fusion toxin DAB_{389}IL-2: The amphipathic helical region of the transmembrane is essential for the efficient delivery of the catalytic domain to the cytosol of target cells. *J Biol Chem*, 1993; 90: 8524-8528.

Vendeville A, Rayne F, Bonhoure A, Bettache N, Montcourrier P, Beaumelle B.HIV-1 Tat enters T cells using coated pits before translocating from acidified endosomes and elicitinbiological responses. *Mol Biol Cell.* 2004 May;15(5):2347-60

7

Pattern Recognition Receptors and Infectious Diseases

Ardi Liaunardy Jopeace[1], Chris B. Howard[1], Ben L. Murton[1], Alexander D. Edwards[2] and Tom P. Monie[1]
[1]Department of Biochemistry, University of Cambridge and
[2]School of Pharmacy, University of Reading
United Kingdom

1. Introduction

1.1 The innate immune system

Our bodies are under constant attack from pathogens. Despite this continual bombardment, under normal circumstances we remain healthy for most of our lives. This protection against infectious and harmful agents is provided by our immune system. The immune system can be broken into two elements: adaptive immunity and innate immunity. Adaptive immunity is a specific response targeted against particular pathogens through, for example, cytotoxic T cells and antibody production. The adaptive immune system has the potential to raise a defence against any invading pathogen. However, this is a relatively slow and energy expensive process. Innate immunity in contrast provides a non-specific response against any pathogen via a variety of components and processes. These include: barrier functions, complement, natural killer (NK) cells, antimicrobial peptides, mucosal secretions, pattern recognition receptors (PRRs) and the commensal micro-organisms. Innate immunity is responsible for clearing the majority of pathogen exposures that would result in infection before the adaptive system is even involved. This chapter will focus upon the role of one particular arm of the innate immune response to infectious diseases - Pattern Recognition Receptors. It will broadly address the mechanisms by which PRRs recognise the pathogens, the effects this has and the types if response it has. It will also bring in examples of evasion strategies used by pathogens to avoid detection and touch on the impact of polymorphisms in the receptors. Finally we will discuss the role of PRRs in a key defence against infectious diseases, vaccination.

1.2 Targets for innate immune recognition by PRRs

PRRs are protein molecules encoded in the genome and not subject to rearrangement or variation during the lifetime of an individual. PRRs function as molecular sensors of infection and are predominantly found on critical immune cells such as macrophages and dendritic cells (DC). However, other cell types likely to come into contact with pathogens, for example epithelial cells, also express subsets of these receptors. Given the absence of functional rearrangement how do PRRs recognise pathogens from diverse families possessing such diverse biology and patterns of infection?

Firstly, the innate immune system is designed to recognise biological components that are common to many pathogens. These are known as pathogen-associated molecular patterns (PAMPs). This means, for example, that a receptor is able to respond to all bacteria that have common components in their cell walls rather than a specific protein that is found on only one type of micro-organism (Table 1).

Secondly, there are a number of families of receptors, and many receptors in each family (Section 2, Table 1). This limited diversity allows the innate immune system to respond, not only to different PAMPs, but also PAMPs found in either the extracellular space or an intracellular environment. By having multiple sites for detection of diverse targets, it is unlikely that any given pathogen will be able to evade all of the levels of detection.

Thirdly, and most importantly, the receptors are able to mount a coordinated response to pathogen infection because of extensive cross-talk and communication between the different signalling pathways. This again minimises the possibility of a pathogen being able to evade the innate immune response. Overall, the innate immune response is primarily designed to induce inflammation at the site of infection, recruit inflammatory cells and mediators and begin to potentiate the adaptive immune system. The coordinated nature of the innate response ensures that any response initiated is robust enough to meet the threat.

Stimulatory Pathogen Associated Molecular Pattern (PAMP)	Pattern Recognition Receptor (PRR)	Signalling Adapter Protein	Transcriptional or Cellular Pathway Activated
Toll-like receptors (TLRs)			
Bacterial cell wall components	TLR2 homo/heterodimers	MyD88	NFκB / AP1
LPS	TLR4 (plasma membrane)	MyD88	NFκB / AP1
LPS	TLR4 (endosome)	TRIF	IRF3 / NFκB / AP1
Flagellin	TLR5	MyD88	NFκB / AP1
dsRNA	TLR3	TRIF	IRF3 / NFκB / AP1
ssRNA	TLR7	MyD88	IRF7 / NFκB
Nod-like receptors (NLRs)			
iE-DAP	NOD1	RIP2	NFκB
MDP	NOD2	RIP2/CARD9	NFκB / AP1
e.g. Pore-forming toxins, nucleic acid	NLRP3	ASC	Caspase-1 activation
Retinoic acid-inducible gene I-like receptors (RLRs)			
dsRNA	RIG-I	MAVS	IRF3 / AP1 / NFκB
C-type lectin receptors (CLRs)			
β-glucans	Dectin-1	Syk	NFκB

Table 1. Pattern Recognition Receptor (PRR) Activation and Outputs. The activation and signalling of PRRs is a complex, multi-factorial process. Activatory ligands (blue column) are recognised by specific PRRs (pink column). This leads to the recruitment of adaptor signalling proteins (lilac column) and the activation of intracellular signalling cascades. The net result is the up-regulation of transcriptional activators or specific cellular processing events (green column).

1.3 Innate immune signalling overview

PRR activation and signalling is a complex multifactorial process that results in remarkably similar outcomes (Figure 1). For example: upregulation of NFκB (Nuclear Factor kappa B) and IRF (interferon (IFN) regulatory factor) family transcription factors; stimulation of the stress kinase pathways (e.g. mitogen-activated protein kinases (MAPK)); and activation of caspase-1 (Figure 1). Ultimately this results in up-regulation of pro-inflammatory cytokines, chemokines and anti-viral proteins. PRRs are activated by PAMPs. Endogenous molecules, such as ATP and heat shock proteins, can also act as ligands for some PRRs. These endogenous ligands are collectively known as damage associated molecular patterns (DAMPs). PRR activation results in conformational changes in the proteins, activates intracellular signalling pathways to amplify the signal and initiates the innate response (Figure 1). Assembly of the downstream signalling complex is reliant on the involvement of specific adapter proteins to recruit signalling components and act as molecular scaffolds for complex assembly. PRRs use specific adaptors and different adaptor proteins result in the activation of different signalling pathways (see Section 2; Table 1).

1.4 Physiological outcomes of innate immune activation

The targets of the transcription factors produced as a result of PRR stimulation are pro-inflammatory effectors, the most important of which are tumour necrosis factor (TNF), interleukin (IL)-1 and IL-6. The pro-inflammatory signals modify the permeability of the vasculature around a site of infection to increase recruitment of specialised immune cells, such as monocytes and macrophages. This leads to the classic signs of infection; redness, heat, swelling and pain. At a cellular level these effectors can regulate cellular death in localised areas of infection, but also coordinate events in the whole body through the activation of the acute-phase response. The production of anti-viral type I IFNs induces apoptosis in infected cells, thereby removing the virus from the system, but also triggers resistance to viral infection in neighbouring cells and so helps restrict the spread of infection.

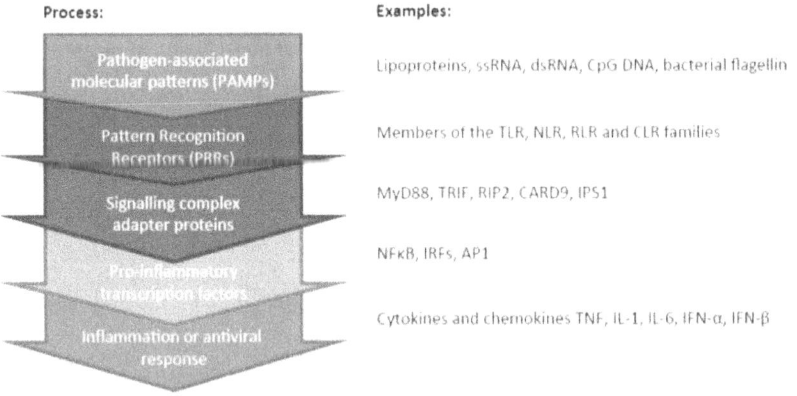

Fig. 1. Overview of innate immune signalling pathways and components. Activation begins with recognition of a stimulatory ligand, such as a pathogen-associated molecular pattern and results in an inflammatory or antiviral response from the cell.

The cellular and molecular changes associated with PRR activation are both complex and subtle. They create a response that can be shaped to deal with the specific nature of the infection. In macrophages many genes that modify their direct involvement in fighting infection and help repair damaged tissues are activated in response to PRR stimulation. Other cells, including monocytes, neutrophils, T-cells and B-cells can also be recruited to either directly help with the immune response or aid in the activation of the adaptive immune system.

2. Pattern recognition receptor families

PRRs are classified into four main families: Toll-like receptors (TLRs); Nucleotide binding leucine rich repeat (NLR) containing receptors, also known as NOD-like receptors; Retinoic acid-inducible gene I (RIG-I)-like receptors; and the C-type lectin receptors. The following sections provide brief details on the general signalling strategy of each of these families as well as specific examples of stimulatory ligands and physiological responses.

2.1 Toll-like receptors (TLRs)

TLRs are type 1 membrane proteins. They were the first components discovered in what we now regard as the innate immune system. TLRs use leucine-rich repeats (LRRs) to detect and bind ligand (Monie et al., 2009). LRRs have a conserved structural backbone which provides a scaffold on which variation can be built (Figure 2). Hence, LRRs from different receptors recognise a diverse range of PAMPs. In humans, TLR1, 2, 4, 5, 6 and 10 project their LRRs into the extracellular space, whereas TLR3, 7, 8 and 9 are compartmentalised to sample the contents of the endosomes.

TLRs signal in dimeric complexes after ligand binding (Figures 2 and 3). In general these are homodimeric complexes except for TLR2 which forms a heterodimer with TLR1 or TLR6. It has also been reported that TLR4 is capable of forming a signalling complex with TLR6. However, in this instance the receptor is involved in sterile inflammation and, in conjunction with CD36 responds to endogenous danger signals rather than PAMPs (Stewart et al., 2009). It is conceivable that following activation multiple dimeric TLR receptors cluster together in specific regions of the cellular membrane in order to augment signalling. Extracellular TLRs generally recognise components found on the outer surfaces of pathogens, such as lipoproteins and flagellin. Endosomal TLRs meanwhile recognise nucleic acids such as CpG-DNA, double-stranded RNA (dsRNA) and single stranded RNA (ssRNA).

The cytoplasmic Toll/IL-1 receptor (TIR) domain (Figure 2) mediates downstream signalling through adaptor recruitment. Based upon adaptor usage TLR signalling can be divided into two categories; those that signal through the protein myeloid differentiation factor 88 (MyD88) and those that don't. MyD88 is recruited to the TIR domains of an activated TLR and results in the formation of a multiprotein complex termed the myddosome (Figure 3). The myddosome contains a number of IL-1R-associated kinases (IRAKs) which direct signalling down specific pathways. Firstly, degradation of the inhibitory protein IκB (inhibitor of kappa B) releases the transcription factor NFκB; and secondly, the MAP (mitogen activated protein) kinase pathway activates the c-fos/jun transcription factor. These signals combine to drive expression of pro-inflammatory cytokines from NFκB and AP1 responsive genes respectively. The endosomal TLRs use the same pathway to activate NFκB and members of the IRF-family of transcription factors that activate expression of type I interferons needed to combat viral infection.

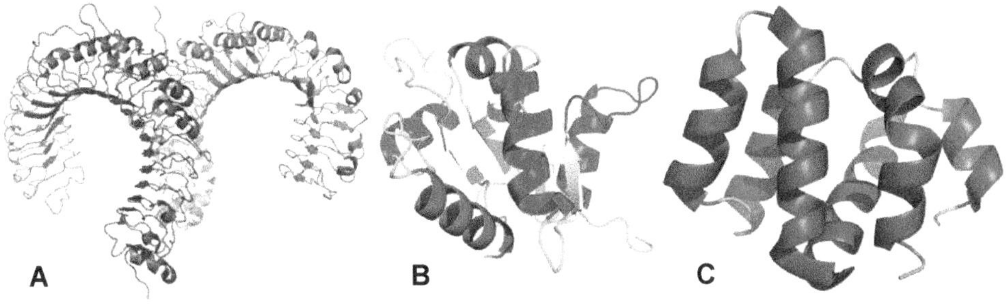

Fig. 2. Selected secondary structures of functional domains from PRRs. (A) Leucine rich repeat (LRR) containing ectodomains of TLR1 (blue) and TLR2 (purple). The synthetic ligand PAM3CYK4 (orange) stimulates heterodimerisation and formation of a signalling competent complex. (B) Toll/IL-1 receptor (TIR) domain of TLR2. The central beta-sheet core (yellow) is surrounded by five alpha helices. The BB loop, between the second beta-sheet and second alpha helix, is coloured blue. The BB loop is a key region of the TIR domain for downstream signalling activation and adaptor recruitment. (C) The caspase activation and recruitment domain (CARD) of the NLR family member NOD1. The CARD domain is a six-helix bundle involved in protein-protein interactions.

The MyD88-independent pathways use the adapter TIR-related adaptor protein inducing IFNβ (TRIF) in combination usually with the adaptor protein TRAM (TRIF-related adaptor molecule). This pathway is used to drive expression of IFN-β either in response to dsRNA detection by TLR3, or TLR4 signalling from the endosome rather than the plasma membrane. There is however significant cross-talk between the pathways. Adaptor proteins have recently been shown to be important in the susceptibility to infectious disease. This is exemplified by the adaptor Mal (MyD88-adaptor like), which is involved in recruitment of MyD88 to the TIR domain of TLR2 and TLR4. In this instance heterozygotic carriage of a single nucleotide polymorphism that results in the amino acid change serine to leucine at residue one-hundred-and-eighty in the TIR domain appears to be protective against the development of sepsis, invasive pneumococcal disease, bacteremia, malaria and tuberculosis (Ferwerda et al., 2009a; Khor et al., 2007)

2.2 Nucleotide binding leucine rich repeat containing receptors (NLRs)

The NLRs are a large family of cytoplasmic PRRs, of which there are at least 23 members. They share a characteristic domain organisation comprising of an N-terminal protein interaction domain, a central nucleotide binding region and C-terminal leucine-rich repeats (Figure 2). Currently the precise method of receptor activation by all the different ligands remains to be elucidated for the NLR family. There are two main groups in the NLR family based on the nature of their N-terminal domain. These are the NLRC sub-family who possess caspase activation and recruitment domain (CARDs) (Figure 2), and the Pyrin domain containing NLRP sub-family.

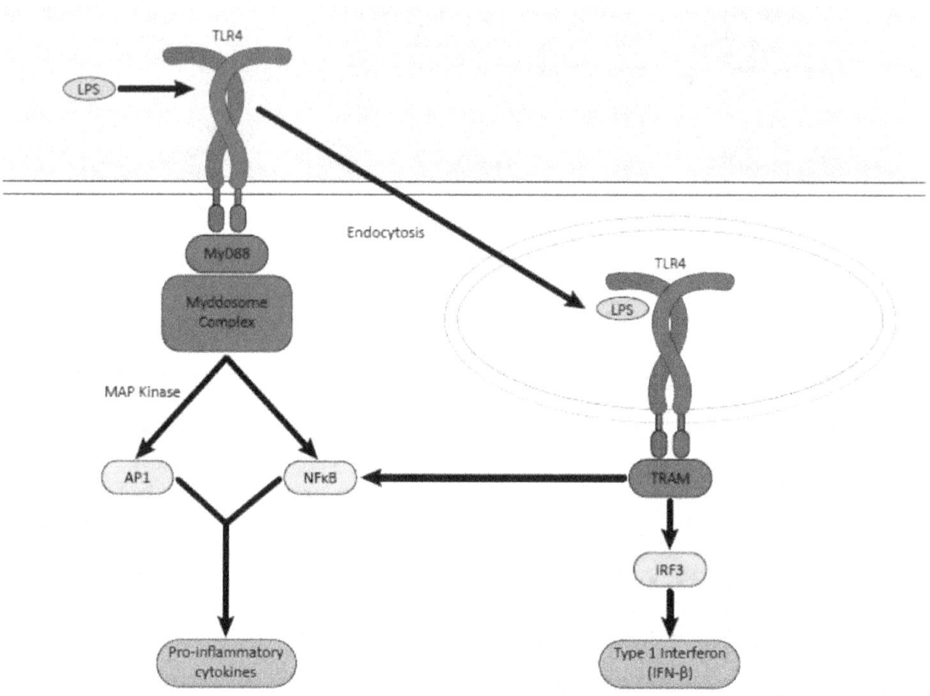

Fig. 3. Simplified schematic of TLR signalling exemplified by TLR4. Ligands are coloured blue, receptors are red, adaptor proteins purple, pro-inflammatory transcription factors green, and cellular outputs orange.

NLR signalling pathways can be broadly split into two: 1) upregulation of NFκB and activation of pro-inflammatory genes; 2) Inflammasome formation, caspase-1 activation and secretion of IL-1β and IL-18 (Figure 4). The first pathway is utilised by the prototypical NLRC family members NOD1 and NOD2. These receptors bind to PAMPs derived from bacterial peptidoglycan (Table 1). The activated NLRs signal through the adapter Receptor Interacting Protein 2 (RIP2) to drive the release of NFκB into the nucleus by the same processes employed by TLRs. In a further demonstration of PRR cross-talk, Nod2 also activates the MAP kinase pathway using a different adapter, CARD9, to upregulate pro-inflammatory gene expression from AP1 dependent promoters. The inflammasome forming NLRs consist, to date, of NLRP1, NLRP3 and NLRC4. The NLRP family members recruit the protein ASC (apoptosis-associated speck-like protein containing a CARD) through homotyoic Pyrin:Pyrin interactions. ASC also possesses a CARD domain which recruits pro-caspase 1 to the inflammasome complex. Self-cleavage of pro-caspase 1 releases active caspase-1 which subsequently cleaves pro-IL-1β and pro-IL-18 into their mature forms for secretion from the cell. Both IL-1β and IL-18 are proinflammatory and they play crucial roles in host defence against pathogens. IL-1β is responsible for the generation of systemic and local immune responses by causing fever, activating lymphocytes and recruiting them along with neutrophils to the site of infection. IL-18 lacks the pyrogenic nature of IL-1β but is involved in induction of IFN-γ production by T-cells and NK cells to drive T-helper cell type 1 (Th1) responses during adaptive immunity development. The NLRC4 inflammasome can activate caspase-1 in an ASC-dependent and -independent manner. Pro-IL-1β and pro-IL-18 are both expressed in an NFκB dependent manner. Hence their cellular levels are increased by TLR and NLR activation. The inflammasome can then be activated in response to a diverse selection of ligands, increasing the levels of IL-1β and IL-18 and amplifying the initial response to many PAMPs.

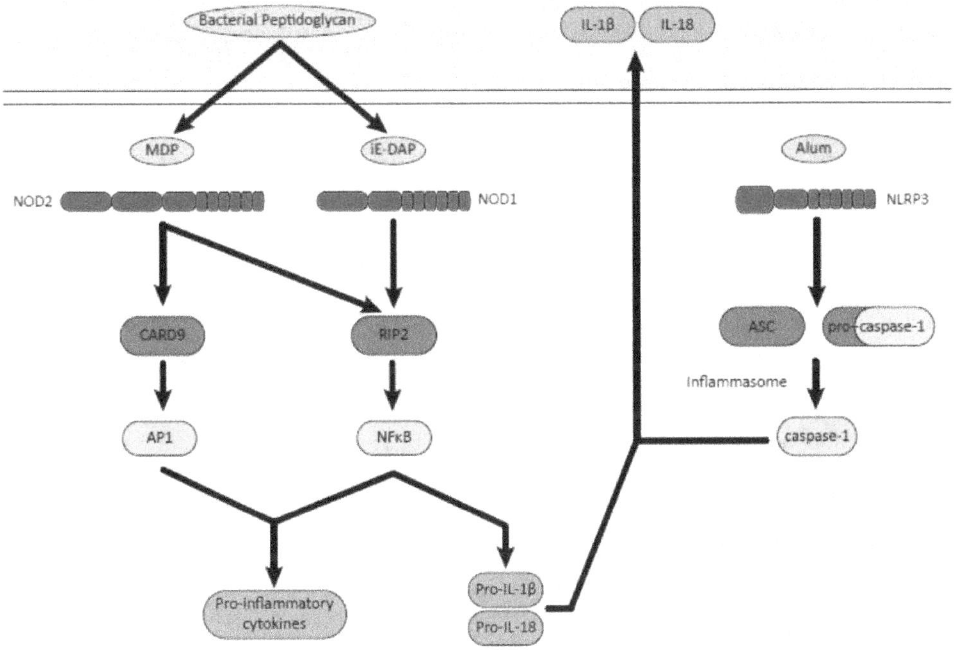

Fig. 4. Simplified representation of NLR family member signalling. Ligands are coloured blue, receptors are red, adaptor proteins purple, pro-inflammatory transcription factors green, and cellular outputs orange. Caspase-1 activation ultimately results in cell death through the process of pyroptosis.

2.3 Retinoic acid-inducible gene I-like receptors (RLRs)

RLRs are a small family of PRRs that detect intracellular RNA. RLRs use CARDs to interact with downstream signalling components. Activation results in expression of type I IFNs and other pro-inflammatory cytokines. In conjunction with endosomal TLRs the RLRs provide a robust antiviral response. RIG-I recognises short uncapped dsRNA or ssRNA, whereas melanoma differentiation-associated 5 (MDA5) detects longer dsRNA such as poly (I:C). Both proteins signal by forming CARD:CARD interactions with MAVS (mitochondrial antiviral signalling protein; also known as IFN-β-promoter stimulator 1 (IPS-1)) which is localised on the exterior membrane of the mitochondria. This activates the IRF transcription factors, but again leads to co-stimulation of the MAP kinase pathway as seen in the signalling of the other PRRs. The RLRs are also involved in sensing and triggering a response to cytoplasmic DNAs which can be transcribed by RNA polymerase III into dsRNA.

2.4 C-type lectin receptors (CLRs)

CLRs are characterised by the presence of a C-type lectin domain. Over 1000 proteins in the human genome could be described as CLRs, however, only a few specifically modulate the innate immune response. CLRs are involved in diverse, often regulatory, roles within the immune system, such as antigen presentation and phagocytosis. Dectin-1 and dectin-2 are the best characterised CLRs and signal through their immunoreceptor tyrosine-based activation motif (ITAM). The ITAM domain activates the spleen tyrosine kinase (Syk) which upregulates many of the pathways triggered by the other PRRs.

2.5 Summary

It is clear that although there is much diversity in the range of PAMPs that can be detected by PRRs, there is a common signalling strategy geared towards causing inflammation to both contain and then remove the infection. The mechanism of activation and signalling cascades involved in this process are highly complex and contain a significant level of overlap, redundancy and cross-talk. A more comprehensive discussion of these processes can be found in a variety of excellent review articles and the references they contain (Davis et al., 2011; Kawai and Akira, 2011; Loo and Gale, 2011; Osorio and Reis e Sousa, 2011).In the following sections we will see that although pathogens usually activate a number of PRRs, they have adapted their modes of attack so as to bypass the innate immune system, and hence be able to colonise the body.

3. Pattern recognition receptor responses to pathogens

The previous section highlighted the diversity of PRRs available to respond to PAMPs. To demonstrate the importance of PRRs in the response to infectious diseases we have chosen four major pathogens; the bacteria *Salmonella spp.*, the virus Influenza A, the fungi *Candida albicans*, and the parasite *Schistosoma mansoni*. Here we describe the importance of PRRs in the recognition of these pathogens and induction of an innate immune response against them. As will become apparent the innate immune system has evolved so that multiple PRRs recognise different PAMPs from the same pathogen.

Pathogens, like higher organisms, also undergo evolutionary pressure to survive. In essence this can be viewed as a host-pathogen arms race. Successful pathogens are able to evade, limit, or manipulate detection by PRRs, and in some cases, utilise PRR signalling pathways for their own benefit. Pathogen survival can be augmented in a number of ways. These include targeting the recognition receptor, the signalling transduction event, and the key effector proteins of the innate immune system (Hajishengallis and Lambris, 2011). The innate immune system is a common target for immune evasion strategies for two primary reasons. Firstly, it is the initial host defence encountered by the pathogens upon infection. Secondly, the innate immune system is essential for the development of adaptive immunity. Consequently, by exploiting the innate immune system, pathogens can undermine the whole immune response of the host. Many different mechanisms are employed by pathogens to subvert immune signalling. These include: the use of immunomodulatory proteins; receptor antagonists; the induction of immunosuppression; activation of host immune inhibitory receptors; reduced expression, or alteration, of the PAMP; and manipulation of PRR crosstalk. In short successful pathogens are able to survive for longer in, and colonise, the host through maintenance of a careful balance between innate immune activation and suppression. In addition to identifying the key PRR-pathogen interactions we will provide examples highlighting the ability of these organisms to survive in the host and evade the innate immune response.

3.1 PRRs and Salmonella

3.1.1 *Salmonella* is a Gram-negative bacterium that causes food-borne diseases

Salmonella is a Gram-negative (Figure 5), rod-shaped, flagellated, bacterium which invades, and replicates and survives within, immune cells such as macrophages (Coburn et al., 2007). There are over 2500 serotypes of *Salmonella enterica. S. enterica typhi* and *S. enterica typhimurium* cause typhoid fever and enterocolitis respectively in humans. These diseases affect millions of people globally causing around 600,000 deaths annually, mostly in infants and immunocompromised patients.

Salmonella is transmitted via the faeco-oral route following ingestion of contaminated food, water or animal products, or close contact with an infected individual. Infection predominantly occurs in the epithelial lining of the intestine with intestinal epithelial cells (IECs) and macrophages being key cells for both bacterial uptake and immunity. IECs act not only as physical barriers to infection, but also contribute to the innate immune response following PRR activation. Bacterial uptake by macrophages (and dendritic cells) results in stimulation of a wide range of PRRs and can also serve as a route to systemic infection. The pathophysiology of *Salmonella* infections is strongly connected to the strong inflammatory response from the host. Interaction between host PRRs and *Salmonella* virulence factors influence the pathology, morbidity, and mortality at different stages of infection.

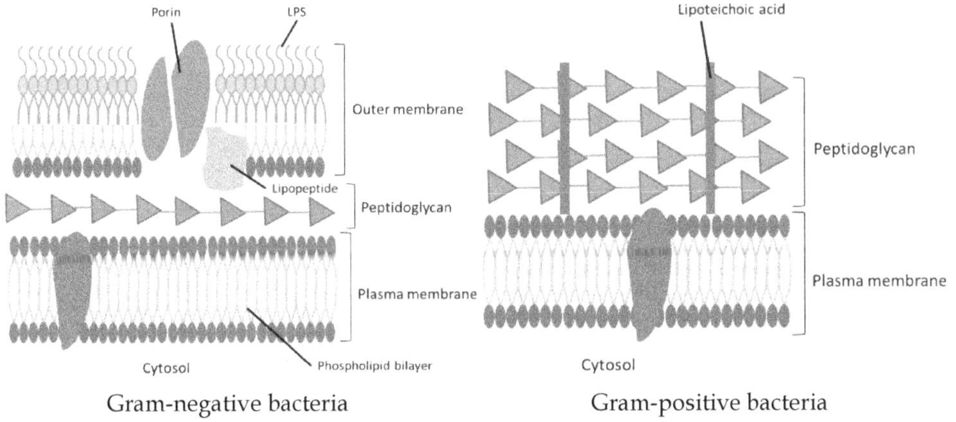

Fig. 5. Schematic of the cell wall structure of Gram-negative (left-hand image) and Gram-positive (right-hand image) bacteria highlighting the key components of each type of bacterial wall. Salmonella is a rod-shaped Gram-negative bacterium. Two key PAMPs associated with Salmonella are LPS and lipopeptide which activate TLR4 and TLR2 respectively. In addition, the surface of Salmonella possesses flagella, another potent immunostimulatory molecule.

3.1.2 *Salmonella* PAMPs and PRR activation

Salmonella is recognised by a wide range of PRRs: TLR1, 2, 4, 5, 6, and 9; NLRC4; NLRP3; NOD1 and NOD2 (Hold et. al., 2011). Of these the key PRRs are TLR2, TLR4, TLR5 and NLRC4. Cell culture studies and mouse models have identified several *Salmonella* PAMPs responsible for PRR activation. Of particular importance are LPS, lipoproteins and flagellin (Figure 5). Flagellin provides an interesting example of a ligand that is able to activate two distinct receptors (TLR5 and NLRC4) leading to distinct immune responses (Franchi et al., 2006; Hayashi et al., 2001).

LPS and lipoproteins lead to classical activation of TLR4 and TLR2 signalling pathways respectively (Section 2.1). The importance of TLR2 signalling is influenced by the severity of infection, playing a key role at high multiplicities of infection. In contrast, the role of TLR4 appears essential at all levels of Salmonella infection (Spiller et al., 2008; Talbot et al., 2009). TLR4 activation by LPS requires several co-receptors such as: myeloid-differentiation 2 (MD2), cluster of differentiation 14 (CD14), and LPS-binding protein (LBP). The TLR4 signalling pathway is different from all other TLRs as its activation results in two separate signalling cascades: MyD88-dependent and MyD88-independent pathways which result in NF-κB activation and IFN-β and NFκB activation respectively (Figure 3). This activation is regulated temporally and spatially as it is been suggested that MyD88-dependent signalling occurs first on the plasma membrane, following which the receptor complex is endocytosed after which it will sequentially activate the MyD88-independent pathway. This is a classic example of the use of subcellular localisation of the receptor signalling complex to determine use of downstream adaptor proteins and the specifics of the signalling pathway activated. The importance of TLR4 in the response to *Salmonella* is highlighted by observations that mice possessing defects in TLR4 are incapable of mounting a normal immune response to *Salmonella typhimurium* infection (Talbot et al., 2009). It appears that the relative importance of different TLR and adaptor proteins in combating *Salmonella* is dependent upon the bacterial load. For example, the adaptor protein Mal only appears important at low multiplicities of infection (Kenny et al., 2009). This may well be a deliberate ploy on the part of the host to manage the severity of the response at a level which reflects the severity of infection.

TLR5 recognises monomeric flagellin. TLR5 is expressed on the basolateral surface, not the apical surface, of polarised epithelial cells so only responds to flagellin that has breached the epithelial barrier. This is likely to be a host strategy to stop inappropriate immune activation by flagellated commensal bacteria in the lumen (Gewirtz et al., 2001; Hayashi et al., 2001) . Once the bacterium has breached the epithelial barrier flagellin can then be detected by the baso-laterally located receptor. In addition, TLR5 is found expressed on the surface of immune cells such as macrophages and DCs.

The mechanism of flagellin recognition by TLR5 is interesting as only monomeric flagellin is recognised. This is because the TLR5 binding site is buried in the functional flagellar filament. This is one of the bacterium's ways of evading the host immune system. A single filamentous flagella consists of 11 protofilaments, each of which contains four globular domains (D0-D3) (Figure 6). The recognition site for TLR5 is contained in the N-terminal D1 domain. This region is essential for motility and is consequently highly conserved (Smith et al., 2003). Mutations within D1 have been shown to abolish recognition by TLR5, bacterial motility, and to disrupt protofilament assembly. In particular differences in amino acids 89-

96 have been implicated in the ability of some species of bacteria to evade immune detection by TLR5 (Andersen-Nissen et al., 2005).

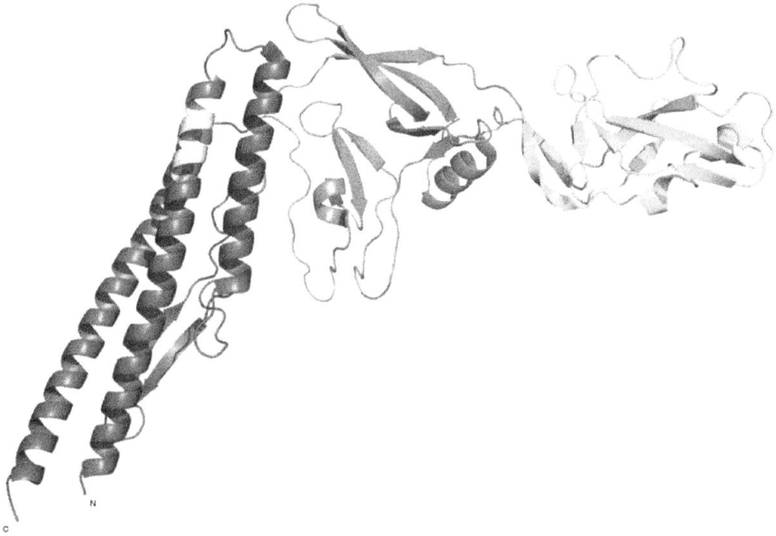

Fig. 6. Crystal structure of FliC flagellin from *S. typhimurium* (pdb entry 1io1). Domain colouring is: D1 - light purple; D2 - blue; D3 - green; the yellow region in D1 corresponds to amino acids 89-96.

Prior to detection by TLR5, flagella has to be depolymerised into its monomeric form. Direct contact between the bacterium and the host cell triggers the *de novo* synthesis and secretion of monomeric flagellin into the host cell via T3SS (Subramanian and Qadri, 2006). This process is triggered by the bacterium sensing lysophospholipids produced by the host cells upon infection and is important for initial inflammatory and innate immune responses by IECs. Following activation TLR5 forms a homodimer and initiates MyD88-dependent signalling cascades (Figure 3) as part of the innate immune response. One effect of this is to recruit neutrophils and macrophages to the site of infection.

Once *Salmonella* has breached the epithelia it can be phagocytosed by macrophages. The bacterium can reside and replicate inside a Salmonella containing vesicle. Fragments of flagellin enter into the cytoplasm, probably via a type III secretion system, from where it stimulates the NLR family receptor NLRC4 (Franchi et al., 2006). NLRC4 is also activated by the protein PrgJ, a component of the type III secretion system expressed by the *Salmonella* pathogenicity island (SPI)-1 (Miao et al., 2010). The mechanisms of NLRC4 activation by bacteria such as Salmonella are complex and seem to follow some form of temporal cascade. The net effect is that activation of NLRC4 leads to inflammasome formation, caspase-1 activation and secretion of IL-1β and IL-18. In addition, caspase-1 activation via NLRC4 can trigger macrophage death through pyroptosis. Pyroptosis is a caspase-1 dependent, programmed cell death event that has features of both apoptosis and necrosis. The process of pyroptosis results in the release of pro-inflammatory cellular contents and also serves to limit intracellular bacterial replication (Roy and Zamboni, 2006) (Figure 4).

3.1.3 Modulation of the innate immune response by *Salmonella*

Salmonella is capable of infecting, surviving, and multiplying within macrophages. This requires multiple virulence proteins which are predominantly encoded on the SPI-2 pathogenicity island. These factors enable the bacterium to resist the oxidative burst and maturation of phagosomes and lysosomes. In fact the bacterium modifies these endocytic vacuoles and generates an environment conducive to bacterial replication - the salmonella containing vacuole (SCV) (Figure 7).

In addition to acting as a trigger of NLRC4 signalling (Section 3.1.2) the T3SS allows proteins to be injected into the cell cytoplasm that modulate cellular function. A major role of these proteins is to alter cytoskeletal function and permit bacterial entry. In addition, *Salmonella* also secretes an immunomodulatory protein SipB. The precise role and mechanism of action of SipB is unknown. However, the protein is capable of interacting with caspase-1 and consequently altering the signalling pathways involved in caspase-1 activation and downstream functionality (Hersh et al., 1999). Other bacteria also produce proteins that modulate immune signalling. For example, it has recently been shown that *Escherichia coli* and *Brucella melitensis* produce TIR domain containing virulence factors that inhibit TLR signalling by directly blocking MyD88 adaptor protein function through a homotypic TIR-TIR interaction (Cirl et al., 2008).

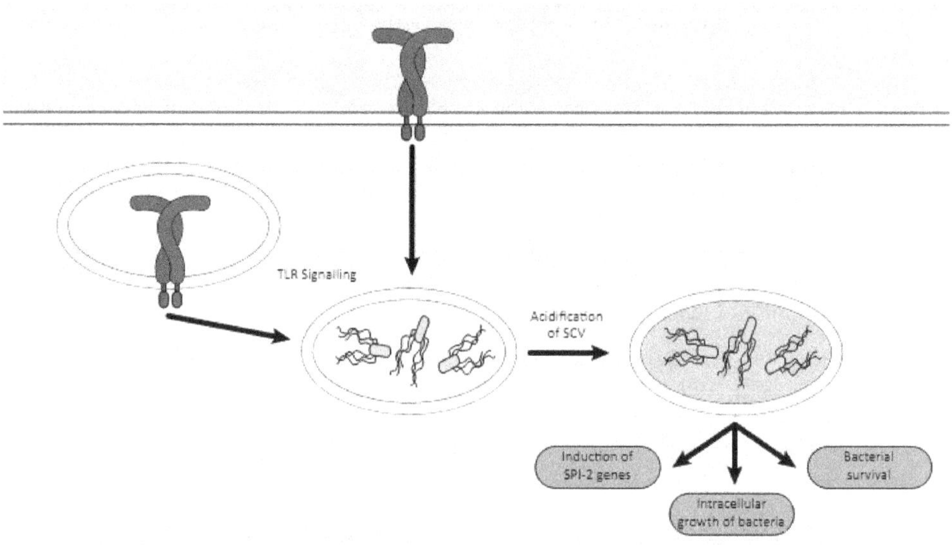

Fig. 7. Formation of a *Salmonella* containing vacuole (SCV) promotes *Salmonella* survival and virulence inside host macrophages. SCV formation appears to be dependent on functional TLR signalling and requires acidification to activate expression of the *Salmonella* pro-survival genes.

3.1.4 Altering PAMP properties as a way to evade immune detection

Salmonella flagellin is a readily available and common target recognised by both extracellular, TLR5, and intracellular, NLRC4, PRRs. Although many PAMPs cannot be altered and changed in order to evade the immune response this is not the case for flagellin. *Salmonella* has been found to downregulate flagellin expression once it is inside macrophages, although how quickly this happens is unclear. A loss of flagellin expression will obviously reduce the potential for immune stimulation, but it has yet to be determined whether this occurs in a timeframe that will influence PRR activation. As TLR5 recognises monomeric flagellin mechanisms that increase flagellum stability and reduce the release of monomeric subunits will also reduce immune activation.

Some other flagellated bacteria have adopted a mechanism in which they express flagellin lacking the proinflammatory regions found in Salmonella FliC (Section 3.1.2). The classic example is *Helicobacter Pylori*. *H.pylori* express the flagellin proteins FlaA and FlaB. These subunits retain the ability to assemble motile flagella, but lack the TLR5 stimulatory regions. This was elegantly demonstrated by experiments in which the comparable sequence from *H.pylori* flagellin was substituted into *Salmonella* FliC. The mutant flagellin lost the ability to activate TLR5.

3.2 PRRs and viral PAMPs

Viruses are more abundant than bacteria; they are also very diverse genetically and evolve rapidly. Viruses are obligate parasites and can only survive and replicate inside host cells. They have different virulence components and simpler structural features in comparison to bacteria. The requirement on the host cell for replication makes viral nucleic acids the key viral PAMPs. Consequently, only a subset of PRRs can detect them. These include: NLRP3; NOD2; TLR3, 7, 8, and 9; and the RIG-I like receptors (Kanneganti, 2010; Perry et al., 2005) (Table 2).

PAMP	PRR	Adapter	Cytokines
Toll-like receptors (TLRs)			
dsRNA	TLR3	TRIF	IFN-β/ pro-inflammatory
G/U rich ssRNA	TLR7	MyD88	IFN-α/ pro-inflammatory
G/U rich ssRNA	TLR8	MyD88	IFN-α
unmethylated CpG DNA motifs	TLR9	MyD88	IFN-α
Nod-like receptors (NLRs)			
ssRNA	NOD2	MAVS	Type I IFNs
Viral RNA	NLRP3	ASC	IL-1β/IL-18
Retinoic acid-inducible gene I-like receptors (RLRs)			
5′ triphosphate ssRNA	RIG-I	MAVS/ASC/CARD9	Type-I IFNs/ IL-1β

Table 2. Natural viral PAMPs are recognised by PRRs and stimulate cytokine production. Viral nucleic acids generally differ from host nucleic acids through the presence of specific motifs and also their subcellular localisation. Viral nucleic acid (blue column) is recognised by specific PRRs (pink column) and this leads to receptor activation. The activated receptor recruits specific adaptor proteins and initiates signalling cascades. The net result of this is the secretion of cytokines.

The host response to viral infection results in the production of anti-viral agents such as type I IFNs that interfere with viral replication and survival inside host cells, and pro-inflammatory cytokines such as IL-1β and IL-18. Type I IFNs are the key players in innate immune response against viral infection. We will expand the discussion on role of PRRs in viral infection by considering the example of influenza virus.

3.2.1 Recognition of influenza by TLRs

Influenza is a negative-sense ssRNA virus that causes pulmonary inflammation and chronic lung diseases. The symptoms vary from fever and inflammation to death, depending on the strain of the virus and the host response. Influenza enters host cells by endocytosis following recognition of sialic acid residues by the viral haemagglutinin protein. This is followed by pH-dependent fusion of the viral and endosomal membranes allowing release of the viral core into the cytosol. The exact sequence of events that subsequently leads to recognition of influenza by PRRs is still largely unknown. Influenza PAMPs can be recognised by a variety of PRRs (Figure 8 and Table 2). However, the majority of immunopathology appears to result from TLR7, NLRP3 and RIG-I activation (Ichinohe, 2010). Plasmacytoid dendritic cells (pDCs) are the major cell-type responsible for mounting an immune response to influenza through the secretion of high amounts of type I IFNs and proinflammatory cytokines (Perry et al., 2005). Macrophages, nasal airway epithelial cells and monocytes have also been found to respond to influenza. Secreted type I IFNs interact with IFN receptors causing expression of type I IFN-stimulated genes with antiviral properties. For example, increased expression of RIG-I like receptors and proteins involved in the inhibition of viral transcription and trafficking. Type I IFNs also influence the development of adaptive immunity such as increasing expression of costimulatory molecules on macrophages and DCs, aiding maturation of DCs, and the activation of T and NK cells.

pDCs are professional antigen presenting cells. Following endocytic uptake of virus particles the virus is degraded and can contact endosomal PRRs. The presence of ssRNA in the endosome activates TLR7 (Lund et al., 2004) which signals in a MyD88-dependent manner to activate IRF3 and IRF7 transcription factors for the expression of type I IFNs. ssRNA recognition by TLR7 appears to require endosomal acidification before the receptor can form a homodimer and initiate the signalling pathways. TLR7 and MyD88 are both required for the type I IFN response to influenza ssRNA in pDCs. Studies have shown that mice deficient in either TLR7 or MyD88 are unable to respond to influenza virus (Diebold et al., 2004; Lund et al., 2004). TLR7 is also expressed in other cell types such as macrophages and conventional DCs, however TLR7 activation in these cell types only result in expression of proinflammatory cytokines. This difference is due to different signalling adaptor proteins present in these different cell types. Human naïve B cells and effector memory $CD4^+$ T cells also express and signal through TLR7 activation (Wang et al., 2006).

The TLR7 response to influenza ssRNA is independent of viral replication. In contrast, there is evidence that dsRNA can induce type I IFN production via a TLR7- and MyD88-independent pathway that requires viral replication (Guillot et al., 2005). Even though influenza is a ssRNA virus, dsRNA molecules are synthesised during the replicative stage of the virus. Certainly TLR3 recognises endosomal dsRNA from influenza virus (Guillot et al., 2005). The downstream signalling proceeds not through MyD88, but the adaptor TRIF to activate IRF3 and late-phase NF-κB. The importance of dsRNA recognition in influenza infection is supported by the observation that the influenza protein NS1, which sequesters viral dsRNA, inhibits type I IFN induction upon viral infection (Lu et al., 1995).

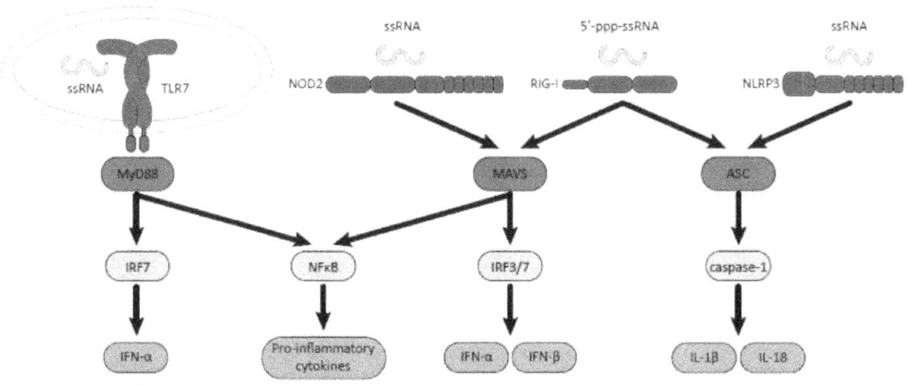

Fig. 8. Cytoplasmic and endosomal PRRs that recognise PAMPs from ssRNA virus such as influenza. Different PRRs can activate different pathways, and some pathways are shared by several PRRs.

3.2.2 Recognition of influenza by NLR and RLRs

Influenza can be recognised by the NLRP3 inflammasome, RIG-I and potentially NOD2 (Kanneganti, 2010). Activation of these signalling pathways results in the activation of caspase-1, IL-1β and IL-18; the production of inflammatory cytokines; and the secretion of type I IFNs via MAVS engagement. Each of these receptors is located in the cytoplasm and hence responds to the presence of RNA, 5′-phosphate ssRNA, or ssRNA within the cytoplasm. This contrasts to TLR7 which responds to ssRNA in the endosomal compartment. In the case of NLRP3 it is unknown whether viral RNA is a directly activating ligand for the receptor. Indeed it is more likely in this instance that the presence of viral RNA in the cytoplasm leads to a homeostatic disruption that in turn activates NLRP3, stimulates inflammasome formation, and initiates a protective innate immune response.

NOD2 and NLRP3 elicit different immune responses to viral RNA (Fig. 6). NLRP3 stimulation leads to activation of caspase 1 and subsequent processing of the pro forms of IL-1β and IL-18 via inflammasome formation. Both IL-1β and IL-18 are important in the clearance of influenza infection as mice which lack the IL-1 receptor and consequently can't respond to these cytokines show impaired viral clearance and increased mortality (Schmitz et al., 2005). Unlike NLRP3, NOD2 does not form an inflammasome. The primary role of NOD2 seems to be the detection of the bacterial peptidoglycan fragment muramyl dipeptide and signalling through NF-κB regulated pathways. However, more recently NOD2 has been reported to respond to viral ssRNA (Sabbah et al., 2009). Viral ssRNA results in activation of an alternative MAVS-dependent NOD2 signalling cascade in which NOD2 relocalises to the mitochondria and ultimately activates IRF3. This leads to the induction of an antiviral type I IFN response. A loss of NOD2 led to an increase in the susceptibility of mice to influenza infection, a reduction in IRF3 phosphorylation and a diminishment of the type I IFN response (Sabbah et al., 2009).

RIG-I can also signal in a MAVS-dependent manner to generate a type I IFN response (Kanneganti, 2010). Interestingly RIG-I has also been reported to stimulate the production of pro-IL-1β production in a MAVS-CARD9-NFkB dependent manner; as well as inducing pro-IL-1β processing and secretion in an ASC-dependent inflammasome manner (Kanneganti, 2010; Pichlmair et al., 2006). This therefore provides a single receptor example of cross-talk along multiple signalling pathways in order to maximise the anti-viral and inflammatory reponse.

3.2.3 Subversion of the innate immune response by influenza

Viruses have long been known to utilise multiple strategies to evade the immune response, persist in the host, or allow reinfection. In the case of influenza virus the influence of antigenic drift in the surface haemaglutinin and neurominidase proteins allows evasion of the adaptive antibody response thereby limiting the protective effects of vaccination and facilitating influenza epidemics. Antigenic shift is a more extreme, and less common, evasion strategy in which viruses from different species undergo recombination to create a new potentially pandemic viral strain. Commonly recombination occurs between human and avian viral strains.

Influenza virus also employs various strategies to disrupt the innate immune response; either by interfering with PRR mediated detection of viral components, or through modulation of signalling cascades. The viral non-structural protein (NS)1 is a good example of a protein that targets a specific signalling pathways to avoid detection. NS1 has the potential to inhibit the activation of caspase 1 and the production of type I IFNs. Interestingly there does appear to be strain-dependent variation in activity of NS1 in this respect. The N-terminal region of NS1 appears to be important for the inhibition of inflammasome-dependent immune responses; specifically through inhibition of caspase-1 activation, and hence IL-1β and IL-18 production (Kanneganti, 2010). NS1 has also been reported to inhibit RIG-I-MAVS-dependent antiviral signalling (Bowie and Unterholzner, 2008). Pichlmair and colleagues, reported that NS1 binds directly to RIG-I and inhibits its activation, thereby reducing type I IFN production (Pichlmair et al., 2006). However, the exact molecular mechanism of how NS1 inhibits RIG-I signalling is not clear. This interaction may directly antagonise RIG-I function, or it could involve other proteins that are required for proper signalling. For example, NS1 also sequesters dsRNA so that they cannot be detected by dsRNA-recognising PRRs such as TLR3 and PKR. More recently, Gack and co-workers showed that NS1 inhibits RIG-I signalling by inhibiting activation of ubiquitin ligase tripartite motif (TRIM)25; a crucial component of the RIG-I signalling cascade required for activation of RIG-I through ubiquitination within the CARD domain (Gack et al., 2007).

3.3 PRRs and *Candida albicans*

3.3.1 *Candida albicans*

The yeast *Candida albicans* is a common human commensal that colonises mucocutaneous surfaces of the oral cavity, gastrointestinal tract and vagina. *Candida albicans* is often a benign member of the mucosal flora. However, under specific host conditions, such as a change in immune status or commensal species, *Candida albicans* can proliferate in a saprophytic state and become an opportunistic pathogen. This usually results in mucosal diseases, but on occasion the infection may become systemic and life-threatening. A specific example is nosocomial candidiasis in hospital patients with a compromised immune system. *Candida albicans* can differentiate in yeast, pseudohyphal and hyphal forms. The hyphal form is often linked to disease as it facilitates infection of epithelial cells and tissue damage. In addition to hyphae *Candida* species enhance their pathogenicity through biofilm formation and secretion of proteases and toxins. The balance between the commensal and pathogenic state is what makes *Candida albicans* a useful study case for looking at the interplay between host PRRs and PAMPs, and the dynamics that lead to protection/tolerance or infection.

3.3.2 Induction of an immune response by *Candida albicans*

It is hypothesised that the initial interaction between the host immune cell and specific *C.albicans* PAMPs is critical for deciding whether the immune response is protective or invasive. Studies suggest that a prolonged anti-inflammatory response against *C. albicans*, including increased production of IL-10, IL-4 and differentiation of regulatory/suppressive T cell subsets facilitates invasion and the initial development of disease. In the absence of IL-10 there is a switch to a protective response by the innate immune system. This includes stimulation of inflammatory cytokines such as IL-12, TNFα, and IL-6; and progression towards a Th17 response leading to IL-17 and IL-22 production to clear the infection. Further evidence for the role of IL-10 as a modulator of yeast infection is suggested by animal models. IL-10 deficient mice are protected against the toxic effects of *C.albicans* infection and show a decline in inflammatory markers associated with yeast infections. In contrast, inclusion of IL-4 and IL-10 in a gastrointestinal model of yeast infection facilitates invasion rather than protection.

Interaction studies between host immune cells and *Candida albicans* have identified various PRRs that recognise yeast derived PAMPs, and facilitate protective responses via the pro-inflammatory pathway. Most yeast and fungal PAMPs have been identified in the cell wall, a complex matrix consisting of glucans, mannans, mannoproteins and glycolipids. Several receptors including TLR4 and the C-type lectins Dectin-2, Mincle and the macrophage mannose receptor bind to mannans of *Candida* species. Dectin-1, lactosylceramide complement receptor-3 and scavenger receptors recognise β-glucans of *Candida.*

3.3.3 TLR sensing of *Candida albicans*

TLRs are involved in the immune response against *C. albicans* as well as other fungal agents, particularly TLR2 and to a lesser extent TLR4. Both pathogenic and commensal forms of *C. albicans* are involved in TLR-dependent signalling, in addition to other commensal yeasts such as *Saccromyces cerevisiae*. TLR2 recognises phospholipomannan components of the fungal cell wall. TLR4 is activated by α-mannans on *C. albicans* and initiates the production of IL-12 by host immune cells and a subsequent protective Th1 response. TLR4 polymorphisms Asp299Gly/Thr399Ile are associated with an increased susceptibility to *C. albicans* infection in the bloodstream, with an increase in IL-10 levels being the contributing factor (Van der Graaf et al., 2006). In addition to a pro-inflammatory response, TLR2 activation may also lead to the production of IL-10 and generation of T regulatory cells and a non-protective Th2 response. This is supported by data on TLR2 KO mice which are more resistant to *Candida* infection. The TLR2 polymorphism R753G gives rise to patients with enhanced *Candida* sepsis, suggesting that TLR2 is an important PRR for regulation of *Candida* infections (Woehrle et al., 2008). Indeed, TLR2 signalling complexes may modulate the Th1/Th2 (IL-10) balance in response to fungi by switching between pro- and anti-inflammatory responses. TLR signalling occurs in crosstalk with the carbohydrate specific PRRs, the C-type and S-type lectins, to regulate *C. albicans* infection.

3.3.4 CLR recognition of *Candida albicans*

CLRs such as Dectin-1, Dectin-2, Mincle, DC-SIGN (SIGNR1, mouse homolog) and mannose receptor (MR) are key PRRs in the immune response against fungi. The interaction of CLRs with PAMPs is mediated via carbohydrate recognition domains (CRD), which facilitate internalisation, degradation and antigenic presentation. CLRs signal via the Syk pathway to initiate an inflammatory response using an ITAM motif in their cytoplasmic tail. Some CLRs such as Dectin-2, lack an ITAM motif and instead utilise adaptor molecules such as the Fc receptor γ chain and the DNAX-activating protein (DAP12) which have an ITAM motif for signalling.

Dectin-1, which is expressed in neutrophils, macrophages and DCs, is a specific receptor for β-1,3 glucans, located in the cell walls of fungi, such as *Saccharomyces cerevisiae* (zymosan) and *Candida albicans*. Dectin-1 signalling pathways are not completely understood. It is proposed that Dectin-1 mediated responses may require crosstalk with TLRs, NLRs, tetraspanins and the DC-SIGN receptor. Dectin-1 binds and internalises β-glucans, and mediates its own signalling pathway which includes the production of reactive oxygen species (ROS) also termed an oxidative burst, activation of NFκβ and secretion of proinflammatory cytokines. Following ligand recognition via the CRD, Dectin-1 is phosphorylated by the tyrosine kinase Src, which recruits Syk to the ITAM motif to activate MAPKs and NFAT. This Syk interaction also mediates formation of the CARD9-Bcl10-Malt1 complex, which stimulates NFκβ and the secretion of proinflammatory cytokines. This ultimately leads to a Th17 T cell response. Th17 cells are particularly important for anti-microbial immunity at the epithelial and mucosal barriers and produce cytokines such as IL-17 and IL-22 which stimulate anti-microbial proteins. A lack of Th17 cells leaves the host susceptible to invasion by opportunistic pathogens such as *C.albicans*.

A recent study suggests that Malt-1 activation of the NFκβ subunit C-Rel is important for induction of Th17 enhancing cytokines IL1β and IL23. It was also evident that Dectin-1 activates all components of the NFκβ complex, whereas Dectin-2 specifically activates C-Rel (Gringhuis et al., 2011). Recent studies suggest that Dectin-1 NFκβ activation is induced by zymosan, whereas hyphal forms of *C.albicans* activate NFκβ via Dectin-2. Hyphae stimulation in *C.albicans* also facilitates association of CARD-9 with Bcl10, in a Dectin-2 specific manner (Bi et al., 2010). This is a good example of how different PRRs of the host have distinguished between pathogenic (hyphae producing) and commensal forms of *Candida albicans.*

The ability of Dectin-1 to activate Th17 responses assists in the prevention of fungal infection. Loss of Dectin-1 in KO mice and Dectin-1 polymorphisms in humans makes the host more susceptible to infection (Ferwerda et al., 2009b). In *C.albicans* infection, β-glucans may also stimulate Th17 and regulatory T cell responses via a Dectin-1/TLR2 crosstalk, in addition to the Dectin-1 specific pro-inflammatory cytokine response (Gantner et al., 2003; LeibundGut-Landmann et al., 2007). This Dectin-1/TLR2 response also involves the production of prostaglandin E2, which upregulates Th17 dependent cytokines IL-6 and IL-23 (Smeekens et al., 2010). Dectin-1 also synergises with TLR2 and TLR4 for the production of TNFα and there is evidence to suggest that Dectin-1 and TLR2/6 pathways crosstalk to enhance responses by each receptor. Furthermore, Dectin-1 activation also upregulates pro-IL-1β for subsequent activation by the NLRP3 inflammasome (Cheng et al., 2011).

Dectin-1 also associates with Galectin-3, an S-type lectin that binds to β-1,2 mannosides present in the cell wall of *Candida albicans,* an interaction that is required for proinflammatory responses in fungi. The Dectin1-Galectin-3 complex modulates TNFα levels, whereby a decrease in galectin-3 corresponds to a decrease in TNFα. Mutant *C.albicans* expressing more β-glucan on the cell wall surface had reduced galectin-3 binding and a reduction in the protective pro-inflammatory response. Hence, association between Galectin-3 and Dectin-1 can modulate the proinflammatory response to help distinguish between pathogenic and nonpathogenic fungi (Esteban et al., 2011).

Dectin-2 recognises several fungal species including *C.albicans* and interacts with PAMPs of high mannose content, specifically α-linked mannans and zymosan. Dectin-2 also activates NFκβ and a Th17 response via the Syk-CARD9 pathway, as well as MAPKs via a CARD9 independent pathway. However unlike Dectin-1, it couples to Syk indirectly utilising the ITAM motif of the Fc receptor. A recent study has suggested that it is Dectin-2, rather than Dectin-1, that is more involved in the Th17 response to *C.albicans* and their hyphae, with IL-1β and IL-23 induction being Dectin-2 dependent. DCs from Dectin-2 KO mice show a limited cytokine response to α-mannans (Saijo et al., 2010).

Macrophage inducible C-type lectin (Mincle) binds to yeast cell wall components, specifically α-linked mannans, and like Dectin-2 also uses the Fc receptor to signal in a Syk-CARD9 dependent matter. Mincle has also been linked to TLR2 responses. DC-SIGN and its mouse homolog (SIGNR1) recognises complex mannoside structures on the surface of yeast facilitating internalisation. SIGNR1 specifically binds zymosan as well as live and heat killed *C.albicans.* SIGNR1 has also been reported to modulate TLR4 dependent signalling and to itself induce a proinflammatory response against *C.albicans* (Takahara et al., 2011). SIGNR1 may also interact with Dectin-1 to enhance Syk dependent pathways.

There is recent evidence to suggest that the interaction of *candida albicans* with glucan (Dectin-1) and mannan (Dectin-2) specific receptors, works in combination with the adaptor protein MyD88 to activate phospholipase A_2 and the production of eicosanoids, which are important modulators of inflammation (Suram et al., 2010).

3.4 PRRs and *Schistosoma mansoni*

3.4.1 Schistosoma infection and immunity

The parasitic worm Schistosoma represents the fourth most prevalent helminth infection worldwide affecting 200 million people. In schistosomiasis, the human parasitic disease caused by helminths, the parasite takes on various forms during its lifecycle, which presents a variety of PAMPs to the host and contribute to the developing host immune response. The lifecycle of *S.mansoni* in mammalian hosts begins when the larval stage (cercariae) is released from an intermediate host (snail; genus *Biomphalaria)* and then infects host cells, where it transforms into adult worms. Hosts infected with these parasites accumulate hundreds of intravascular worms which secrete various antigenic molecules into the blood which continuously trigger the host inflammatory response and facilitate prolonged colonisation. During *S.mansoni* infection, the adult worms can survive for many years, where they evade the host immune response, by establishing a balance between host activation and immune suppression. The adult worms also produce hundreds of eggs daily over a life period of 5 to 30 years. A Th2 anti-inflammatory response is triggered by the presence of eggs as well as soluble antigens secreted by the eggs, whereas a Th1 inflammatory specific response is more likely when adult worms interact with host immune cells.

3.4.2 Recognition of *Schistosoma mansoni* by PRRs

Schistosoma mansoni produces various glycoconjugates (glycoproteins and glycolipids) that interact with PRRs of the innate immune system and potentially modulate the function of host immune cells (Figure 9). The mouse model of schistosomiasis identified that Schistosoma glycoconjugates containing Lacto-N-fucopentaose III (LNFPIII) induce a Th2 response in collaboration with TLR4. Also the schistosomal tegument has been reported to activate inflammatory responses in DCs via a TLR4/MyD88 pathway. Schistosomiasis is also associated with high levels of endotoxemia and elevated levels of high mobility group 1 (HMGB1) protein, which is a ligand for TLR2, TLR4 and the RAGE receptor.

Lysophosphatidylserine (Lyso-PS) and dsRNA from the eggs of *S.mansoni* also activate TLR2 and TLR3 inflammation pathways respectively. Soluble schistosomal egg antigens (SEA) inhibit TNFα and IL-6 secretion originating from TLR signalling pathways. This TLR suppression occurs at the same time as NLRP3 activation and IL-1β production (Ritter et al., 2010). SEA binds to the Dectin-2/FcRγ complex and signals via the Syk pathway to induce ROS and potassium efflux, known effectors of the inflammasome NLRP3. *S.mansoni* infection of mice without inflammasome components ASC and NLRP3 failed to induce an inflammatory response indicated by the lowered IL-1β levels and the downregulation of T cell responses.

CLRs also recognise glycans associated with schistosomes using one or more CRD (Figure 9). The CLRs DC-SIGN, macrophage galactose type lectin (MGL) and MR on human DCs, bind specific glycans on the SEA of *S.mansoni*. This binding facilitates internalisation of the SEA and promotion of a Th2 response. DC-SIGN can also bind to the larval form of *S.mansoni* via glycolipids. Human DCs primed with adult worm glycolipids switch towards a Th1 immune response and induce an inflammatory cytokine cascade. DC-SIGN binds to fucose components of the glycolipid of the worm and helps activate TLR4 signalling and inflammation (van Stijn et al., 2010). It is proposed that DC-SIGN recruits glycolipids and then presents them to TLR4, via a TLR4-DC-SIGN complex in lipid rafts.

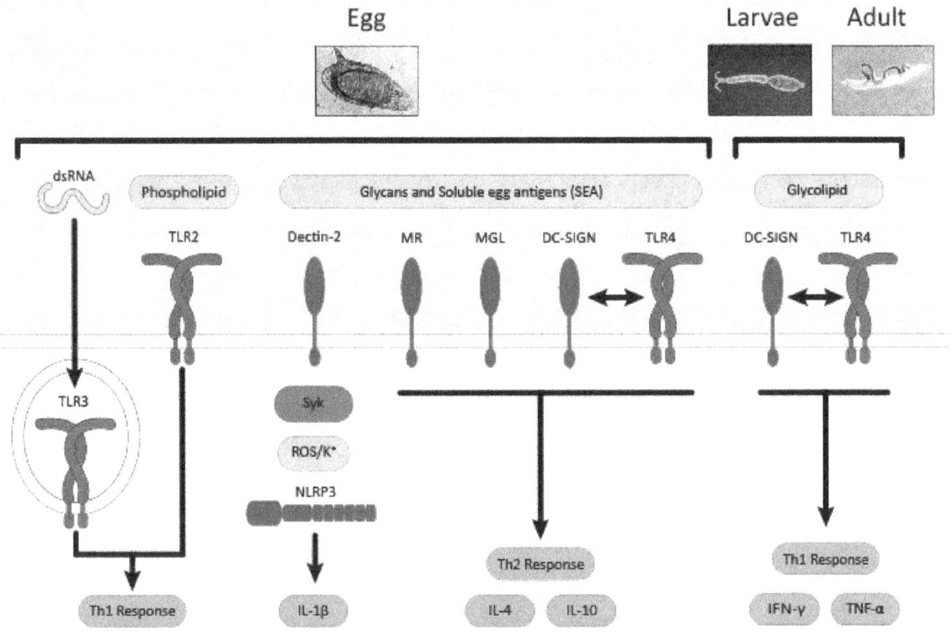

Fig. 9. PRRs involved in the immune response against schistosomal PAMPs at different stages of the schistosomes lifecycle. The activation of a Th1 (inflammatory) and a Th2 (humoral) response demonstrates the ability of the parasite to regulate infection. Pictures of schistosoma egg, larvae and adult reproduced with the permission of David Dunne.

4. The role of PRRs in immunisation against infectious disease

Immunisation is a crucial and highly successful defence against many infectious diseases including: measles, tetanus, diphtheria, rubella, polio and tuberculosis. Over recent years it has become apparent that PRRs play a major and crucial role in the processes of immune priming and polarization. These new findings have been applied to vaccine research in two major areas: firstly to determine the molecular mechanism of action of known vaccines and adjuvants; and secondly new adjuvant components have been developed that target specific PRRs in a quest towards rationally designed 'customised' vaccines.

4.1 The role of PRRs in current vaccines

PRRs are important for the priming of adaptive immune responses (Section 3.3). It is not surprising that many current vaccines also function, at least in part, by activating PRRs. Studies with knock-out mice have shown that PRRs are critical for the optimal function of several known vaccines. However, PRRs are not necessary for all vaccines to induce protective immune responses, and several vaccines instead trigger alternative pro-inflammatory pathways that appear to primarily recognize tissue or cellular injury rather than PAMPs.

Although much is known about the PAMP content of many vaccines, the role of PRRs in triggering protective immunity is more challenging to determine for three reasons. Firstly, individual PAMPs can be efficiently identified by measuring innate activation of cells such as DC *in vitro* whereas induction of immunity can only be measured *in vivo* with corresponding increase in cost and difficulty of interpretation. Secondly, the presence of multiple PAMPs and corresponding PRRs that coordinate host responses means that study of immunity in single knockouts often leads to partial phenotypes. Thirdly, many important human vaccines- particularly live attenuated vaccines - show host-species specific activity, preventing the direct study in PRR knockout mice.

4.1.1 Evidence of PAMP content and PRR activation by traditional vaccines

Traditionally, vaccines belong to one of three types: live attenuated vaccines, such as the eponymous *vaccinia,* are infectious agents in their own right, and prime protective immunity but lack pathogenicity; inactivated vaccines contain whole infectious agents that have been inactivated - for example by heat or chemical sterilization - to prevent infection, but still provoke protective immunity without replication; subunit vaccines contain a purified protective antigen combined with an adjuvant i.e. a formulation that promotes an immune response against the subunit. Of these three types, it is clear that both live attenuated and inactivated vaccines closely resemble pathogens - and therefore contain many PAMPs and trigger multiple PRRs. Subunit vaccines, in contrast, only contain PAMPs if they are co-purified with the antigenic subunit, if the antigenic subunit is itself PRR agonistic, or if the adjuvant activates PRRs (see 4.1.2, 4.1.3 and 4.1.4).

4.1.2 PRR activation by live attenuated vaccines

Our oldest vaccines are live attenuated pathogens. Yet they are also the most poorly understood due to the complex interplay between parasite and host. Live attenuated vaccines contain a plethora of PAMPs. For example, live attenuated bacterial vaccines such as *Mycobacterium tuberculosis* BCG and live oral Typhoid Fever vaccine are rich in well known PAMPs such as bacterial DNA, lipopolysaccharides and lipopeptides. Two major challenges in characterizing PRR triggering by live attenuated viral vaccines are the fact that PAMP content and location changes during the infectious cycle (e.g. production of different types of nucleic acids, viral entry into host cells); and the presence of PRR inhibitors can obscure signaling.

Vaccinia is one of the best studied live attenuated vaccines. The importance of PRRs in vaccinia virus sensing became clear very early on with the discovery that its genome encodes inhibitors of IL-1 and TLR signaling (Bowie et al., 2000). Host responses to vaccinia are complex. Pathways act separately and synergistically, and there are diverse responses from different cell types. Studies of viral-induced cytokine production from cells from knockout mice have started to unpick this complexity and demonstrated that vaccinia can trigger multiple PRR including TLR2/TLR6, (Delaloye et al., 2009; Zhu et al., 2007), the RLR MDA-5 (Delaloye et al., 2009), and TLR8 (Martinez et al., 2010). The inflammasome component NALP3 is also required for maximal cytokine responses (Delaloye et al., 2009).

Although the rich PAMP content of live attenuated vaccines has been characterised, understanding fully how PRR triggering induces protective adaptive immunity still remains a challenge. For example, MyD88-/- mice show reduced protection from experimental tuberculosis after vaccination with BCG (Fremond et al., 2004). And studies of the mouse Typhoid model *Salmonella* typhimurium suggest that TLRs and MyD88 are required in a range of cell types for optimal function of oral live attenuated bacterial vaccines (Dougan et al., 2011). Likewise, although the precise PRR requirement for protective immunity to vaccinia cannot be determined due to the lack of appropriate (or safe) models, TLR2 and MyD88 knockout mice do show partial reduction in MVA-specific T cell responses and CD8+ T cell IFNγ secretion (Zhu et al., 2007).

4.1.3 PRR activation by inactivated vaccines

Inactivated vaccines are generally simpler to study because they have a fixed content, do not undergo metabolic changes, and in general do not subvert host signaling. Furthermore, a great deal is known about the PAMP content of inactivated organisms since killed microbes have been of great use for decades as a source of 'natural' PAMPs in the identification and study of PRRs.

Recently, a major pathway for viral nucleic acid recognition - viral ssRNA triggering TLR7 - was initially identified by study of IFNα production by pDC in response to heat-inactivated influenza virus (Diebold et al., 2004) (Section 3.2.1). Indeed, in the absence of TLR7 whole inactivated influenza virus vaccine loses immunogenicity (Geeraedts et al., 2008). This study highlighted in particular the importance of TLR7 in driving a particular class of immune response - specifically Th1 immunity - reinforcing the notion that PRR triggering controls immune response polarization as well as magnitude. In contrast, split virus or subunit vaccines, which are less potent but considered safer, showed little TLR7 dependence presumably as a result of loss of the packaged viral ssRNA that potently stimulates TLR7 during production (Geeraedts et al., 2008). Of course these studies into the PRR requirements of vaccines have been performed in mouse models and to date the importance of PRR signaling for protective immunity in humans has yet to be determined, and may show different patterns.

Evidence for the need for TLR signaling for the activity of inactivated bacterial vaccines comes from the whole cell Pertussis vaccine. Although this vaccine contains a wide range of bacterial PAMPs, TLR4 and TRIF but not TLR2 knockout mice showed reduced immunity. This suggests that LPS is more critical than lipopeptides for induction of adaptive responses in this instance (Fransen et al., 2010).

4.1.4 PRR triggering by subunit vaccines

At first sight, subunit vaccines should not contain PAMPs because the critical microbial 'subunit' should be an antigen, i.e. target for adaptive - not innate - immune responses. But although simpler and purer than whole inactivated vaccines, many current human subunit vaccines still contain microbe-derived PAMPs either co-purified with the antigen or in some cases the antigenic subunit is itself a PRR agonist. Thus, meningitis vaccines based on purified outer membrane vesicle preparations of Neisseria meningitides contain both LPS and TLR2-stimulatory lipopeptides, and require TLR4 and TRIF signaling for optimal immune priming (Fransen et al., 2010). As well as PAMPs co-purified with antigenic subunits, many non-protein protective antigens such as polysaccharides or lipoproteins can directly trigger PRR. For example, the outer-surface lipoprotein (OspA) subunit of Borrelia burgdorferi activates TLR2 and has been used as an effective human vaccine against Lyme disease. This particular antigenic PAMP not only shows reduced immunogenicity in TLR2 knockout mice, but human hyporesponsiveness to the vaccine is associated with low TLR1 expression (Alexopoulou et al., 2002).

4.1.5 PAMP-free triggering of PRRs by adjuvants

The sections above have introduced the importance of TLRs in the development of immunity following vaccination. It is now becoming apparent that other PRRs, and stimulation of alternative proinflammatory pathways, can be important for vaccine functionality. There is evidence that some vaccine adjuvants can induce long-lasting and protective immune responses independently of TLR-based signalling pathways (Gavin et al., 2006; Nemazee et al., 2006). Furthermore, the majority of recently developed human adjuvant formulations, such as emulsions (Reed et al., 2009), do not obviously contain microbial components and are therefore unlikely to contain PAMPs. The NLRP3 inflammasome has been shown to be activated by the common adjuvant alum, however it is currently debatable as to whether this activation is required for the adjuvant activity of alum (De Gregorio et al., 2009; Franchi and Nunez, 2008; Li et al., 2008; McKee et al., 2009). Several other PAMP-free adjuvant formulations, including oil emulsions, saponins and microparticles made from biodegradeable polymer poly(lactic-co-glycolic acid) also trigger NALP3-dependent immune activation (Williams et al., 2010). In addition, the Syk/CARD9 pathway is activated by the potent adjuvant additive, trehalose 6,6-dibehenate, a synthetic mimic of a mycobacterial cell wall component (Werninghaus et al., 2009).

4.2 Implications of PRR research findings for the development of new vaccines

There is still a large demand for better vaccines in order to reduce costs, improve potency and efficacy, to tackle diseases which currently lack a vaccine (e.g. Human Immunodeficiency Virus) and to respond quickly to new challenges from infectious diseases (e.g. pandemic influenza). Understanding how PRRs contribute to protective immunity and how this can be modulated are key if vaccines are to improve.

One area of particular importance to vaccine development is the need to rationally design new adjuvants with greater potency than current ones such as alum (Mbow et al., 2010; Reed et al., 2009; Leroux-Roels, 2010). Selective triggering of different PRRs and DC subsets are thought to be major points of control of immune polarization (Iwasaki and Medzhitov, 2004; Kapsenberg, 2003). It follows therefore that not only are new adjuvants needed, but these must be engineered to stimulate the correct PRR on the optimal cell type. The most clinically relevant illustration of the benefits of adding PRR agonists to increase adjuvant activity is GSK's adjuvant AS 04, which incorporates the TLR4 agonist monophosphoryl lipid A (MPLA) to alum (Didierlaurent et al., 2009). The human papilloma virus virus-like particle vaccine Cervarix is formulated with AS 04, which may account for its apparent increased potency compared to Gardasil, a similar VLP vaccine that uses alum without MPLA (Einstein et al., 2009). Interestingly MPLA appears to preferentially activate TLR4 signalling through the TRIF:TRAM pathway and not Mal:MYD88 (Mata-Haro et al., 2007).

Without doubt the role of synthetic PRR-specific agonists as additives to vaccine adjuvants will become a developing and increasingly important field of research. Of course given the potent immunostimulatory properties of PRR agonists care will have to be taken to avoid potentially damaging, or fatal, systemic effects.

4.2.1 TLR agonists in adjuvants

As well as the benefits of adding MPLA to alum, a wide range of TLR agonists have been shown to promote immunity when added to antigens. These include TLR2-stimulatory lipopeptides such as MALP-2, the TLR5 agonist flagellin, TLR9-stimulatory CpG oligos, small molecule TLR7/8 agonists such as imidazoquinolines, the TLR3 agonist polyI:C and various modified RNA and DNA oligos that can act on TLR3,7 and/or 9. TLR triggering, such as by CpG oligos or imidazoquinolines, frequently promotes Th1 responses (Schnare et al., 2001), but there are a number of exceptions, including Th2 induction by lipopeptides and flagellin that trigger TLR2 and TLR5 respectively (Didierlaurent et al., 2004; Redecke et al., 2004). It has become clear that for maximal potency and benefits the TLR agonist requires linking in some way with the target antigen. For example, agonists have been covalently coupled to proteins; synthesized directly in combination with the TLR agonist; or antigen and PRR agonists can be immobilised together on a particulate scaffold. The importance of linking PRR agonists with antigen was demonstrated in a recent study where peptides were co-encapsulated with a TLR9 agonist using the biodegradeable polymer PLGA; only when antigen and CpG oligonucleotides were present in the same PLGA microsphere was an effective cytotoxic T cell response achieved (Schlosser et al., 2008).

4.2.2 Combinatorial PRR triggering

Just as most microbes contain a number of different PAMPs and trigger several PRR, there is a need to combine PRR triggers in adjuvants for synergistic effects, and to closely mimic pathogens. The best studied example of synergistic PRR signaling comes from the activation of TLR2 combined with signaling through the CLEC dectin-1 (Gantner et al., 2003; Underhill, 2007). PRR signaling also synergises with other proinflammatory pathways. Major examples include the interplay between T cell feedback signals through CD40 expressed on PRR-stimulated DC (Schulz et al., 2000), and the requirement of NALP3 for maximal response to various PRR including vaccinia (Delaloye et al., 2009).

5. Conclusions

Without doubt PRRs have a crucial role to play in the detection of, and response to, infectious diseases. The repertoire and versatility of the host in detecting PAMPS and associated danger signals is outstanding and continually expanding. In fact this is only matched by the steps taken by pathogens to circumvent these defence strategies. As research progresses in this field it is becoming increasingly apparent that although the outputs of PRR activation are broadly similar - i.e. pro-inflammatory cytokine induction, caspase-1 processing and IFN induction - the mechanisms by which this takes place are actually remarkably subtle. There is significant crosstalk between TLR, NLR, CLR and RLR signalling pathways. In addition, there is clear redundancy in function between different receptors that helps to ensure appropriate recognition of, and response to, pathogens. The complexity of the signalling crosstalk is only likely to increase as our understanding of these systems improves.

Another key area in which PRR recognition of infectious diseases is becoming increasingly important is the development of adaptive immunity. The innate response seems to play a vital role in directing the nature of the adaptive response, particularly in relation to driving development of particular T-cell subsets. This is a rapidly developing area and the search for rational vaccine design makes it critical to infectious disease research. The study of the cellular and molecular biology of PRRs has provided a strong theoretical and experimental foundation for the rational design of vaccine adjuvants. This new understanding must be harnessed to provide a complete toolkit for custom adjuvant design. However, in common with other biomedical disciplines, clinical uptake typically lags behind scientific discovery and we wait to see how best this knowledge can be transferred to provide clinical benefit.

6. Acknowledgements

The work in our group is funded by The Wellcome Trust (TPM; WT0805090MA) and the Biotechnology and Biological Sciences Research Council (TPM; RG52820). We thank David Dunne for the images of *Schistosoma* eggs, larvae and adult worms used in Figure 9.

7. References

Alexopoulou, L., Thomas, V., Schnare, M., Lobet, Y., Anguita, J., Schoen, R.T., Medzhitov, R., Fikrig, E., and Flavell, R.A. (2002). Hyporesponsiveness to vaccination with Borrelia burgdorferi OspA in humans and in TLR1- and TLR2-deficient mice. Nat Med *8*, 878-884.

Andersen-Nissen, E., Smith, K.D., Strobe, K.L., Barrett, S.L., Cookson, B.T., Logan, S.M., and Aderem, A. (2005). Evasion of Toll-like receptor 5 by flagellated bacteria. Proc Natl Acad Sci U S A *102*, 9247-9252.

Bi, L., Gojestani, S., Wu, W., Hsu, Y.M., Zhu, J., Ariizumi, K., and Lin, X. (2010). CARD9 mediates dectin-2-induced IkappaBalpha kinase ubiquitination leading to activation of NF-kappaB in response to stimulation by the hyphal form of Candida albicans. J Biol Chem *285*, 25969-25977.

Bowie, A., Kiss-Toth, E., Symons, J.A., Smith, G.L., Dower, S.K., and O'Neill, L.A. (2000). A46R and A52R from vaccinia virus are antagonists of host IL-1 and toll-like receptor signaling. Proc Natl Acad Sci U S A *97*, 10162-10167.

Bowie, A.G., and Unterholzner, L. (2008). Viral evasion and subversion of pattern-recognition receptor signalling. Nat Rev Immunol *8*, 911-922.

Cheng, S.C., van de Veerdonk, F.L., Lenardon, M., Stoffels, M., Plantinga, T., Smeekens, S., Rizzetto, L., Mukaremera, L., Preechasuth, K., Cavalieri, D., *et al.* (2011). The dectin-1/inflammasome pathway is responsible for the induction of protective T-helper 17 responses that discriminate between yeasts and hyphae of Candida albicans. J Leukoc Biol *90*, 357-366.

Cirl, C., Wieser, A., Yadav, M., Duerr, S., Schubert, S., Fischer, H., Stappert, D., Wantia, N., Rodriguez, N., Wagner, H., *et al.* (2008). Subversion of Toll-like receptor signaling by a unique family of bacterial Toll/interleukin-1 receptor domain-containing proteins. Nat Med *14*, 399-406.

Coburn, B., Grassl, G.A., and Finlay, B.B. (2007). Salmonella, the host and disease: a brief review. Immunol Cell Biol *85*, 112-118.

Davis, B.K., Wen, H., and Ting, J.P. (2011). The inflammasome NLRs in immunity, inflammation, and associated diseases. Annu Rev Immunol *29*, 707-735.

De Gregorio, E., D'Oro, U., and Wack, A. (2009). Immunology of TLR-independent vaccine adjuvants. Curr Opin Immunol *21*, 339-345.

Delaloye, J., Roger, T., Steiner-Tardivel, Q.G., Le Roy, D., Knaup Reymond, M., Akira, S., Petrilli, V., Gomez, C.E., Perdiguero, B., Tschopp, J., *et al.* (2009). Innate immune sensing of modified vaccinia virus Ankara (MVA) is mediated by TLR2-TLR6, MDA-5 and the NALP3 inflammasome. PLoS Pathog *5*, e1000480.

Didierlaurent, A., Ferrero, I., Otten, L.A., Dubois, B., Reinhardt, M., Carlsen, H., Blomhoff, R., Akira, S., Kraehenbuhl, J.P., and Sirard, J.C. (2004). Flagellin promotes myeloid differentiation factor 88-dependent development of Th2-type response. J Immunol *172*, 6922-6930.

Didierlaurent, A.M., Morel, S., Lockman, L., Giannini, S.L., Bisteau, M., Carlsen, H., Kielland, A., Vosters, O., Vanderheyde, N., Schiavetti, F., *et al.* (2009). AS04, an aluminum salt- and TLR4 agonist-based adjuvant system, induces a transient localized innate immune response leading to enhanced adaptive immunity. J Immunol *183*, 6186-6197.

Diebold, S.S., Kaisho, T., Hemmi, H., Akira, S., and Reis e Sousa, C. (2004). Innate antiviral responses by means of TLR7-mediated recognition of single-stranded RNA. Science *303*, 1529-1531.

Dougan, G., John, V., Palmer, S., and Mastroeni, P. (2011). Immunity to salmonellosis. Immunol Rev *240*, 196-210.

Einstein, M.H., Baron, M., Levin, M.J., Chatterjee, A., Edwards, R.P., Zepp, F., Carletti, I., Dessy, F.J., Trofa, A.F., Schuind, A., *et al.* (2009). Comparison of the immunogenicity and safety of Cervarix and Gardasil human papillomavirus (HPV) cervical cancer vaccines in healthy women aged 18-45 years. Hum Vaccin *5*, 705-719.

Esteban, A., Popp, M.W., Vyas, V.K., Strijbis, K., Ploegh, H.L., and Fink, G.R. (2011). Fungal recognition is mediated by the association of dectin-1 and galectin-3 in macrophages. Proceedings of the National Academy of Sciences *108*, 14270-14275.

Ferwerda, B., Alonso, S., Banahan, K., McCall, M.B., Giamarellos-Bourboulis, E.J., Ramakers, B.P., Mouktaroudi, M., Fain, P.R., Izagirre, N., Syafruddin, D., *et al.* (2009a). Functional and genetic evidence that the Mal/TIRAP allele variant 180L has been selected by providing protection against septic shock. Proc Natl Acad Sci U S A *106*, 10272-10277.

Ferwerda, B., Ferwerda, G., Plantinga, T.S., Willment, J.A., van Spriel, A.B., Venselaar, H., Elbers, C.C., Johnson, M.D., Cambi, A., Huysamen, C., *et al.* (2009b). Human dectin-1 deficiency and mucocutaneous fungal infections. N Engl J Med *361*, 1760-1767.

Franchi, L., Amer, A., Body-Malapel, M., Kanneganti, T.D., Ozoren, N., Jagirdar, R., Inohara, N., Vandenabeele, P., Bertin, J., Coyle, A., *et al.* (2006). Cytosolic flagellin requires Ipaf for activation of caspase-1 and interleukin 1beta in salmonella-infected macrophages. Nat Immunol *7*, 576-582.

Franchi, L., and Nunez, G. (2008). The Nlrp3 inflammasome is critical for aluminium hydroxide-mediated IL-1beta secretion but dispensable for adjuvant activity. Eur J Immunol *38*, 2085-2089.

Fransen, F., Stenger, R.M., Poelen, M.C., van Dijken, H.H., Kuipers, B., Boog, C.J., van Putten, J.P., van Els, C.A., and van der Ley, P. (2010). Differential effect of TLR2 and TLR4 on the immune response after immunization with a vaccine against Neisseria meningitidis or Bordetella pertussis. PLoS One *5*, e15692.

Fremond, C.M., Yeremeev, V., Nicolle, D.M., Jacobs, M., Quesniaux, V.F., and Ryffel, B. (2004). Fatal Mycobacterium tuberculosis infection despite adaptive immune response in the absence of MyD88. J Clin Invest *114*, 1790-1799.

Gack, M.U., Shin, Y.C., Joo, C.H., Urano, T., Liang, C., Sun, L., Takeuchi, O., Akira, S., Chen, Z., Inoue, S., *et al.* (2007). TRIM25 RING-finger E3 ubiquitin ligase is essential for RIG-I-mediated antiviral activity. Nature *446*, 916-920.

Gantner, B.N., Simmons, R.M., Canavera, S.J., Akira, S., and Underhill, D.M. (2003). Collaborative induction of inflammatory responses by dectin-1 and Toll-like receptor 2. J Exp Med *197*, 1107-1117.

Gavin, A.L., Hoebe, K., Duong, B., Ota, T., Martin, C., Beutler, B., and Nemazee, D. (2006). Adjuvant-enhanced antibody responses in the absence of toll-like receptor signaling. Science *314*, 1936-1938.

Geeraedts, F., Goutagny, N., Hornung, V., Severa, M., de Haan, A., Pool, J., Wilschut, J., Fitzgerald, K.A., and Huckriede, A. (2008). Superior immunogenicity of inactivated whole virus H5N1 influenza vaccine is primarily controlled by Toll-like receptor signalling. PLoS Pathog *4*, e1000138.

Gewirtz, A.T., Navas, T.A., Lyons, S., Godowski, P.J., and Madara, J.L. (2001). Cutting edge: bacterial flagellin activates basolaterally expressed TLR5 to induce epithelial proinflammatory gene expression. J Immunol *167*, 1882-1885.

Gringhuis, S.I., Wevers, B.A., Kaptein, T.M., van Capel, T.M., Theelen, B., Boekhout, T., de Jong, E.C., and Geijtenbeek, T.B. (2011). Selective C-Rel activation via Malt1 controls anti-fungal T(H)-17 immunity by dectin-1 and dectin-2. PLoS Pathog *7*, e1001259.

Guillot, L., Le Goffic, R., Bloch, S., Escriou, N., Akira, S., Chignard, M., and Si-Tahar, M. (2005). Involvement of toll-like receptor 3 in the immune response of lung epithelial cells to double-stranded RNA and influenza A virus. J Biol Chem *280*, 5571-5580.

Hajishengallis, G., and Lambris, J.D. (2011). Microbial manipulation of receptor crosstalk in innate immunity. Nat Rev Immunol *11*, 187-200.

Hayashi, F., Smith, K.D., Ozinsky, A., Hawn, T.R., Yi, E.C., Goodlett, D.R., Eng, J.K., Akira, S., Underhill, D.M., and Aderem, A. (2001). The innate immune response to bacterial flagellin is mediated by Toll-like receptor 5. Nature *410*, 1099-1103.

Hersh, D., Monack, D.M., Smith, M.R., Ghori, N., Falkow, S., and Zychlinsky, A. (1999). The Salmonella invasin SipB induces macrophage apoptosis by binding to caspase-1. Proc Natl Acad Sci U S A *96*, 2396-2401.

Ichinohe, T. (2010). Respective roles of TLR, RIG-I and NLRP3 in influenza virus infection and immunity: impact on vaccine design. Expert Rev Vaccines *9*, 1315-1324.

Iwasaki, A., and Medzhitov, R. (2004). Toll-like receptor control of the adaptive immune responses. Nat Immunol *5*, 987-995.

Kanneganti, T.-D. (2010). Central roles of NLRs and inflammasomes in viral infection. Nat Rev Immunol *10*, 688-698.

Kapsenberg, M.L. (2003). Dendritic-cell control of pathogen-driven T-cell polarization. Nat Rev Immunol *3*, 984-993.

Kawai, T., and Akira, S. (2011). Toll-like receptors and their crosstalk with other innate receptors in infection and immunity. Immunity *34*, 637-650.

Kenny, E.F., Talbot, S., Gong, M., Golenbock, D.T., Bryant, C.E., and O'Neill, L.A.J. (2009). MyD88 Adaptor-Like Is Not Essential for TLR2 Signaling and Inhibits Signaling by TLR3. J Immunol *183*, 3642-3651.

Khor, C.C., Chapman, S.J., Vannberg, F.O., Dunne, A., Murphy, C., Ling, E.Y., Frodsham, A.J., Walley, A.J., Kyrieleis, O., Khan, A., *et al.* (2007). A Mal functional variant is associated with protection against invasive pneumococcal disease, bacteremia, malaria and tuberculosis. Nat Genet *39*, 523-528.

LeibundGut-Landmann, S., Gross, O., Robinson, M.J., Osorio, F., Slack, E.C., Tsoni, S.V., Schweighoffer, E., Tybulewicz, V., Brown, G.D., Ruland, J., *et al.* (2007). Syk- and CARD9-dependent coupling of innate immunity to the induction of T helper cells that produce interleukin 17. Nat Immunol *8*, 630-638.

Leroux-Roels, G. (2010). Unmet needs in modern vaccinology: adjuvants to improve the immune response. Vaccine *28 Suppl 3*, C25-36.

Li, H., Willingham, S.B., Ting, J.P., and Re, F. (2008). Cutting edge: inflammasome activation by alum and alum's adjuvant effect are mediated by NLRP3. J Immunol *181*, 17-21.

Loo, Y.M., and Gale, M., Jr. (2011). Immune signaling by RIG-I-like receptors. Immunity *34*, 680-692.

Lu, Y., Wambach, M., Katze, M.G., and Krug, R.M. (1995). Binding of the influenza virus NS1 protein to double-stranded RNA inhibits the activation of the protein kinase that phosphorylates the elF-2 translation initiation factor. Virology *214*, 222-228.

Lund, J.M., Alexopoulou, L., Sato, A., Karow, M., Adams, N.C., Gale, N.W., Iwasaki, A., and Flavell, R.A. (2004). Recognition of single-stranded RNA viruses by Toll-like receptor 7. Proc Natl Acad Sci U S A *101*, 5598-5603.

Martinez, J., Huang, X., and Yang, Y. (2010). Toll-like receptor 8-mediated activation of murine plasmacytoid dendritic cells by vaccinia viral DNA. Proc Natl Acad Sci U S A *107*, 6442-6447.

Mata-Haro, V., Cekic, C., Martin, M., Chilton, P.M., Casella, C.R., and Mitchell, T.C. (2007). The vaccine adjuvant monophosphoryl lipid A as a TRIF-biased agonist of TLR4. Science *316*, 1628-1632.

Mbow, M.L., De Gregorio, E., Valiante, N.M., and Rappuoli, R. (2010). New adjuvants for human vaccines. Curr Opin Immunol *22*, 411-416.

McKee, A.S., Munks, M.W., MacLeod, M.K., Fleenor, C.J., Van Rooijen, N., Kappler, J.W., and Marrack, P. (2009). Alum induces innate immune responses through macrophage and mast cell sensors, but these sensors are not required for alum to act as an adjuvant for specific immunity. J Immunol *183*, 4403-4414.

Miao, E.A., Mao, D.P., Yudkovsky, N., Bonneau, R., Lorang, C.G., Warren, S.E., Leaf, I.A., and Aderem, A. (2010). Innate immune detection of the type III secretion apparatus through the NLRC4 inflammasome. Proceedings of the National Academy of Sciences *107*, 3076-3080.

Monie, T.P., Bryant, C.E., and Gay, N.J. (2009). Activating immunity: lessons from the TLRs and NLRs. Trends Biochem Sci *34*, 553-561.

Nemazee, D., Gavin, A., Hoebe, K., and Beutler, B. (2006). Immunology: Toll-like receptors and antibody responses. Nature *441*, E4; discussion E4.

Osorio, F., and Reis e Sousa, C. (2011). Myeloid C-type lectin receptors in pathogen recognition and host defense. Immunity *34*, 651-664.

Perry, A.K., Chen, G., Zheng, D., Tang, H., and Cheng, G. (2005). The host type I interferon response to viral and bacterial infections. Cell Res *15*, 407-422.

Pichlmair, A., Schulz, O., Tan, C.P., Naslund, T.I., Liljestrom, P., Weber, F., and Reis e Sousa, C. (2006). RIG-I-mediated antiviral responses to single-stranded RNA bearing 5'-phosphates. Science *314*, 997-1001.

Redecke, V., Häcker, H., Datta, S.K., Fermin, A., Pitha, P.M., Broide, D.H., and Raz, E. (2004). Cutting Edge: Activation of Toll-Like Receptor 2 Induces a Th2 Immune Response and Promotes Experimental Asthma. The Journal of Immunology *172*, 2739-2743.

Reed, S.G., Bertholet, S., Coler, R.N., and Friede, M. (2009). New horizons in adjuvants for vaccine development. Trends Immunol *30*, 23-32.

Ritter, M., Gross, O., Kays, S., Ruland, J., Nimmerjahn, F., Saijo, S., Tschopp, J., Layland, L.E., and Prazeres da Costa, C. (2010). Schistosoma mansoni triggers Dectin-2, which activates the Nlrp3 inflammasome and alters adaptive immune responses. Proc Natl Acad Sci U S A *107*, 20459-20464.

Roy, C.R., and Zamboni, D.S. (2006). Cytosolic detection of flagellin: a deadly twist. Nat Immunol *7*, 549-551.

Sabbah, A., Chang, T.H., Harnack, R., Frohlich, V., Tominaga, K., Dube, P.H., Xiang, Y., and Bose, S. (2009). Activation of innate immune antiviral responses by Nod2. Nat Immunol *10*, 1073-1080.

Saijo, S., Ikeda, S., Yamabe, K., Kakuta, S., Ishigame, H., Akitsu, A., Fujikado, N., Kusaka, T., Kubo, S., Chung, S.H., *et al.* (2010). Dectin-2 recognition of alpha-mannans and induction of Th17 cell differentiation is essential for host defense against Candida albicans. Immunity *32*, 681-691.

Schlosser, E., Mueller, M., Fischer, S., Basta, S., Busch, D.H., Gander, B., and Groettrup, M. (2008). TLR ligands and antigen need to be coencapsulated into the same biodegradable microsphere for the generation of potent cytotoxic T lymphocyte responses. Vaccine *26*, 1626-1637.

Schmitz, N., Kurrer, M., Bachmann, M.F., and Kopf, M. (2005). Interleukin-1 is responsible for acute lung immunopathology but increases survival of respiratory influenza virus infection. J Virol *79*, 6441-6448.

Schnare, M., Barton, G.M., Holt, A.C., Takeda, K., Akira, S., and Medzhitov, R. (2001). Toll-like receptors control activation of adaptive immune responses. Nat Immunol *2*, 947-950.

Schulz, O., Edwards, A.D., Schito, M., Aliberti, J., Manickasingham, S., Sher, A., and Reis e Sousa, C. (2000). CD40 triggering of heterodimeric IL-12 p70 production by dendritic cells in vivo requires a microbial priming signal. Immunity *13*, 453-462.

Smeekens, S.P., van de Veerdonk, F.L., van der Meer, J.W., Kullberg, B.J., Joosten, L.A., and Netea, M.G. (2010). The Candida Th17 response is dependent on mannan- and beta-glucan-induced prostaglandin E2. Int Immunol *22*, 889-895.

Smith, K.D., Andersen-Nissen, E., Hayashi, F., Strobe, K., Bergman, M.A., Barrett, S.L., Cookson, B.T., and Aderem, A. (2003). Toll-like receptor 5 recognizes a conserved site on flagellin required for protofilament formation and bacterial motility. Nat Immunol *4*, 1247-1253.

Spiller, S., Elson, G., Ferstl, R., Dreher, S., Mueller, T., Freudenberg, M., Daubeuf, B., Wagner, H., and Kirschning, C.J. (2008). TLR4-induced IFN-gamma production increases TLR2 sensitivity and drives Gram-negative sepsis in mice. J Exp Med *205*, 1747-1754.

Stewart, C.R., Stuart, L.M., Wilkinson, K., van Gils, J.M., Deng, J., Halle, A., Rayner, K.J., Boyer, L., Zhong, R., Frazier, W.A., *et al.* (2009). CD36 ligands promote sterile inflammation through assembly of a Toll-like receptor 4 and 6 heterodimer. Nat Immunol *11*, 155-161.

Subramanian, N., and Qadri, A. (2006). Lysophospholipid sensing triggers secretion of flagellin from pathogenic salmonella. Nat Immunol *7*, 583-589.

Suram, S., Gangelhoff, T.A., Taylor, P.R., Rosas, M., Brown, G.D., Bonventre, J.V., Akira, S., Uematsu, S., Williams, D.L., Murphy, R.C., *et al.* (2010). Pathways regulating cytosolic phospholipase A2 activation and eicosanoid production in macrophages by Candida albicans. J Biol Chem *285*, 30676-30685.

Takahara, K., Tokieda, S., Nagaoka, K., Takeda, T., Kimura, Y., and Inaba, K. (2011). C-type lectin SIGNR1 enhances cellular oxidative burst response against C. albicans in cooperation with Dectin-1. Eur J Immunol *41*, 1435-1444.

Talbot, S., Tötemeyer, S., Yamamoto, M., Akira, S., Hughes, K., Gray, D., Barr, T., Mastroeni, P., Maskell, D.J., and Bryant, C.E. (2009). Toll-like receptor 4 signalling through MyD88 is essential to control <i>Salmonella enterica</i> serovar Typhimurium infection, but not for the initiation of bacterial clearance. Immunology *128*, 472-483.

Underhill, D.M. (2007). Collaboration between the innate immune receptors dectin-1, TLRs, and Nods. Immunol Rev *219*, 75-87.

Van der Graaf, C.A., Netea, M.G., Morre, S.A., Den Heijer, M., Verweij, P.E., Van der Meer, J.W., and Kullberg, B.J. (2006). Toll-like receptor 4 Asp299Gly/Thr399Ile polymorphisms are a risk factor for Candida bloodstream infection. Eur Cytokine Netw *17*, 29-34.

van Stijn, C.M., Meyer, S., van den Broek, M., Bruijns, S.C., van Kooyk, Y., Geyer, R., and van Die, I. (2010). Schistosoma mansoni worm glycolipids induce an inflammatory phenotype in human dendritic cells by cooperation of TLR4 and DC-SIGN. Mol Immunol *47*, 1544-1552.

Wang, J.P., Liu, P., Latz, E., Golenbock, D.T., Finberg, R.W., and Libraty, D.H. (2006). Flavivirus activation of plasmacytoid dendritic cells delineates key elements of TLR7 signaling beyond endosomal recognition. J Immunol *177*, 7114-7121.

Werninghaus, K., Babiak, A., Gross, O., Holscher, C., Dietrich, H., Agger, E.M., Mages, J., Mocsai, A., Schoenen, H., Finger, K., *et al.* (2009). Adjuvanticity of a synthetic cord factor analogue for subunit Mycobacterium tuberculosis vaccination requires FcRgamma-Syk-Card9-dependent innate immune activation. J Exp Med *206*, 89-97.

Williams, A., Flavell, R.A., and Eisenbarth, S.C. (2010). The role of NOD-like Receptors in shaping adaptive immunity. Curr Opin Immunol *22*, 34-40.

Woehrle, T., Du, W., Goetz, A., Hsu, H.Y., Joos, T.O., Weiss, M., Bauer, U., Brueckner, U.B., and Marion Schneider, E. (2008). Pathogen specific cytokine release reveals an effect of TLR2 Arg753Gln during Candida sepsis in humans. Cytokine *41*, 322-329.

Zhu, J., Martinez, J., Huang, X., and Yang, Y. (2007). Innate immunity against vaccinia virus is mediated by TLR2 and requires TLR-independent production of IFN-beta. Blood *109*, 619-625.

8

Diphtheria Disease and Genes Involved in Formation of Diphthamide, Key Effector of the Diphtheria Toxin

Shanow Uthman[1], Shihui Liu[2], Flaviano Giorgini[1], Michael J. R. Stark[3], Michael Costanzo[4] and Raffael Schaffrath[1,5]

[1]Department of Genetics, University of Leicester, Leicester,
[2]Laboratory of Bacterial Diseases, NIAID, NIH, Bethesda, MD,
[3]Wellcome Trust Centre for Gene Regulation & Expression, University of Dundee,
[4]The Donnelly Centre, University of Toronto, Toronto, Ontario,
[5]Institut für Biologie, Mikrobiologie, Universität Kassel, Kassel,
[1]UK
[2]USA
[3]Scotland
[4]Canada
[5]Germany

1. Introduction

Within shared ecological niches, secretion of lethal protein toxins by microorganisms is a common strategy to ensure positive selection and survival of the toxin producing killer strains amongst other microbial competitors including bacteria, yeast and fungi (Schmitt & Schaffrath, 2005). Frequently, toxin production and secretion are traits that are genetically associated with extrachromosomal elements such as linear DNA killer plasmids and double-stranded RNA mycoviruses from yeast and fungi or episomal and prophage DNA integrated into the chromosome of the microbial toxin producer (reviewed by Meinhardt et al., 1997; Schaffrath & Meinhardt, 2005; Leis et al., 2005). The latter scenario is predominantly found in bacterial species and accounts for lysogenic conversions, phenomena in which phenotypes of the microbial host including pathogenicity, growth performance and production of virulence factors and toxins can be significantly affected by expression of prophage encoded genes. Prominent examples for phage-dependent toxin expression and disease formation include exotoxin-associated scarlet fever by *Streptocoocus pyogenes* (Johnson et al., 1986; Broudy et al., 2001), dysentery causing Shiga toxins Stx1 and Stx2 from *Shigella dysenteriae* (Newland et al., 1985; Willshaw et al., 1985; Huang, et al., 1986), phage CTXφ encoded cholera toxin from *Vibrio cholera* (Waldor & Mekalanos, 1996; Faruque & Nair, 2002) and diphtheria toxin encoded on a beta prophage from lysogens of *Corynebacterium diphtheriae* (Holmes & Barksdale, 1969; Bishai & Murphy 1988). Together with tRNase ribotoxins and anticodon nucleases from prokaryal and eukaryal microbes that have been shown to be encoded by transposable elements as well as circular and non-conventional linear DNA plasmids (Tokunaga et al., 1990; Kaufmann, 2000; Schaffrath & Meinhardt, 2005; Schaffrath et al., 1999), all of these genetic constellations implicate scenarios in which killer phenotypes have been evolved and spread by way of viral DNA transduction pathways or other forms of horizontal gene transfer. In support of this notion, certain cytoplasmic killer plasmids and their associated toxin phenotypes can be transferred between distinct yeast genera by means of cytoduction (Gunge 1983; Sugisaki et al., 1985) and horizontal transfer of the diphtheria toxin encoding *tox* gene from phages has been assigned to *in situ* lysogenic conversion of non-toxigenic to virulent corynebacteria (Freeman, 1951).

With regards to individual toxin response pathways in sensitive target cells, the specific cellular components being targeted by individual microbial protein toxins, not surprisingly, vary significantly depending on the nature of the essential cellular process that is targeted by the toxin in question (Schmitt & Schaffrath, 2005). For instance, microbial toxins capable of inhibiting the process of protein biosynthesis not only have been shown to target individual steps of mRNA translation (e.g. initiation, elongation and termination) but also to attack different components of the ribosomal machinery or associated factors required for mRNA translation (e.g. proteins, mRNAs, tRNAs and rRNAs). In this review, we will focus on one such microbial protein toxin that targets the essential process of mRNA translation and protein biosynthesis: diphtheria toxin (DT) from the Gram-positive bacterium *Corynebacterium diphtheriae* (for previous reviews, see Pappenheimer, 1977, 1984; Murphy, 1996). For DT to unfold its lethal action, the toxin needs to hijack a post-translationally modified residue known as diphthamide in its target protein EF2 (eukaryotic translation elongation factor 2). Next and by virtue of its enzymatic activity, DT ADP-ribosylates its target protein, an irreversible modification that inactivates the essential function of EF2 in mRNA translation. Eventually, EF2 inactivation by DT causes depletion of *de novo* protein biosynthesis and results in the death of the target cell including the model eukaryote and budding yeast *Saccharomyces cerevisiae* (reviewed by Collier, 2001; Todar 2004; Ratts & Murphy, 2005). Here, we review recent advances in the molecular biology of DT and present new insights into DT mode of action and DT response pathway components. An attractive idea emerging from research into DT mode of action is to take its basic molecular biology and apply it to biomedical intervention schemes against tumour cells, microbial pathogens or other biomedically and biotechnically relevant cell systems whose proliferation heavily relies on mRNA translation and protein biosynthesis (White-Gilbertson et al., 2009; Uthman et al., 2011). Such strategies are particularly informed by the use of chimeric DT fusion proteins that combine the lethal ADP-ribosylation activity of DT with a specific cell surface receptor domain for target cell or tissue specificity (Kreitman, 2006, 2009).

2. History and discovery of the diphtheria pathogen

Since the discovery in 1884 by German bacteriologists and physicists Edwin Klebs (1834–1912) and Friedrich Löffler (1852–1915), that *Corynebacterium diphtheriae* (also known as the *Klebs-Löffler* bacillus) is the causative agent of diphtheria (Fig. 1), diphtheria has arguably developed into one of the prototypic, toxigenic and infectious human diseases. Soon after Löffler speculated that organ damage during diphtheria was the consequence of a bacterial toxin, French Pierre-Paul-Émile Roux (1853-1933) and Swiss-French Alexandre Émile Jean Yersin (1863-1943) showed elegantly at the Pasteur Institute that the major bacterial virulence factor was indeed a potent exotoxin (Roux & Yersin, 1888). Upon sterile-filtration of *C. diphtheriae* cultures, they injected toxin-containing, cell free supernatants into laboratory animals and found that disease symptoms (including the eventual death of the animals) were developed in a manner indistinguishable from animals infected with the bacterium alone or even from infected humans. In addition, they proved that toxin-containing urine obtained from children infected with *C. diphtheriae* was sufficient to induce the disease symptoms seen in the above laboratory animals.

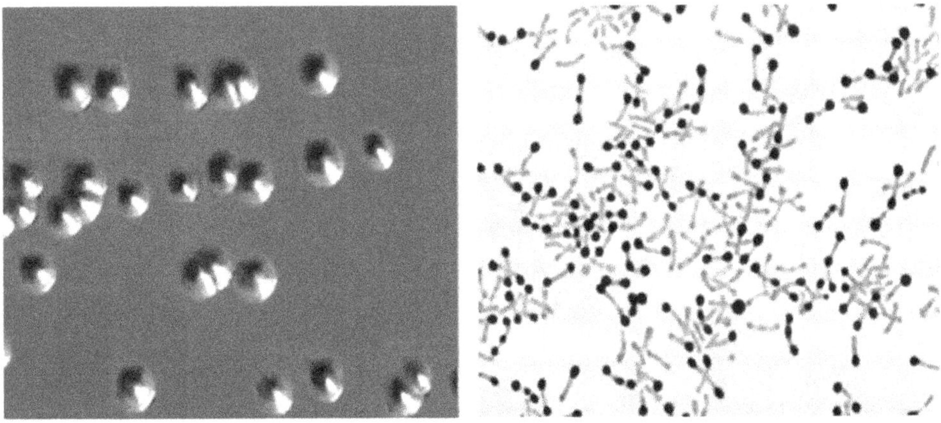

Fig. 1. *Corynebacterium diphtheriae*, the causative agent of the diphtheria disease. Formation of *C. diphtheriae* colonies is shown on blood agar (left panel) according to the CDC (Centers for Disease Control and Prevention, USA). Stained cells of *C. diphtheriae* (right panel). Their barred appearance is due to metachromatic granules which contain polyphosphate. Permission by Professor Kenneth Todar, University of Wisconsin, USA, to show the photographs (Todar, 2004) is gratefully acknowledged by the authors.

Löffler was the first to show that the pathogen could selectively be cultured from nasopharyngeal infections, indicating that diphtheria spreads within the upper respiratory tract. The disease causes a sore throat, low fever and an adherent green grey membrane on the tonsils, pharynx, and nasal cavities. This thick and fibrinous pseudomembrane, which can severely obstruct airways and suffocate patients, is the result of a combination of bacterial and host effects in response to pathogen cell growth and toxin production as well as the host's immune response and necrosis of the underlying host cell tissue. In 1890, German scientists Emil Adolf von Behring (1854–1917) and Paul Ehrlich (1854–1915) began to study the immunization of horses against diphtheria in order to generate a serum for medical use in humans. Considered to be Ehrlich's first bacteriological achievement attracting world-wide renown, the transformation of diphtheria antitoxin into an effective protective preparation was successfully used during an epidemic in Germany. Rather controversially, however, only von Behring was awarded the first Nobel Prize in Medicine in 1901 for developing a serum therapy against diphtheria.

3. Manifestations, pathogenesis and epidemiology of diphtheria

There are two disease forms, cutaneous and nasopharyngeal diphtheria (Fig. 2). The latter may vary from mild pharyngitis to hypoxia and suffocation with symptoms including fever of more than 39.5°C (~103°F) and profound swelling of the neck upon cervical lymph node infections (also known as bull neck diphtheria). Ultimately, diphtheria may cause life-threatening complications including loss of motor function and difficulty in swallowing and/or congestive heart failure as a result of diphtheria toxin (DT) induced myocarditis (~20% of cases) and peripheral motor neuropathy (~10% of cases) (Fig. 2) (Solders et al., 1989; Havaldar et al., 2000). Diphtheritic skin lesions in the milder form of cutaneous diphtheria are also covered by the typical pseudomembrane (see above). Eventually, DT distribution by way of the circulatory system may reach distant organs and cause paralysis (Fig. 2). Asymptomatic nasopharyngeal carriage is common in regions where diphtheria is endemic. In susceptible individuals, toxigenic strains cause disease by multiplying and secreting DT in either nasopharyngeal or skin lesions (Fig. 2). The diphtheritic lesion is often covered by the pseudomembrane which is composed of fibrin, bacteria, and inflammatory cells (Fig. 2).

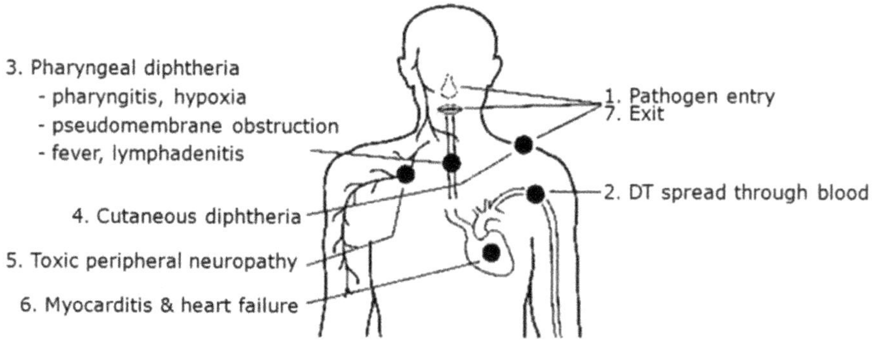

Fig. 2. Pathogenesis of the diphtheria disease. The illustration summarizes clinical manifestations of both pharyngeal and cutaneous diphtheria as well as the spread of the disease which involves blood-borne diphtheria toxin (DT) rather than distribution and dissemination of the pathogen *C. diphtheriae*. Systemic complications are indicated by the occurrence of toxic peripheral neurotrophy and toxic myocarditis eventually causing congestive heart failure. The scheme represents a modified version inspired by a comprehensive diphtheria review (Murphy, 1996)

Diphtheria pathogenesis is largely determined by the capacity of virulent *C. diphtheriae* biotypes (see below) to produce the deadly DT and to colonize and multiply in skin lesions or nasopharyngeal cavities. Since both determinants are encoded by the bacterium carrying a lysogenic beta prophage (Freeman, 1951; Bishai & Murphy, 1988), virulence results from the combined effects of the bacterial and phage genomes (Fig. 3). Even though avirulent *C. diphtheriae* strains seldom associate with the disease, it has been documented that non-toxigenic strains may acquire virulence following lysogenic conversion *in situ* (see below). Although it is clear that events other than production and secretion of DT promote host tissue colonization, detailed knowledge about *C. diphtheriae* factors involved in virulence is scarce. Putative roles in the colonization process have been discussed for a sialic acid splitting neuraminidase from the pathogen and for a corynebacterial cell surface component known as cord factor, i.e. 6,6'-di-O-mycoloyl-α, α-D-trehalose (reviewed by Murphy, 1996). The emergence of continuously changing lysotypes in the pathogen's population is likely due to their ability to compete more efficiently in segments of the nasopharyngeal ecologic niche. Thus, a given lysotype may persist for a while only to be replaced during later stages in the infection by another one that is more adapted to its niche.

Diphtheria is a contagious disease; although toxigenic strains have been isolated from horses, the pathogen *C. diphtheriae* is usually spread by direct physical contact among humans, namely by droplets or through inhaling aerosols of infected individuals. In addition, *in situ* conversion of avirulent strains to pathogenic ones may involve lateral gene transfer following bacterial lysis and release of the DT encoding phage gene (Freeman, 1951; Holmes & Barksdale, 1969). In regions of active immunization programs, isolated focal outbreaks can be associated with carriers who returned from visits to regions still endemic for diphtheria. In the US, Europe and elsewhere, diphtheria was a disease typical of children before mass immunization with diphtheria toxoid. Today, virulent biotypes of *C. diphtheriae* are rarely isolated and clinical diphtheria has largely been eradicated from industrialized nations through global vaccination schemes. Due to effective Diphtheria–Pertussis–Tetanus (DPT) vaccines, the number of diphtheria cases among school-aged children in the US has significantly dropped from 52 in 1980-2000 to 3 in 2000-2007 (Atkinson et al., 2007). For adults, however, vaccine boosts, are strongly advocated since immunity wears off with age and 30-60% of adults are estimated to be at risk, in particular, persons travelling to countries in which diphtheria has not been fully eradicated but poses a constant endemic health-threat. In the 1980s and 1994, public health breakdown in Sweden and Russia caused epidemic clinical diphtheria (Rappuoli et al., 1988) with officials recording more than 80,000 cases including 2,000 deaths. Focal outbreaks reported thereafter were almost certainly associated with diphtheria carriers who returned from Russia to Europe and the US.

4. Host defence, diagnosis and control

Recognition that systemic organ damage associated with diphtheria is due to the action of the lethal DT rather than dissemination of blood borne pathogens led to the development of a highly successful toxoid vaccine in which inactivated DT that remains antigenic is able to raise an immune response. The toxoid is prepared by incubating DT with formaldehyde at 37° C under alkaline conditions. Although immunization with the toxoid has made diphtheria a rare disease, diphtheria outbreaks do still occur in non-immunized and immune-compromised groups. Control of diphtheria, therefore, depends upon adequate immunization with antigenically intact yet inactivated diphtheria toxoid. Immunization against diphtheria should begin in the second month of life with a series of three primary doses spaced 4 to 8 weeks apart, followed by a fourth dose approximately 1 year after the last primary inoculation. Diphtheria toxoid is widely used as a component in the DPT vaccine (see above). Epidemiologic surveys have shown that immunization against diphtheria is approximately 97% effective. Although mass immunization against diphtheria is practiced in the United States and Europe and there is an adequate immunization rate in children, a large proportion of the adult population may have antibody titers that are below the protective level. The adult population should be reimmunized with diphtheria toxoid every 10 years (see above). Indeed, booster immunization with diphtheria-tetanus toxoids should be administered to persons traveling to regions with high rates of endemic diphtheria (Central and South America, Africa, Asia, Russia and Eastern Europe). In recent years, the use of highly purified toxoid preparations for immunization has minimized the occasional severe hypersensitivity reaction.

Although antibiotics (e.g. penicillin and erythromycin) are used as part of the treatment of patients who present with diphtheria, prompt passive immunization with diphtherial antitoxin is most effective in reducing the fatality rate. The long half-life of specific antitoxin in the circulation is an important factor in ensuring effective neutralization of diphtheria toxin; however, to be effective, the antitoxin must react with the toxin before it becomes internalized into the cell. Protection and immunity towards diphtheria involves an antibody response to DT following clinical disease or a formaldehyde-inactivated diphtheria toxoid following immunization. Immunization with diphtheria toxoid is extraordinarily effective. Diphtheria patients must be promptly treated with antitoxin to neutralize circulating DT.

Clinical diagnosis of diphtheria requires bacteriologic laboratory confirmation of toxigenic *C. diphtheriae* in throat or lesion cultures. For primary isolation, a variety of media may be used including Löffler, Müller-Miller tellurite or Tinsdale tellurite agars. Sterile cotton-tipped applicators are used to swab the pharyngeal tonsils or their beds. Calcium alginate swabs may be inserted through both nares to collect nasopharyngeal samples for culture. Since diphtheritic lesions are often covered with a pseudomembrane (see above) the surface of the lesion may have to be carefully exposed before swabbing with the applicator. In addition to the determination of biotype and lysotype of *C. diphtheriae* isolates, it is possible to use molecular biology techniques in the study of diphtheria outbreaks and pathogen identification. The latter may involve restriction endonuclease digestion patterns of *C. diphtheriae* chromosomal DNA as well as the use of the cloned DT gene (*tox*; see below) or specific corynebacterial insertion sequences as genetic probes (von Hunolstein et al., 2003).

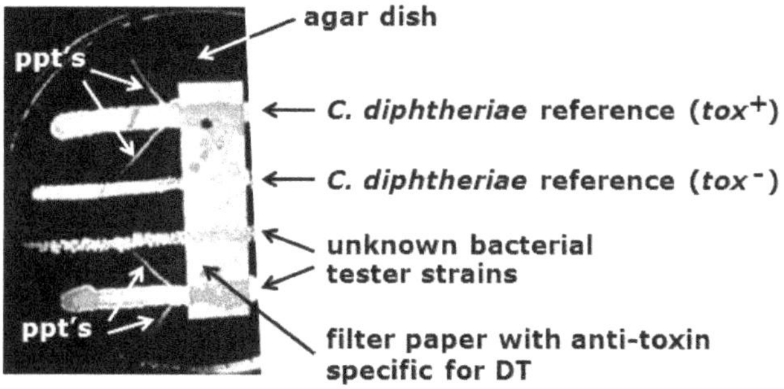

Fig. 3. The Elek immunodiffusion test. Shown is an agar plate with an antitoxin soaked filter that is inoculated with known toxigenic (*tox*⁺) and non-toxigenic (*tox*⁻) isolates of *C. diphtheriae* and unknown bacterial tester strains. The thin white lines (arrows) represent anti-toxin/DT precipitates ("ppt's") indicating bacterial DT production. Permission to show Rahul Gladwin's blog data (http://www.rahulgladwin.com/noteblog/bacteriology/what-is-an-eleks-test.php) is acknowledged.

For many years, the Schick test has been established to assess immunity to diphtheria toxin, although today it has been replaced in many regions by serologic tests for specific antibodies to diphtheria toxin. In the Schick test, 0.0124 microgram of diphtheria toxoid in 0.2 millilitre is injected intradermally at a control site and a small amount of diphtheria toxin (ca. 0.8 nanogram in 0.2 millilitre) is injected intradermally into the forearm (test site). Usually, after 48 and 96 hours respecitively, readings are taken with non-specific skin reactions generally peaking by 48 hours. After 96 hours, an erythematous reaction with some possible necrosis at the test site indicates non-sufficient antitoxic immunity for neutralization of DT to occur (≤ 0.03 IU/millilitre). Inflammation at either test or control sites after 48 hours is indicative for a hypersensitivity reaction to the antigen preparation. In many instances, DT is only partially purified prior to inactivation with formaldehyde (see above) and as a result, preparations of toxoid may contain other corynebacterial products, which may elicit a (false positive) hypersensitivity reaction in some individuals.

Following initial isolation, *C. diphtheriae* may be identified as *mitis*, *intermedius*, or *gravis* biotype (see below) on the basis of physiological parameters including carbohydrate fermentation profiles and hemolysis on sheep blood agar plates. The toxigenicity of *C. diphtheriae* strains is determined by a variety of *in vitro* and *in vivo* tests. The most common *in vitro* assay for toxigenicity is the Elek immunodiffusion test (Fig. 3), which is based on the double diffusion of DT and antitoxin in an agar medium. A sterile, antitoxin-saturated filter paper strip is embedded in the culture medium and *C. diphtheriae* isolates are streak-inoculated at a 90° angle to the filter paper. The production of DT can be readily detected within 18 to 48 hours by the formation of a toxin-antitoxin precipitating band in the agar. Alternatively, many eukaryotic cell lines (e.g. African green monkey kidney or Chinese hamster ovary) are sensitive to DT, enabling *in vitro* tissue culture tests to be used for detection of toxin and DT-dependent ADP ribosylation of the cellular target protein, eukaryotic translation elongation factor 2 (EF2, see below). Several highly sensitive *in vivo* tests for DT have also been described (e.g. guinea pig challenge test, rabbit skin test). Clinical diagnosis depends upon culture-proven toxigenic *C. diphtheriae* infection of the skin, nose, or throat combined with clinical signs of nasopharyngeal diphtheria, i.e. dysphagia, sore throat, bloody nasal discharge, formation of pseudomembranes etc.

5. The diphtheria pathogen *Corynebacterium diphtheriae*

5.1 *C. diphtheriae* and diphtheria toxin (DT) production

Diphtheria is caused by *Corynebacterium diphtheriae*, in particular its pathovarieties or biotypes *gravis*, *intermedius* and *mitis* (reviewed by Murphy, 1996). The bacterial cells are Gram-positive, club-shaped, non-motile and non-capsulated (Fig. 1). Cultures grown in tissue or *in vitro* often contain typical cell wall spots that may affect the Gram reaction and are composed of characteristic polymetaphosphate inclusions; these are stainable with methylene-blue and appear as purple granules (Fig. 1). Although the three biotypes differ in colony morphology, growth performance and virulence, they all share the ability to secrete the lethal protein: diphtheria toxin (DT). Intriguingly, DT is specified for by *tox*, a gene carried on one of a family of related corynebacteriophages integrated into the host chromosome of *C. diphtheriae* (Fig. 4) (for review, see Bishai & Murphy 1988). That DT is encoded by the prophage gene was demonstrated when non-pathogenic strains of *C. diphtheriae* became lysogenically converted upon infection with a bacterial virus known as beta phage (Freeman, 1957; Holmes & Barksdale, 1969). Moreover, mutant phages gave rise to nontoxic material that cross-reacted with diphtheria antitoxins, albeit being significantly shorter than full-length DT (Uchida et al., 1971).

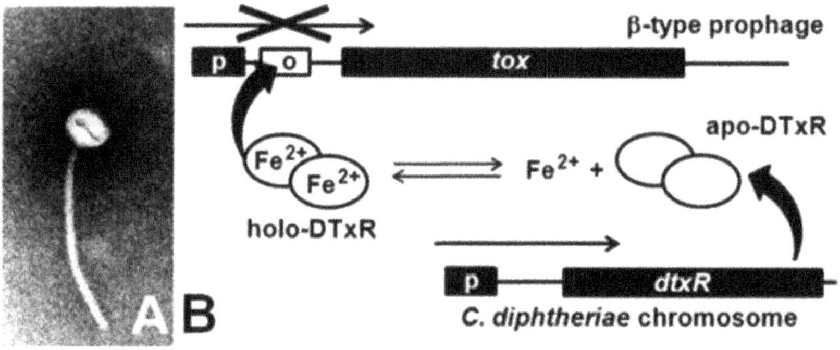

Fig. 4. Phage origin of *tox*, the structural gene encoding diphtheria toxin (DT), and model for *tox* gene regulation in the bacterial host *C. diphtheriae*. (A) Electron micrograph of the beta corynebacteriophage (for review, see Calendar, 1988) which carries the DT gene *tox* and upon infection and genomic integration converts non-toxigenic strains of *C. diphtheriae* into virulent ones. (B) Model of regulated *tox* gene expression by the repressor DTxR. Regulation of the phage *tox* gene depends on DTxR, a Fe^{2+}-binding and iron-responsive repressor dimer that is encoded by the *dtxR* gene on the *C. diphtheriae* genome (Tao, et al., 1994). This is why expression of the *tox* gene depends on the physiological state of the microbial host: under low iron conditions, Fe^{2+} ions dissociate from DTxR and liberate the *tox* gene operator from occupation by DTxR. This leads to *tox* gene derepression and DT can be expressed and secreted into the culture medium. In the presence of iron and upon binding Fe^{2+} ions, the holo-form of DTxR is recruited to the operator region upstream of *tox* and thereby prevents transcription of the DT gene by RNA polymerase to occur (D'Aquino et al., 2005). Upon depletion of Fe^{2+} from the medium, the holo-repressor complex (holo-DTxR) dissociates into its inactive apo-form (apo-DTxR) and the *tox* gene is relieved from transcriptional repression. The authors acknowledge permission by Professor Kenneth Todar, University of Wisconsin, USA, to reproduce a modified version of the electron micrograph (Todar, 2004) representing corynebacteriophage beta.

For optimal growth, some *C. diphtheriae* pathogens require thiamine or biotin and cultivation of most biotypes of *C. diphtheriae* depend on supplementation with nicotinic and pantothenic acids. In addition to being restricted to lysogenic bacteria, expression of the DT gene *tox* is controlled by an iron-responsive host repressor termed DTxR (Fig. 4) (Tao, et al., 1994). Thus, even though the *tox* gene is of viral origin, its regulation at the level of transcriptional repression/activation is coupled to the iron metabolism of the bacterial host (Tao, et al., 1994; D'Aquino et al., 2005). Therefore, optimal DT production is preferably achieved under conditions of low iron levels using culture medium that has been thoroughly deferrated. As for a physiological role of DT, the *tox* gene itself is not essential for the phage cycle and both synthesis and release of DT are not coupled to phage-induced lysis of *C. diphtheriae* cells. Also, it remains to be seen whether the lethal protein, which may account for ~5% of total protein expression in *C. diphtheriae*, benefits the bacterial life style in one way or another.

Nonetheless, by killing epithelial cells from infected pharyngeal niches, DT may contribute to colonization and virulence of the bacterial pathogen.

As early as 1887, Löffler described avirulent cells of *C. diphtheriae* from healthy individuals that were indistinguishable from virulent ones isolated from patients. It is now known that avirulent strains can be converted to virulent ones following infection with *tox* carrying corynebacteriophages *in vitro* and *in situ*. To this end, genetic drift of DT including horizontal gene transfer has not been described so that DT production appears to be confined to the three biotypes of *C. diphtheriae*. In addition to *C. diphtheriae*, other species of the genus *Corynebacterium* may occasionally cause infection of the nasopharnyx and the skin. These include *C. ulcerans*, *C. pseudotuberculosis*, *C. pseudodiphtheriticum* and *C. xerosis* with the latter two being capable of producing pyrazinamidase, an intriguing enzyme which converts pyrazinamide (also used in prodrug treatment of *Mycobacterium tuberculosis*) to pyrazinoic acid (McClatchy et al., 1981). In veterinary medicine, *C. renale* and *C. kutscheri* are important pathogens which cause respectively, pyelonephritis in cattle and latent infections in mice.

5.2 DT, an A/B prototype toxin with ADP-ribosyltransferase activity

In sensitive species of humans, monkeys or rabbits, DT is extremely potent with as little as 100 nanograms of DT per kilogram of body weight being lethal. Protein structural analysis has revealed that DT, which is a 535 amino acid residue protein, is organized into individual protein domains with three distinct pathological functions: an N-terminal catalytic ADP-ribosyltransferase domain (i), a receptor binding domain for docking onto target cells (ii) and a transmembrane domain for subcellular delivery of the catalytic domain (iii) (Fig. 5) (Collier & Kandel, 1971; Gill & Pappenheimer, 1971; Gill & Dinius, 1971). Similar to the plant toxin ricin or *Pseudomonas* exotoxin A (ETA), DT is a prototype member of the classical A/B family of toxins (Lord & Roberts, 2005; Sandvig et al., 2005). In their secreted exo-forms, they mature by partial proteolysis into the N-terminal and C-terminal fragments A and B, respectively, which are held together by a disulfide bridge. While fragment B carries the receptor binding domain and the transmembrane motif (see above), segment A harbours the catalytic domain of DT.

Cell intoxication by DT is a multi-step process (Fig. 6) and involves (1) DT docking onto the cell surface receptor, (2) DT uptake and internalization by receptor-mediated endocytosis, (3) acidification of the endocytic vesicle by an ATP-driven proton pump, (4) uncoupling of fragment A from the A/B toxin and (5) delivery of the cytotoxic domain from the lumen of the endocytic vesicle into the cytosol (reviewed by Collier, 2001 and Ratts & Murphy, 2005). Next, by virtue of its catalytic activity, fragment A of DT targets the eukaryotic translation elongation factor 2 (EF2) for NAD^+-dependent ADP-ribosylation (Fig. 6) (Collier & Cole, 1969; Pappenheimer, 1977). The resulting post-translational modification of EF2 by DT inhibits the essential elongation function of EF2 during *de novo* protein synthesis and eventually, leads to cell death (Fig. 6) (Van Ness et al., 1980; Sitikov et al., 1984). DT is an extremely potent agent and it has been demonstrated that subcellular import of a single molecule of its ADP-ribosylating domain toxin is sufficient for cell death induction. Studies on archaeal and eukaryal cells, which can both be killed by DT, demonstrate that the ADP-ribosylation reaction of DT is conserved and requires an exotic and highly modified histidine residue (Kimata & Kohno, 1994) in the EF2 target protein which is also known as diphthamide (Fig. 7). Intriguingly, the EF2 analogues from the bacterial pathogens undergo no such diphthamide modification, which explains why *C. diphtheriae* cells are auto-immune and protected against their own ADP-ribosylase killer toxin (reviewed by Collier, 2001 and Ratts & Murphy, 2005).

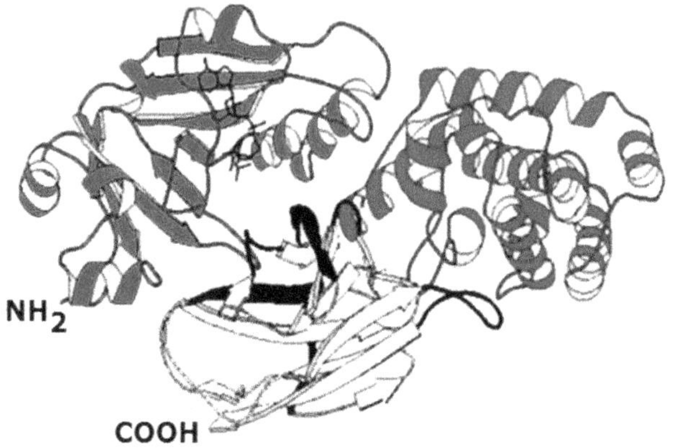

Fig. 5. MolScript-based ribbon diagram highlighting the modular domain organization of the DT monomer. The amino and carboxyl termini of full length DT are indicated (NH_2 and COOH, respectively). The domain in red represents the N-terminal ADP-ribosyltransferase catalytic centre which accounts for cytotoxic ADP-ribosylation and inactivation of the DT target protein EF2; the yellow motif illustrates the C-terminal binding domain important for cell surface attachment and receptor-mediated endocytosis of DT; the protein domain in blue is the transmembrane motif responsible for endosome insertion and subsequent subcellular release of the cytotoxic ADP-ribosylase domain. Permission by Professor Kenneth Todar, University of Wisconsin, USA, to reproduce a modified version of the illustration (Todar, 2004) is gratefully acknowledged.

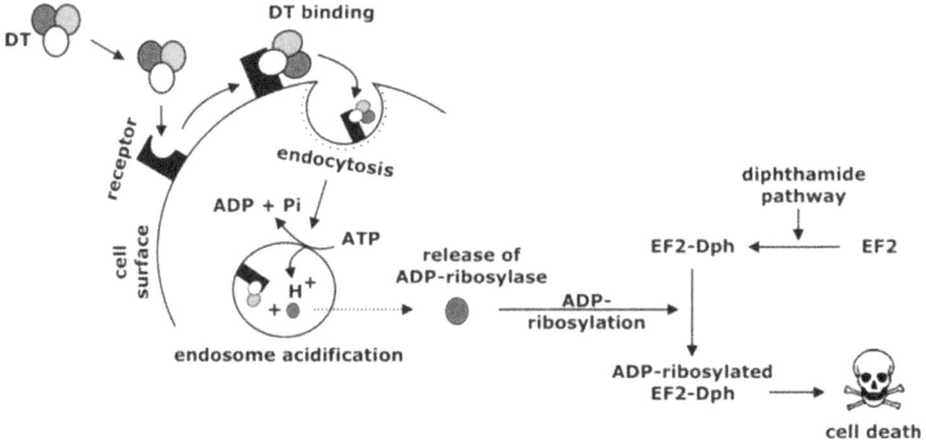

Fig. 6. Schematic diagram of eukaryotic target cell intoxication by DT. The toxin (with domain colour coding as introduced in Fig. 5) binds to its cell surface receptor by virtue of

its receptor binding (yellow) domain and is internalized by receptor-mediated endocytosis using clathrin-coated endosomes. Upon endosome acidification by a proton pump ATPase (pH ~5.1) located in the membrane of endocytic vesicles, the catalytic ADP-ribosylase domain (red) of DT becomes uncoupled from the receptor binding (yellow) and transmembrane (blue) domains. The catalytic domain is delivered to the cytosol and targets diphthamide-modified EF2 for ADP-ribosylation. This results in EF2 inactivation, inhibition of protein synthesis and eventually, death of the target cell. Scheme depiction has been inspired by previous DT reviews (for details see, Murphy, 1996; Collier, 2001; Todar 2004; Ratts & Murphy, 2005).

6. Diphthamide modification of eukaryotic translation elongation factor 2 (EF2)

6.1 Posttranslational biosynthesis of diphthamide on EF2

Diphthamide synthesis on EF2 operates through a complex pathway, which has been conserved among lower and higher eukaryotes (Chen et al., 1985; Moehring et al., 1984; Liu et al., 2004). In the budding yeast *Saccharomyces cerevisiae,* diphthamide biosynthesis requires at least five genes, *DPH1-DPH5* (Liu et al., 2004), two mammalian homologues of which (*DPH1/OVCA1* & *DPH3/KTI11*) are intriguingly involved in embryonic development and cell proliferation in rodents and humans (Fichtner & Schaffrath, 2002; Chen & Behringer, 2004; Fichtner et al., 2003; Liu & Leppla, 2003; Nobukuni et al., 2005; Liu et al., 2006). Though complex in nature, the diphthamide pathway has been shown to be molecularly dissectable. In *S. cerevisiae,* genetic screens selecting for resistance towards DT led to the isolation of diphthamide mutants that corresponded to five individual complementation groups (*dph1-dph5*) (Chen et al., 1985).

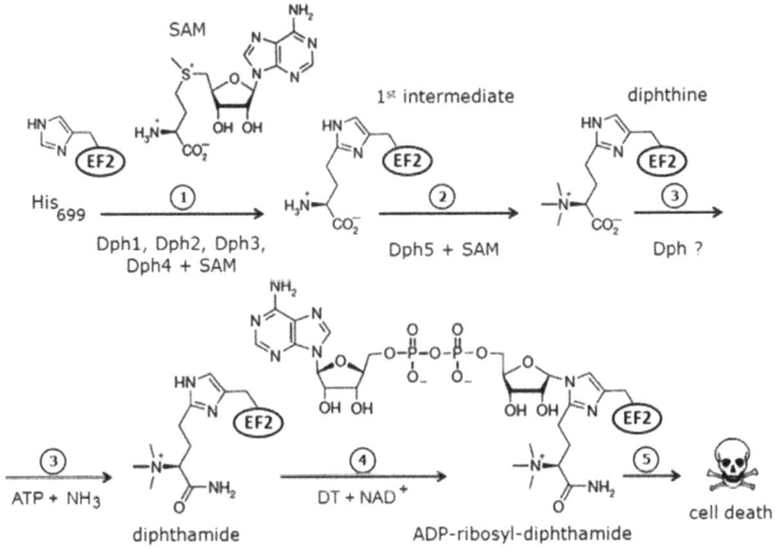

Fig. 7. Diphthamide modification on eukaryotic translation elongation factor 2 (EF2) in budding yeast operates through a multi-step pathway. The diphthamide pathway, modified

after Zhang et al. (2010), involves known and elusive (?) steps with the intermediates 2-(3-carboxyl-3-aminopropyl)-histidine and diphthine being generated. Abbreviations used: S-adenosylmethionine (SAM); adenosine triphosphate (ATP); nicotinamide adenine dinucleotide (NAD^+). The pathway culminates in diphthamide-driven ADP-ribosylation of EF2 (ADP-ribosyl-diphthamide) by DT and other bacterial ADP-ribosylase toxins, including *Pseudomonas* exotoxin A or *Vibrio cholerae* cholix toxin (Zhang et al., 2008; Jørgensen et al., 2008) all of which induce cell death.

Diphthamide biosynthesis involves stepwise modifications starting with the transfer of the 3-amino-3-carboxypropyl (ACP) group from S-adenosylmethionine (SAM) to the C-2 position of the imidazole ring in the target histidine residue (EF2 His_{600} from the archaeon *Pyrococcus horikoshii;* EF2 His_{699} from budding yeast; EF2 His_{715} in mammals) (Fig. 7). In yeast, this step depends on the diphthamide factors Dph1, Dph2, and Dph3 which all interact with each other (Fichtner et al., 2003; Liu et al., 2004; Bär et al., 2008) as well as Dph4, a J-protein (Webb et al., 2008) potentially chaperoning the Dph1-Dph3 complex. Eventually, Dph1-Dph4 action generates the first intermediate of the diphthamide modification pathway: 2-[3-carboxyl-3-aminopropyl]-histidine (Fig. 7) (Zhang et al., 2010). Next, the ammonium group of the intermediate undergoes trimethylation yielding the second intermediate diphthine (Fig. 7). This step is at least in part catalyzed by the protein methyltransferase Dph5 and requires three molecules of the methyl donor SAM (Fig. 7) (Chen & Bodley, 1988; Mattheakis et al., 1992). Finally, the carboxyl group of diphthine undergoes amidation (Fig. 7) in a process that is potentially catalyzed rather than spontaneous or non-enzymatic and likely to involve an as of yet unassigned ATP-dependent amidase (Fig. 7) (Liu et al., 2004). Once fully modified, the N-1 position of the diphthamide-imidazole ring (Fig. 7) is the site for NAD^+-dependent ADP-ribosylation by DT. Intriguingly, other microbial ADP ribosylase toxins including *Pseudomonas* exotoxin A [ETA] (Zhang et al., 2008) and *Vibrio cholera* cholix toxin (Jørgensen et al., 2008) are known to target the dipththamide residue of EF2 in a highly similar, if not identical, manner. Eventually, ADP-ribosyl-diphthamide, the resulting terminal modification, irreversibly inactivates the translation elongation function of EF2 (Fig. 7) (Sitikov et al., 1984).

As for the elusive and terminal amidation step, no DT resistant yeast mutants have been identified to date, probably because diphthine is a substrate (though poor) for ADP-ribosylating toxins. Provided terminal amidation was an enzymatically catalysed process rather than a spontaneous one (see above), amidase-deficient mutants may still display DT sensitivity, which is why the amidase in question may have repeatedly escaped identification in the above screens for DT resistance. It will be interesting to see whether this also holds true for screens involving EF2 inhibitors or antagonists that are not related to DT but share with DT a common requirement for diphthamide modification of EF2. This is of particular interest in the light of recent evidence that *dph1, dph2, dph3, dph4* and *dph5* deletion mutants from yeast not only are protected against DT (Fig. 8) but are also all resistant to growth inhibition by sordarin (Fig. 8) (Bär et al., 2008; Botet et al., 2008). The latter is an ascomycetous glycoside (Hauser & Sigg, 1971) whose antifungal activity obviously depends on diphthamide, but that operates by selectively blocking the EF2-ribosome complex rather than inhibiting EF2 by ADP-ribosylation (Dominguez et al., 1999).

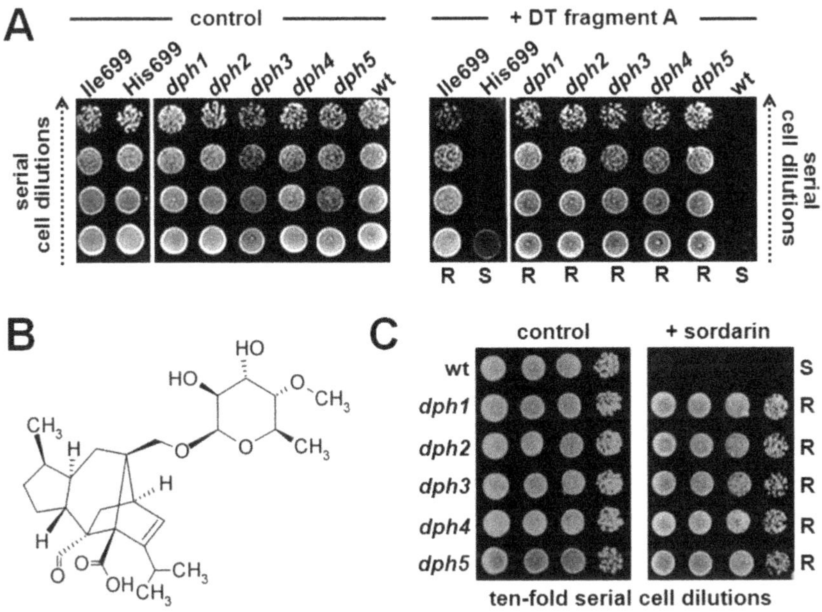

Fig. 8. Diphthamide modification is essentially required for growth inhibition of yeast cells by DT and by the antifungal sordarin. (A) DT resistance due to defects in diphthamide synthesis on EF2. Yeast cells with an EF2 diphthamide target residue substitution (His699Ile) (Kimata & Kohno, 1994) and diphthamide mutants (*dph1*, *dph2*, *dph3*, *dph4* and *dph5*) (Chen et al., 1985) resist (R) against conditional expression of the lethal DT fragment A while wild-type cells (wt; His699) remain sensitive (S) to the ADP-ribosylase and are killed (right panel). Empty vector control (left panel) shows the growth control in the absence of DT. (B) Chemical formula of sordarin, an EF2-specific antifungal and ribosome inhibitor. (C) Like DT, sordarin action requires diphthamide synthesis on EF2. Wild-type (wt) parental strain W303 and its diphthamide mutants (*dph1*-*dph5*) were cultivated in the absence (control) or presence of the antifungal (+ sordarin). A resistant (R) cell response is distinguished from sensitivity (S).

A

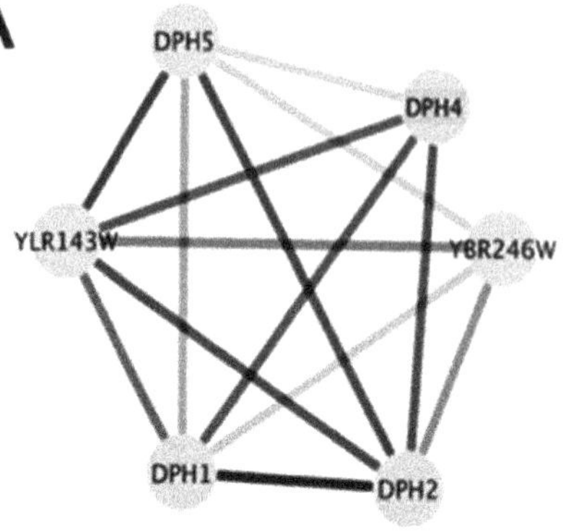

B

Gene	correlation score*
DPH2	0.314
DPH4	0.248
YLR143w	0.234
DPH5	0.182
YBR246w	0.158

* **profiles correlated to *dph1* traits**

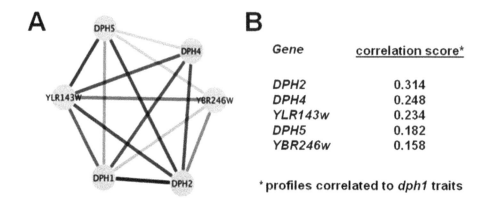

Fig. 9. Based on synthetic genetic array (SGA) analysis, yeast Open Reading Frames (ORFs) *YLR143w* and *YBR246w* represent loci that are potentially related to the *DPH* genes and the diphthamide pathway. (A) Genetic interaction data (Baryshnikova et al., 2010) indicating relatedness between ORFs *YLR143w* and *YBR246w* and diphthamide synthesis genes *DPH1, DPH2, DPH4* and *DPH5*. (B) Phenotypic clustering (Carette et al., 2009) and phenotypic scores, in relation to dipthamide mutant *dph1*, between *YBR246w* and *DPH5* genes as well as *YLR143w* and *DPH4* suggest both ORFs to be related to *DPH1* and to the diphthamide modification pathway.

In an effort to further analyze the relationships among individual components of the diphthamide pathway, we found that the Dph1, Dph2 and Dph3 proteins form a protein complex whose assembly is crucial for diphthamide formation and consequently for ADP-ribosylation of EF2 by DT (Fig. 10). Strikingly, the *DPH3* gene from budding yeast was shown to be allelic with the locus Killer Toxin Insensitive 11 (*KTI11*) (Butler et al., 1994). *KTI11* was shown to be required for the *Kluyveromyces lactis* tRNAse toxin zymocin to kill other yeast species including *S. cerevisiae* (Fichtner & Schaffrath, 2002). In particular, the Kti11/Dph3 gene product was shown to be involved in a tRNA modification pathway that is essential for the tRNase activity of zymocin to cleave target tRNAs and cause yeast cell death by way of tRNA depletion (Huang et a., 2005; Lu et al., 2006; Jablonowski & Schaffrath, 2007; Jablonowski et al., 2006; Kheir et al., 2011). In addition to interacting with Dph1, Dph2 and EF2 (Fichtner et al., 2003; Bär et al., 2008), Dph3/Kti11 was furthermore shown to communicate with other proteins (Kti13: Zabel et al., 2008) or protein complexes (Rvs161•Rvs167; Elongator complex: Fichtner et al., 2003; Krogan et al., 2006) suggesting multiple roles for Kti11/Dph3 in processes not necessarily limited to the diphthamide modification pathway. In support of such versatility, DelGIP1 (the human homologue of yeast Kti11/Dph3) interacts with deafness locus-associated guanine nucleotide exchange factor (DelGEF) and the DelGIP1•DelGEF protein complex affects exocyst-dependent secretion of proteoglycans (Sjölinder et al., 2002, 2004). Also, our group was able to show that conditional phenotypes and stress-inducible growth defects of a yeast mutant with a single *KTI11/DPH3* gene deletion were more severe and pronounced in relation to rather mild defects of yeast mutants lacking *DPH1* or *DPH2* gene function (Bär et al., 2008), supporting its role in a wider range of cellular functions in yeast. Atomic absorption spectroscopy has recently shown that the Kti11/Dph3 protein folds into a closed compact and globular protein structure with its C-terminal alpha-helix protruding outward (Sun et al., 2005). Moreover, the protein co-ordinates a zinc ion via a $Zn(Cys)_4$ binding module that is highly conserved among Kti11/Dph3 homologues from plants, animals and humans (Proudfood et al., 2008). Presumably, it is this motif that is engaged in the putative electron-carrier activity recently proposed for Kti11/Dph3 by Proudfood et al. (2008). In line with this notion, both single and multiple Cys substitutions of the four critical residues in the potential $Zn(Cys)_4$ binding module cause inactivation of the Kti11/Dph3 variants and traits including resistance to growth inhibition by DT, sordarin and zymocin that are identical to the phenotypes of null-mutants lacking *KTI11/DPH3* gene function (Fichtner & Schaffrath, 2002; Bär et al., 2008).

Strikingly, the multi-step pathway for diphthamide formation and EF2 modification (Fig. 7) has been conserved from lower to higher eukaryotes. Among the five budding yeast diphthamide genes (*DPH1*, *DPH2*, *DPH3*, *DPH4* and *DPH5*) (Fig. 7), there are two mammalian homologues (*DPH1/OVCA1* and *DPH3/KTI11*) that are required for cell proliferation, tumourigenesis and neuronal development in mice and human cells. As a result, defects in *DPH3/KTI11* are associated with neurodegeneration in mice (Liu et al., 2006) and mutations in *OVCA1/DPH1* have identified a tumour suppressor role for this diphthamide-related gene product in the context of ovarian cancer (Chen & Behringer, 2004). In an effort to further study diphthamide function and the interrelation between components of the diphthamide pathway, we found by co-immune precipitation and tandem affinity purification protocols that the Dph1, Dph2 and Dph3 factors form a protein complex, assembly of which is crucial for EF2 ADP-riboslyation by DT (Fichtner et al., 2003; Bär et al., 2008). Moreover, we and others discovered that the Dph1-Dph5 proteins are all required for the cytotoxic activity of sordarin (Bär et al., 2008; Botet et al., 2008), another EF2-related antifungal and translation inhibitor (Justice et al., 1998).

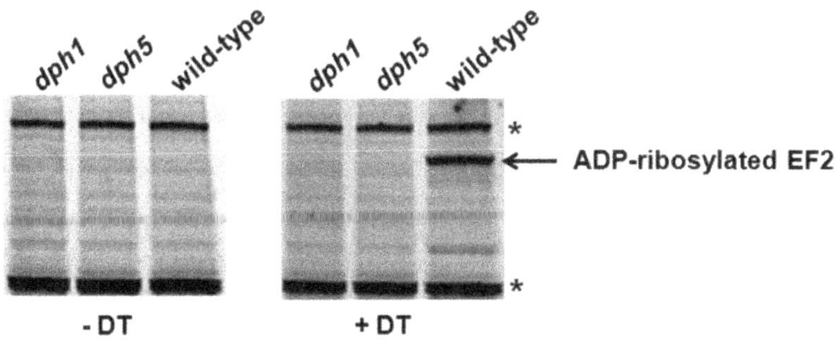

Fig. 10. Yeast diphthamide modification mutants evade ADP-ribosylation of EF2 by DT. Shown are EF2 ADP ribosylation assays on total protein extracts from the indicated yeast strain backgrounds in the absence (left panel) and presence (right panel) of recombinant DT. When using biotin-labeled NAD^+ as donor for the *in vitro* ADP ribosylation assay, wild-type strains display EF2 ADP-ribosylation acceptor activity (indicated by the arrow) whereas diphthamide mutans *dph1* and *dph5* fail to do so. The asterisks denote unspecific signals in proteins irrespective of DT treatment and/or strain backgrounds tested.

In a search for new diphthamide-related factors, two novel and uncharacterized open reading frames (ORFs), YBR246w and YLR143w, have been identified recently as new potential components for diphthamide biosynthesis using genetic screens in human and yeast cells (Botet et al., 2008; Carette et al., 2009). Based on synthetic genetic interaction data deposited at the genetic interaction database (GID; University of Toronto, Canada) (Baryshnikova et al., 2010) and the significance of the phenotypic correlation scores, both budding yeast ORFs are predicted to have EF2-related functions (Fig. 9). In addition, possible effector roles of YBR246w and YLR143w for EF2 specific antifungals including sordarin are becoming evident: when deleted, these new loci not only affect the communication between Dph5 and EF2 but also phenocopy traits (including sordarin resistance) that are typical of *dph1*, *dph2*, *dph3*, *dph4* and *dph5* mutants from yeast (Bär et al., 2008; Botet et al., 2008; Carette et al., 2009). Although being aware that the sordarin phenotype may also be ascribable to defects in EF2-unrelated genes that are required for binding and/or import of the deadly antifungal (Botet et al., 2008), we consider these ORFs to be candidate diphthamide biosynthesis genes. In support of this notion, preliminary data based on *in vitro* EF2 modification assays demonstrate that inactivation of YBR246w and YLR143w eliminates the ADP-ribosylation acceptor activity of EF2 in the presence of DT. Since this is a trait that is specific to the *bona fide* diphthamide synthesis defect of *dph1*, *dph2*, *dph3*, *dph4* and *dph5* mutants (Liu & Leppla, 2003; Liu et al., 2004) (Fig. 10), YBR246w or YLR184w deletion may cause a diphthamide defect, too, which abolishes DT-dependent ADP-ribosylation of EF2.

To sum up, diphthamide incorporation of EF2 is not only pathologically relevant for ADP-ribosylation by DT but also crucial for toxicity of the antifungal sordarin. Physiologically, the dipthamide pathway appears to be important for mRNA translation as well as proper cell proliferation and neural development in eukaryal cells. Surprisingly, our data imply that formation of diphthamide is genetically more complex than originally anticipated (Chen et al., 1985; Liu et al., 2004) and that the pathway may comprise more gene products than the five Dph1-Dph5 members known to date (Carette et al., 2009). For future work, it will be significant to define the roles of new diphthamide candidates and how they may relate to or communicate with the other known pathway members.

6.2 Biological significance for diphthamide modification of EF2

Diphthamide on EF2 is the target for bacterial ADP-ribosylase toxins (DT; ETA; cholix) and also affects toxicity of sordarin and ricin, a ribosome inhibiting protein toxin from plants (Gupta et al. 2008). Although this emphasizes its varied pathological relevance, the physiological significance of diphthamide remains enigmatic and elusive. Nonetheless, the evolutionary conservation of the diphthamide pathway among eukaryotes strongly suggests that diphthamide will be important in processes including mRNA translation. In support of this notion, evidence from research groups including our own has shown that diphthamide defects increase translational frame-shifting (Ortiz et al., 2006; Bär et al., 2008). Moreover, homologues of diphthamide synthesis genes (*DPH1/OVCA1* and *DPH3/KTI11*) affect the proliferation and development of mammalian cells, which is why inactivation of *DPH3/KTI11* is associated with tRNA modification defects and neurodegeneration and mutations in *DPH1/OVCA1* revealed a tumour suppressor role for this diphthamide synthesis gene in ovarian cancer (Chen & Behringer, 2004; Nobukuni et al., 2005; Huang et al., 2005; Liu et al., 2006; Kim et al., 2010).

Whether or not this implies structural or regulatory roles for diphthamide in mRNA translation remains to be seen. The latter, however, is intriguing with the emergence of a cellular ADP-ribosyltransferase that resembles the diphthamide-dependent ADP-ribosylation reaction by DT (Lee & Iglewski, 1984; Jäger et al., 2011). As a result, diphthamide may be envisioned to be used as an on/off switch for endogenous ADP-ribosylation of EF2 and control of mRNA translation and protein synthesis. Irrespective of unclear physiological functions, recent genetic data imply that the diphthamide pathway is more complex than originally anticipated and likely to comprise further components, in addition to Dph1-Dph5 (Carette et al., 2009). For future research, it will be therefore crucial to define the identity of new diphthamide synthesis candidates and provide insights into how they communicate with known members of the pathway.

7. Engineering DT chimera for use in cell-specific proliferation control

Protein engineering is a new and rapidly developing area within the field of molecular biology; it brings together recombinant DNA methodologies and solid phase DNA synthesis in the design and construction of chimeric genes whose products have unique properties. Through a combination of protein engineering and DT structure-function studies, it has been possible to genetically substitute the native DT receptor-binding domain B (Figs. 5 and 6) with a variety of polypeptide hormones and cytokines (e.g. α-melanocyte-stimulating hormone [α-MSH], interleukin [IL] 2, IL-4, IL-6, IL-7, epidermal growth factor, etc) (Foss, 2001; Kreitman, 2006, 2009). The resulting fusion toxins or chimera combine the receptor-binding specificity of the cytokine with the catalytic ADP-ribosylase domain of DT. In each instance, the chimeric proteins have unique properties and selectively attack only those target cells that bear the appropriate target cell receptor on the cell surface. One of these engineered fusion toxins, DAB389IL-2 (ONTAK) (Le Maistre et al., 1992), has been evaluated in clinical trials for the treatment of human lymphomas, in which cells with high affinity IL-2 receptors play a major role in pathogenesis. Administration of ONTAK has been shown to be well tolerated, safe and to induce durable remission from disease in the absence of undesired side effects. Moreover, ONTAK and its predecessor, DAB486IL-2 (Le Maistre et al., 1992) have demonstrated activity in a variety of diseases, including cutaneous T cell lymphoma (CTCL), psoriasis, rheumatoid arthritis and HIV infection. Hence, DT-based fusion toxins are important biological agents for the treatment of certain tumours or disorders in which specific cell surface receptors can be selectively targeted (Hesketh et al., 1993; Van der Spek et al., 1994; Foss, 2001; Kreitman, 2006, 2009) and it is likely that such DT chimera will be providing further and important new biological tools for selected cell targeting and DT-dependent inactivation of protein biosynthesis, a fundamental biological process with key roles for cell cycling and cancer formation (White-Gilbertson et al., 2009).

8. Conclusion

Diphtheria represents one of the best studied bacterial diseases of humans with its etiology, mode of transmission, pathogenic mechanism and molecular basis of DT structure and function being clearly established. Consequently, highly effective methods for treatment and prevention of diphtheria have been developed and many contributions to the fields of medical microbiology, immunology and molecular biology as well as to our understanding of host-bacterial interactions and pathogenesis have been made possible by studying diphtheria and DT. Diphtheria is caused by *C. diphtheriae*, pathovar. *gravis*, *intermedius* and *mitis*, three biotypes that differ in virulence and growth performance but share the ability to secrete the lethal ADP ribosylase toxin DT, the protein product of a lysogenic phage gene. The DT gene *tox* is under control of an iron-responsive repressor (DtxR) so that DT production is limited under conditions of low iron levels and to lysogenic bacteria only. DT is a typical A/B toxin containing two fragments that are proteolytically processed from a single precursor and held together by a disulfide bridge. The A fragment is catalytically active and the B fragment promotes receptor-mediated endocytosis of DT. Upon import, the A subunit is cleaved-off from the B fragment and gets released into the cytoplasm. Here, DT unfolds its toxicity and ADP-ribosylates eukaryotic translation elongation factor 2 (EF2). ADP-ribosylation of EF2 by DT is irreversible, eventually inhibiting mRNA translation and protein synthesis and inducing the death of the target cell. Studies from archaeal and eukaryal target cells demonstrate that the ADP-ribosylase activity of DT requires diphthamide, a highly modified histidine residue in EF2. Intriguingly, the EF2 analogues from *Corynebacteria* lack diphthamide, which explains why the DT producers are immune to their own toxin.

Strikingly, diphthamide formation on EF2 operates through a multi-step pathway that is conserved among archaea and eukaryotes. In the yeast *S. cerevisiae*, it comprises at least five different genes, *DPH1-DPH5*, of which two mammalian homologues (*DPH1/OVCA1* & *DPH3/KTI11*) are required for cell proliferation, tumourigenesis and neuronal development. As a result, defects in *DPH3/KTI11* are associated with neurodegeneration and mutations in *OVCA1/DPH1* have identified a tumour suppressor role for the diphthamide-related product in ovarian cancer. In an effort to further study the diphthamide pathway, we found that the Dph1, Dph2 and Dph3 factors form a protein complex, assembly of which is crucial for EF2 ADP-riboslyation by DT. Moreover, all five Dph1-Dph5 proteins are required for the cytotoxic activity of sordarin, another EF2-related inhibitor. In a search for novel diphthamide-related genes from yeast by use of synthetic genetic array (SGA) analysis and the genetic interaction database (GID), we identified two open reading frames (ORFs: YBR246W; YLR143w) previously implicated in antifungal activity of DT and sordarin. In line with predicted EF2 roles, deletion mutants lacking YBR246W or YLR184w are resistant towards doses of sordarin that are lethal to wild-type yeast cells. Moreover, EF2 modification assays in the presence of DT demonstrate that protein extracts from the deletion strains lack ADP-ribosylation acceptor activity of EF2. This suggests that YBR246W or YLR184w inactivation may have caused a diphthamide biosynthetic defect, which abrogates DT-dependent ADP-ribosylation of EF2. In sum, diphthamide incorporation of EF2 is not only relevant for ADP-ribosylation by DT but also crucial for toxicity of the antifungal sordarin. Physiologically, the dipthamide pathway appears to be important for mRNA translation as well as proper cell proliferation and neural development in eukaryal cells. Surprisingly, our data imply that formation of diphthamide is genetically more complex than originally anticipated and that the pathway may comprise more than the five Dph1-Dph5 gene products known to date.

Finally, the study of diphtheria toxin structure/function relationships has clearly shown DT toxin to be a three-domain protein with individual roles for receptor binding, endocytosis and catalysis (i.e. NAD^+-dependent ADP-ribosylation). Through protein engineering, a rapidly developing area within the field of molecular biology that brings together recombinant DNA methodologies and solid phase DNA synthesis, the design of diphtheria fusion toxin genes has been feasible whose products have unique properties. Thus, it has been possible to genetically substitute the native diphtheria toxin receptor-binding domain with a variety of polypeptide hormones and cytokines so that the resulting fusion toxins combine the receptor-binding specificity of the cytokine with the ADP ribosylase activity of DT. The fusion toxins can selectively intoxicate only those cells which bear the appropriate targeted receptor. It is likely that such DT-based fusion toxins will be important new biological agents for the treatment of tumours/disorders in which specific cell surface receptors may need to be targeted.

9. Acknowledgment

Support to SL by the US National Institute of Allergy and Infectious Diseases Intramural Programme and by the Biotechnology and Biological Sciences Research Council (BBSRC) to MJRS (BB/F0191629/1) and RS (BB/F019106/1) is gratefully acknowledged. SU has been awarded an *OVCA1* PhD studentship through the HOPE Foundation for Cancer Research, UK, and receives support from the Department of Genetics, University of Leicester, UK. RS greatfully acknowledges support from the Feodor Lynen Fellowship (3.1-3. FLF-DEU/1037031) Alumnus Programme of the Alexander von Humboldt Foundation, Bonn, Germany.

10. References

Atkinson, W., Hamborsky, J., McIntyre, L., & Wolfe, S. (eds.) (2007). *Diphtheria*. In: Epidemiology and Prevention of Vaccine-Preventable Diseases (The Pink Book) (10 ed.). Washington DC: Public Health Foundation. pp. 59–70.

Baryshnikova, A., Costanzo, M., Dixon, S., Vizeacoumar, F.J., Myers, C.L., Andrews, B., & Boone, C. (2010). Synthetic genetic array (SGA) analysis in *Saccharomyces cerevisiae* and *Schizosaccharomyces pombe*. *Methods in Enzymology* 470: 145-179.

Bär, C., Zabel. R., Liu, S., Stark, M.J., & Schaffrath, R. (2008). A versatile partner of eukaryotic protein complexes that is involved in multiple biological processes: Kti11/Dph3. *Mol Microbiol* 69: 1221-1233.

Bishai, W.R., & Murphy, J.R. (1988). Bacteriophage gene products that cause human disease. In Calendar, R. (ed.): *The Bacteriophages*. Plenum, New York.

Botet, J., Rodríguez-Mateos, M., Ballesta, J.P., Revuelta, J.L., & Remacha, M. (2008). A chemical genomic screen in *Saccharomyces cerevisiae* reveals a role for diphthamidation of translation elongation factor 2 in inhibition of protein synthesis by sordarin. *Antimicrobial Agents and Chemotherapy* 52: 1623-1629.

Broudy, T.B., Pancholi, V., & Fischetti, V.A. (2001). Induction of lysogenic bacteriophage and phage-associated toxin from group a streptococci during coculture with human pharyngeal cells. *Infection and Immunity* 69: 1440-1443.

Butler, A.R., White, J.H., Folawiyo, Y., Edlin, A., Gardiner, D., & Stark, M.J. (1994). Two *Saccharomyces cerevisiae* genes which control sensitivity to G1 arrest induced by *Kluyveromyces lactis* toxin. *Molecular and Cellular Biology* 14: 6306-6316.

Calendar, R. (1988). *The Bacteriophages*, Plenum, New York.

Carette, J.E., Guimaraes, C.P., Varadarajan, M., Park, A.S., Wuethrich, I., Godarova, A., Kotecki, M., Cochran, B.H., Spooner, E., Ploegh, H.L., & Brummelkamp, T.R. (2009). Haploid genetic screens in human cells identify host factors used by pathogens. *Science* 326: 1231-1235.

Chen, C.M., & Behringer, R.R. (2004). Ovca1 regulates cell proliferation, embryonic development, and tumorigenesis. *Genes and Development* 18: 320-332.

Chen, J.Y., Bodley, J.W. (1988). Biosynthesis of diphthamide in *Saccharomyces cerevisiae*. Partial purification and characterization of a specific S-adenosylmethionine:elongation factor 2 methyltransferase. *Journal of Biological Chemistry* 263: 11692-11696.

Chen, J.Y., Bodley, J.W., & Livingston, D.M. (1985). Diphtheria toxin-resistant mutants of *Saccharomyces cerevisiae*. *Molecular and Cellular Biology* 5: 3357-3360.

Collier, R.J. (2001). Understanding the mode of action of diphtheria toxin: a perspective on progress during the 20th century. *Toxicon* 39: 1793–1803.

Collier, R.J., & Cole, H.A. (1969). Diphtheria toxin subunit active in vitro. *Science* 164: 1179-1181.

Collier, R.J., & Kandel, J. (1971). Structure and activity of diphtheria toxin. I. Thiol-dependent dissociation of a fraction of toxin into enzymically active and inactive fragments. *Journal of Biological Chemistry* 246: 1496-1503.

D'Aquino, J.A., Tetenbaum-Novatt, J., White, A., Berkovitch, F., & Ringe, D. (2005). Mechanism of metal ion activation of the diphtheria toxin repressor DtxR. *Proceedings of the National Academy of Sciences of the United States of America* 102: 18408-18413.

Dominguez, J.M., Gomez-Lorenzo, M.G., & Martin, J.J. (1999). Sordarin inhibits fungal protein synthesis by blocking translocation differently to fusidic acid. *Journal of Biological Chemistry* 274: 22423-22427.

Faruque, S.M., & Nair, G.B. (2002). Molecular ecology of toxigenic *Vibrio cholerae*. *Microbiology and Immunology* 46: 59–66.

Fichtner, L., & Schaffrath, R. (2002). *KTI11* and *KTI13*, *Saccharomyces cerevisiae* genes controlling sensitivity to G1 arrest induced by *Kluyveromyces* lactis zymocin. *Molecular Microbiology* 44: 865-875.

Fichtner, L., Jablonowski, D., Schierhorn, A., Kitamoto, H.K., Stark, M.J., & Schaffrath, R. (2003). Elongator's toxin-target (TOT) function is nuclear localization sequence dependent and suppressed by post-translational modification. *Molecular Microbiology* 49: 1297-1307.

Foss, F.M. (2001). Interleukin-2 fusion toxin: targeted therapy for cutaneous T cell lymphoma. *Annals of the New York Academy of Sciences* 941: 166-176.

Freeman, V.J. (1951). Studies on the virulence of bacteriophage-infected strains of *Corynebacterium diphtheriae*. *Journal of Bacteriology* 61: 675–688.

Gill, D.M., & Dinius, L.L. (1971). Observations on the structure of diphtheria toxin. *Journal of Biological Chemistry* 246: 1485-1491.

Gill, D.M., & Pappenheimer, A.M. (1971). Structure-activity relationships in diphtheria toxin. *Journal of Biological Chemistry* 246: 1492-1495.

Gunge, N. (1983). Yeast DNA plasmids. *Annual Reviews of Microbiology* 37: 253-276.

Gupta, P.K., Liu, S., Batavia, M.P., & Leppla, S.H. (2008). The diphthamide modification on elongation factor-2 renders mammalian cells resistant to ricin. *Cellular Microbiology* 10: 1687-1694.

Hauser, D., & Sigg, H,P. (1971). Isolierung und Abbau von Sordarin. *Helvetica Chimica Acta* 54: 1178-1190.

Havaldar, P.V., Sankpal, M.N., & Doddannavar, R.P. (2000). Diphtheritic myocarditis: clinical and laboratory parameters of prognosis and fatal outcome. *Annals of Tropical Paediatrics* 20: 209–215.

Hesketh, P., Caguioa, P., Koh, H., Dewey, H., Facada, A., McCaffrey, R., Parker, K., Nylen, P., Woodworth, T. (1993). Clinical activity of a cytotoxic fusion protein in the treatment of cutaneous T cell lymphoma. *Journal of Clinical Oncology* 11: 1682-1690.

Holmes, R. K., & Barksdale, L. (1969). Genetic analysis of tox+ and tox- bacteriophages of *Corynebacterium diphtheriae. Journal of Virology* 3: 586-598.

Huang, B., Johansson, M.J., & Byström, A.S. (2005). An early step in wobble uridine tRNA modification requires the Elongator complex. *RNA* 11: 424-436.

Huang, A., De Grandis, S., Friesen, J., Karmali, M., Petric, M., Congi, R., & Brunton, J.L. (1986). Cloning and expression of the genes specifying Shiga-like toxin production in *Escherichia coli* H19. *Journal of Bacteriology* 166: 375-379.

Jablonowski, D., & Schaffrath, R. (2007). Zymocin, a composite chitinase and tRNase killer toxin from yeast. *Biochemical Society Transactions* 35: 1533-1537.

Jablonowski, D., Zink, S., Mehlgarten, C., Daum, G., & Schaffrath, R. (2007). $tRNA^{Glu}$ wobble uridine methylation by Trm9 identifies Elongator's key role for zymocin-induced cell death in yeast. *Molecular Microbiology* 59: 677-688.

Jäger, D., Werdan, K., & Müller-Werdan, U. (2011). Endogenous ADP-ribosylation of elongation factor-2 by interleukin-1β. *Molecular and Cellular Biochemistry* 348: 125-128.

Johnson, L.P., Tomai, M.A., & Schlievert, P.M. (1986). Bacteriophage involvement in group A streptococcal pyrogenic exotoxin A production. *Journal of Bacteriology* 166: 623-627.

Jørgensen, R., Purdy, A.E., Fieldhouse, R.J., Kimber, M.S., Bartlett, D.H. & Merrill, A.R. (2008). Cholix toxin, a novel ADP-ribosylating factor from *Vibrio cholerae. Journal of Biological Chemistry* 283: 10671-10678.

Justice, M.C., Hsu, M.J., Tse, B., Ku, T., Balkovec, J., Schmatz, D., & Nielsen, J. (1998). Elongation factor 2 as a novel target for selective inhibition of fungal protein synthesis. *Journal of Biological Chemistry* 273: 3148-3151.

Kaufmann, G. (2000). Anticodon nucleases. *Trends in Biochemical Sciences* 25: 70-74.

Kheir, E., Bär, C., Jablonowski, D., & Schaffrath, R. (2011). Cell growth control by tRNase ribotoxins from bacteria and yeast. In: Mendez-Vilas A., ed., *Science and Technology against Microbial Pathogens. Research, Development and Evaluation*, World Scientific Publishing Ltd; pp. 398-402.

Kim, S., Johnson, W., Chen, C., Sewell, A.K., Byström, A.S., & Han, M. (2010) Allele-specific suppressors of lin-1(R175Opal) identify functions of MOC-3 and DPH-3 in tRNA modification complexes in *Caenorhabditis elegans. Genetics* 185: 1235-1247.

Kimata, Y., & Kohno, K. (1994). Elongation factor 2 mutants deficient in diphthamide formation show temperature-sensitive cell growth. *Journal of Biological Chemistry* 269: 13497-13501.

Kreitman, R.J. (2006). Immunotoxins for targeted cancer therapy. *Journal of the American Association of Pharmaceutical Scientists* 8: E532-551.

Kreitman, R.J. (2009). Recombinant immunotoxins containing truncated bacterial toxins for the treatment of hematologic malignancies. *BioDrugs* 23: 1-13.

Krogan, N.J., Cagney, G., Yu, H., Zhong, G., Guo, X., Ignatchenko, A., Li, J., Pu, S., Datta, N., Tikuisis, A.P., Punna, T., Peregrín-Alvarez, J.M., Shales, M., Zhang, X., Davey, M., Robinson, M.D., Paccanaro, A., Bray, J.E., Sheung, A., Beattie, B., Richards, D.P., Canadien, V., Lalev, A., Mena, F., Wong, P., Starostine, A., Canete, M.M., Vlasblom, J., Wu, S., Orsi, C., Collins, S.R., Chandran, S., Haw, R., Rilstone, J.J., Gandi, K., Thompson, N.J., Musso, G., St Onge, P., Ghanny, S., Lam, M.H., Butland, G., Altaf-Ul, A.M., Kanaya, S., Shilatifard, A., O'Shea, E., Weissman, J.S., Ingles, C.J., Hughes,

T.R., Parkinson, J., Gerstein, M., Wodak, S.J., Emili, A., & Greenblatt, J.F. (2006). Global landscape of protein complexes in the yeast *Saccharomyces cerevisiae*. *Nature* 440: 637-643.

Lee, H., & Iglewski, W.J. (1984). Cellular ADP-ribosyltransferase with the same mechanism of action as diphtheria toxin and Pseudomonas toxin A. *Proceedings of the National Academy of Sciences of the United States of America* 81: 2703-2707.

Leis, S., Spindler, J., Reiter, J., Breinig, F., & Schmitt, M.J. (2005). *S. cerevisiae*K28 toxin - a secreted virus toxin of the A/B family of protein toxins. In: Schmitt, M.J., Schaffrath, R. (eds.) *Topics in Current Genetics, Microbial Protein Toxins*, vol. 11, Springer-Verlag, Berlin, Heidelberg, New York, pp. 111-132.

Le Maistre, C.F., Craig, F.E., Meneghetti, C., McMullin, B., Parker, K., Reuben, J., Boldt, D.H., Rosenblum, M., & Woodworth, T. (1992). Phase I trial of a 90-minute infusion of the fusion toxin DAB486 IL-2 in hematological cancers. *Cancer Research* 53: 3930-3934.

Liu, S., & Leppla, S.H. (2003). Retroviral insertional mutagenesis identifies a small protein required for synthesis of diphthamide, the target of bacterial ADP-ribosylating toxins. *Molecular Cell* 12: 603-613.

Liu, S., Milne, G.T., Kuremsky, J.G., Fink, G.R., & Leppla, S.H. (2004). Identification of the proteins required for biosynthesis of diphthamide, the target of bacterial ADP-ribosylating toxins on translation elongation factor 2. *Molecular and Cellular Biology* 24: 9487-9497.

Liu, S., Wiggins, J.F., Sreenath, T., Kulkarni, A.B., Ward, J.M., & Leppla, S.H. (2006). Dph3, a small protein required for diphthamide biosynthesis, is essential in mouse development. *Molecular and Cellular Biology* 26: 3835-3841.

Lord, J.L, & Roberts, L.M. (2005). Ricin: structure, synthesis and mode of action. In: Schmitt MJ, Schaffrath R, eds. *Topics in Current Genetics, Microbial Protein Toxins*, vol. 11, Springer-Verlag, Berlin, Heidelberg, New York; pp. 215-233.

Lu, J., Huang, B., Esberg, A., Johansson, M.J., & Byström, A.S. (2006). The *Kluyveromyces lactis* gamma-toxin targets tRNA anticodons. *RNA* 11: 1648-1654.

Mattheakis, L.C., Shen, W.H., & Collier, R.J. (1992). *DPH5*, a methyltransferase gene required for diphthamide biosynthesis in *Saccharomyces cerevisiae*. *Molecular and Cellular Biology* 12: 4026-4037.

McClatchy, J.K., Tsang, A.Y., & Cernich, M.S. (1981). Use of pyrazinamidase activity on Mycobacterium tuberculosis as a rapid method for determination of pyrazinamide susceptibility. *Antimicrobial Agents and Chemotherapy* 20: 556–557.

Meinhardt, F., Schaffrath, R., & Larsen, M. (1997). Microbial linear plasmids. *Applied Microbiology and Biotechnology* 47: 329-336.

Moehring, T.J., Danley, D.E., Moehring, J.M. (1984) *In vitro* biosynthesis of diphthamide, studied with mutant Chinese hamster ovary cells resistant to diphtheria toxin. *Molecular and Cellular Biology* 4: 642-650.

Murphy, J.R. (1996). *Corynebacterium diphtheriae*. In: Baron S, ed. *Medical Microbiology*, 4th edition, Chapter 32, The University of Texas Medical Branch at Galveston, 1996. Available at: http://www.ncbi.nlm.nih.gov/books/NBK7971/

Newland, J.W., Strockbine, N.A., Miller, S.F., O'Brien, A.D., & Holmes, R.K. (1985). Cloning of Shiga-like toxin structural genes from a toxin converting phage of *Escherichia coli*. *Science* 230: 179-181.

Nobukuni, Y., Kohno, K., & Miyagawa, K. (2005). Gene trap mutagenesis-based forward genetic approach reveals that the tumor suppressor *OVCA1* is a component of the biosynthetic pathway of diphthamide on elongation factor 2. *Journal of Biological Chemistry* 280: 10572-10577.

Ortiz, P.A., Ulloque, R., Kihara, G.K., Zheng, H., & Kinzy, T.G. (2006). Translation elongation factor 2 anticodon mimicry domain mutants affect fidelity and diphtheria toxin resistance. *Journal of Biological Chemistry* 281: 32639–32648.

Pappenheimer, A.M. (1977). Diphtheria toxin. *Annual Review of Biochemistry* 46: 69-94.

Pappenheimer, A.M., (1984). Diphtheria. In Germanier, R. (ed.) *Bacterial Vaccines*. Academic Press, San Diego.

Proudfoot, M., Sanders, S.A., Singer, A., Zhang, R., Brown, G., Binkowski, A., Xu, L., Lukin, J.A., Murzin, A.G., Joachimiak, A., Arrowsmith, C.H., Edwards, A.M., Savchenko, A.V., & Yakunin AF. (2008). Biochemical and structural characterization of a novel family of cystathionine beta-synthase domain proteins fused to a Zn ribbon-like domain. *Journal of Molecular Biology* 375: 301-315.

Rappuoli, R., Perugini, M., & Falsen, E. (1988). Molecular epidemiology of the 1984–1986 outbreak of diphtheria in Sweden. *New England Journal of Medicine* 318: 12-14.

Ratts, R., & Murphy, J.R. (2005). Diphtheria toxin, diphtheria-related fusion protein toxins and the molecular mechanism of their action against eukaryotic cells. In: Schmitt MJ, Schaffrath R, eds. *Topics in Current Genetics, Microbial Protein Toxins*, vol. 11, Springer-Verlag, Berlin, Heidelberg, New York; pp. 1-20.

Roux, E., & Yersin, A. (1888) Contribution al'etude de la diphtheriae. *Annales de l'Institut Pasteur* 2: 629-661.

Sandvig, K., Wälchli, S., & Lauvrak, S.U. (2005). Shiga toixns and their mechnaisms of cell entry. In: Schmitt MJ, Schaffrath R, eds. *Topics in Current Genetics, Microbial Protein Toxins*, vol. 11, Springer-Verlag, Berlin, Heidelberg, New York; pp. 35-53.

Schaffrath, R., & Meinhardt, F. (2005) *Kluyveromyces lactis* zymocin and other plasmid-encoded yeast killer toxins. In: Schmitt, M.J., Schaffrath, R. (eds.) *Topics in Current Genetics, Microbial Protein Toxins*, vol. 11, Springer-Verlag, Berlin, Heidelberg, New York, pp. 133-155.

Schaffrath, R., Meinhardt, F., Meacock, P.A. (1999). Molecular manipulation of *Kluyveromyceslactis* linear DNA plasmids: Gene targeting and plasmid shuffles. *FEMS Microbiology Letters* 178: 201-210.

Schmitt, M.J., & Schaffrath, R. (2005) *Microbial Protein Toxins, Topics in Current Genetics*, vol. 11, Springer-Verlag, Berlin, Heidelberg, New York.

Sitikov, A.S., Davydova, E.K., Bezlepkina, T.A., Ovchinnikov, L.P., & Spirin, A.S. (1984). Eukaryotic elongation factor 2 loses its non-specific affinity for RNA and leaves polyribosomes as a result of ADP-ribosylation. *FEBS Letters* 176: 406-410.

Sjölinder, M., Uhlmann, J., & Ponstingl, H. (2002). DelGEF, a homologue of the Ran guanine nucleotide exchange factor RanGEF, binds to the exocyst component Sec5 and modulates secretion. *FEBS Letters* 532: 211-215.

Sjölinder, M., Uhlmann, J., & Ponstingl, H. (2004). Characterisation of an evolutionary conserved protein interacting with the putative guanine nucleotide exchange factor DelGEF and modulating secretion. *Experimental Cell Research* 294: 68-76.

Solders, G, Nennesmo, I., & Persson, A. (1989). Diphtheritic neuropathy, an analysis based on muscle and nerve biopsy and repeated neurophysiological and autonomic function tests. *Journal of Neurology, Neurosurgery and Psychiatry* 52: 876–880.

Sugisaki, Y., Gunge, N., Sakaguchi, K., Yamasaki, M., & Tamura, G. (1985). Transfer of DNA killer plasmids from *Kluyveromyces lactis* to *Kluyveromyces fragilis* and *Candida pseudotropicalis*. *Journal of Bacteriology* 164: 1373-1375.

Sun, J., Zhang, J., Wu, F., Xu, C., Li, S., Zhao, W., Wu, Z., Wu, J., Zhou, C.Z., & Shi, Y. (2005). Solution structure of Kti11p from *Saccharomyces cerevisiae* reveals a novel zinc-binding module. *Biochemistry* 44: 8801-8809.

Tao, X., Schiering, N., Zeng, H.Y., Ringe, D., & Murphy, J.R. (1994). Iron, DtxR, and the regulation of diphtheria toxin expression. *Molecular Microbiology* 14:191-197.
Todar, K. (2004). Web Review of Todar's Online Textbook of Bacteriology. *The Good, the Bad, and the Deadly*. Chapter Diptheria (*Corynebacterium diphtheriae*).
Tokunaga, M., Kawamura, A., Kitada, K., Hishinuma, F. (1990). Secretion of killer toxin encoded on the linear DNA plasmid pGKL1 from *Saccharomyces cerevisiae*. *Journal of Biological Chemistry* 265: 17274-17280.
Uchida, T., Gill, D.M., & Pappenheimer, A.M. (1971). Mutation in the structural gene for diphtheria toxin carried by temperate phage. *Nature - New Biology* 233: 8-11.
Uthman, S., Kheir, E., Bär, C., Jablonowski, D., & Schaffrath, R. (2011). Growth inhibition strategies based on antimicrobial microbes/toxins. In: *Science against Microbial Pathogens: Communicating Current Research and Technological Advances*, Mendez-Vilas A., ed., Formatex, Badajoz, Spain, in press.
Van der Spek, J., Cosenza, L., Woodworth, T., Nichols JC, Murphy J.R. (1994). Diphtheria toxin-related cytokine fusion proteins: elongation factor 2 as a target for the treatment of neoplastic disease. *Molecular and Cellular Biochemistry* 138: 151-156.
Van Ness, B.G., Howard, J.B., & Bodley, J.W. (1980). ADP-ribosylation of elongation factor 2 by diphtheria toxin. NMR spectra and proposed structures of ribosyl-diphthamide and its hydrolysis products *Journal of Biological Chemistry* 255: 10710-10716.
von Hunolstein, C., Alfarone, G., Scopetti, F., Pataracchia, M., La Valle, R., Franchi, F., Pacciani, L., Manera, A., Giammanco, A., Farinelli, S., Engler, K, De Zoysa, A., & Efstratiou, A. (2003). Molecular epidemiology and characteristics of Corynebacterium diphtheriae and Corynebacterium ulcerans strains isolated in Italy during the 1990s. *Journal of Medical Microbiology* 52: 181-188.
Waldor, M.K., & Mekalanos, J.J. (1996). Lysogenic conversion by a filamentous phage encoding cholera toxin. *Science* 272: 1910–1914.
Webb, T.R., Cross, S.H., McKie, L., Edgar, R., Vizor, L., Harrison, J., Peters, J., & Jackson, I.J. (2008). Diphthamide modification of eEF2 requires a J-domain protein and is essential for normal development. *Journal of Cell Science* 121: 3140-3145.
White-Gilbertson, S., Kurtz, D.T., & Voelkel-Johnson, C. (2009). The role of protein synthesis in cell cycling and cancer. *Molecular Oncology* 3: 402-408.
Willshaw, G.A., Smith, H.R., Scotland, S.M., & Rowe, B. (1985). Cloning of genes determining the production of vero cytotoxin by *Escherichia coli*. *Journal of General Microbiology* 131: 3047-3053.
Zabel, R., Bär, C., Mehlgarten, C., & Schaffrath, R. (2008). Yeast alpha-tubulin suppressor Ats1/Kti13 relates to the Elongator complex and interacts with Elongator partner protein Kti11. *Molecular Microbiology* 69: 175-187.
Zhang, Y., Liu, S., Lajoie, G., & Merrill A.R. (2008). The role of the diphthamide-containing loop within eukaryotic elongation factor 2 in ADP-ribosylation by *Pseudomonas aeruginosa* exotoxin A. *Biochemical Journal* 413: 163-174.
Zhang, Y., Zhu, X., Torelli, A.T., Lee, M., Dzikovski, B., Koralewski, R.M., Wang, E., Freed, J., Krebs, C., Ealick, S.E., & Lin, H. (2010). Diphthamide biosynthesis requires an organic radical generated by an iron-sulphur enzyme. *Nature* 465: 891-896.

9

Stem Cells in Infectious Diseases

Ramesh Chandra Rai, Debapriya Bhattacharya and Gobardhan Das
Immunology Group, International Centre for Genetic Engineering and Biotechnology, New Delhi, India

1. Introduction

Stem cells are unspecialized cells found in embryos (blastocyst stage) and in various tissues of adults. They divide mitotically to self renew and can differentiate into different types of cells in appropriate conditions for specific functions. They serve as cell reservoirs for purpose of repair of damaged tissues of the body. Recent research suggests that stem cells especially mesenchymal stem cells have immuno-modulatory characteristics. Due to this property many trials are being conducted with transplantation of MSCs in treating diseases which arise from immunological abuses. These cells have capacity of specific homing and thus can repair infection induced injuries of various organs of body. Evidences suggest that mesenchymal stem cells could on the other hand be a potential target for treatment of tuberculosis.

Even after more than a century of its discovery in 1882 by Robert Koch, *Mycobacterium tuberculosis* (*M. tb*) continues to be one of the leading causes of mortality and morbidity in humans among infectious diseases. One third of global population is latently infected with *M. tb* (World Health Organisation November 2010), and is a cause of around two million deaths each year. The majority of infected individuals remain asymptomatic until there is any perturbation of host immune responses. Currently available vaccine, Bacillus Calmette-Guérin (BCG) is effective only in disseminated TB in young children. On the contrary, its efficacy dramatically varies in adult pulmonary TB depending on ethnicity and geographical locations. Current therapy of TB is very effective and is adopted by internationally recognized Directly Observed Treatment Short course (DOTS) programme. However, this regimen of therapy consists of multiple antibiotics for an extended period of time, and thus incorporates the risk of developing drug resistance. In fact, non-compliance is the central cause for generation of multiple and extensively drug resistant (MDR and XDR) forms of TB (Peter A. Otto *et al.*, 2008). Therefore, there is an urgent need for alternative therapeutic targets and newer strategies for treatment of *Mycobacterium tuberculosis* infections.

Considerable efforts have been made to uncover the strategy used by the harbouring tubercular bacilli to induce persistent/latent infection. Only recently, it has been clearly demonstrated that mesenchymal stem cells (MSCs) play a "Janus" like activity and establish a dynamic equilibrium. MSCs position themselves in between harbouring bacilli and host protective T cells. Therefore, MSCs could be a potential therapeutic target for treatment of latent tuberculosis (Raghuvanshi S. *et al.*, 2010). They are recruited at the site of infection and do not allow *M. tb* to spread but at the same time suppress host immune response mounted against the pathogen, thus preventing complete elimination of pathogen from the host (Raghuvanshi S. *et al.*, 2010). These results shed a light on possible new ways for treating tuberculosis, which has been a major killer of humans for centuries.

2. Stem cells and various diseases

Due to self renewal and multi-lineage differentiation capabilities, transplantation of stem cells has emerged as a very promising way of treatment of many diseases. Stem cell therapy of different diseases involves the local delivery of stem cells to injured/ infected site or their systemic transfusion. Owing the ability to differentiate into various lineages, stem cells hold therapeutic potential for treatment of many non-infectious and infectious diseases.

2.1 Non-infectious diseases

Mesenchymal stem cells can manipulate host immune responses; they have been used for treating/preventing many diseases which arise because of irregularities of immune system or host responses. Also the infused stem cells are able to differentiate to a particular type of cell after reaching the site in response to local signals. Although this notion have not yet been demonstrated very well. Many reports suggest their use in case of cardiovascular, lung fibrosis, neural and orthopaedic diseases (Barry FP and Murphy JM, 2004; Ortiz LA. *et al.*, 2003).

In a study by Teng, YD. *et al.*, 2002, have shown improvement in injured spinal cord by transplanting neural stem cell in adult rat. These approaches can also be extended to treat the conditions of stroke and other neurodegenerative diseases (Barry FP. and Murphy JM, 2004). Recently Lin H. *et al.*, 2011, reported positive therapeutic use of MSCs in different liver diseases and inherited metabolic disorders. They have shown that cytokines produced from MSCs can attenuate inflammatory injury to the liver and prevent apoptosis of liver cells. Also MSCs helped in regaining the proliferation and function of hepatocytes.

2.1.1 Auto-immune diseases

When immune system of human body recognises its own component as non-self, it starts immune response against it. This leads to auto-immune diseases such as inflammatory bowel disease, arthritis etc. In inflammatory bowel disease which includes ulcerative colitis and Crohn's disease, the intestine become inflamed (Melgar S and Shanahan F, 2010; Siegmund B and Zeitz M, 2011). This is due to immune reaction of person's body towards its own intestinal tissues. In case of arthritis especially in rheumatoid arthritis, there is inflammation of joints due to overt immune responses. This leads to damage of joints which is due to inflammation of joint lining tissues. So, objective of treatments will be suppression of immune responses.

2.1.2 Graft Versus Host Diseases (GVHD)

It is a situation when host immune system rejects transplanted organ or part of it as a non-self. Infiltration of MSCs can suppress host immune response and thus can prevent GVHD

(Le Blanc K, *et al.*, 2004; Tse WT, 2003). Prolonged survival of skin graft was observed when MSCs were used (Bartholomew A, *et al.*, 2002). So it can reverse the process of rejection and GVHD when used in transplantation (Bobis S., *et al.*, 2006; Le Blank K and Ringden O., 2005). GVHD was not observed in case of patients with metachromatic leukodystrophy and Hurler's syndrome after MSCs were infused (Koc, O. N. *et al.*, 2002).

In such situations immuno-suppressive effect of MSCs can help in preventing these diseases.

2.2 Infectious diseases

There is growing understanding among scientific community that many of infectious diseases may be cured or controlled using stem cells. Stem cell therapy can also be used in general to fight infections e.g. sepsis, a life threatening condition which arises from spread of an infection throughout the body and body's response to it. Report from Mei SH. *et al.*, 2010; suggest that sepsis could be treated successfully by transplanting mesenchymal stem cells to the patient.

2.2.1 Stem cell therapy for treatment of HIV infection

Stem cell therapy for treatment of HIV is under intensive investigation in recent times. Scientists are trying to reconstitute HIV-resistant lymphoid and myeloid system in experimental mice model to combat HIV infections (Holt, N. *et al.*, 2010; Steven G Deeks and Joseph M McCune, 2010). Holt, N. *et al.* 2010, engineered human hematopoietic cells to disrupt the CCR5 receptors which are utilized by viruses for their entry. When these engineered cells are transplanted to mice, they confer resistance towards the HIV infections. When CCR5 disrupted stem cells transplanted in a HIV patient, patient remained free of virus for 20 months even in absence of antiretroviral therapies (Hütter G *et al.*, 2009).

In a similar kind of approach Kitchen SG. *et al.*, 2009; demonstrated that hematopoietic stem cells could be engineered to target HIV infected cells. They generated CD8+ cytotoxic T cell lymphocytes which express transgenic-human anti-HIV T cell receptor. After cloning and transplantation to mice model, these cells were able to kill cells which were infected with HIV and were displaying its antigens.

2.2.2 Stem cell therapy for treatment of malaria

Malaria, which is characterized by invasion of erythrocytes by *Plasmodium,* leads to extreme perturbation of hematopoiesis. Severe destruction of red blood cells causes anaemia, thus posing pressure on bone marrow to meet the requirement of myeloid cells. Scientists from National Institute for Medical Research, UK, have identified an atypical progenitor cells from malaria infected mice which can give rise to a lineage of cells capable of fighting this disease (Belyaev, NN, 2010). Transplantation of these cells into mice with severe malaria helped mice recover from the disease. Other reports also supports stem cell therapy for malaria treatment (Saei, AA. and Ahmadian, S., 2009). Stem cells can also be engineered to produce erythrocytes with modified hemoglobin as its variants are associated with protection from malaria.

Approaches may differ but stem cells are in focus for treatment of many diseases. The current reports from our lab suggest that tuberculosis could be prevented possibly by targeting mesenchymal stem cells.

3. Tuberculosis and its treatment options

Mycobacterium tuberculosis infects humans through aerial route and thus lungs are the primary organ for its infection. Subsequently infection spreads to other organs of body such as spleen and lymph nodes. Recruitment of macrophages and lymphocytes at the site of infection leads to formation of granuloma which is small area of inflammation due to tissue injury or infection and a hallmark of tuberculosis. Many other diseases are also associated with the formation of granulomas such as sarcoidosis, histoplasmosis, syphilis, Crohn's disease etc. Granulomas are formed when immune cells contains a foreign substance after recognition which could not get cleared by body's immune system. They are characterized by presence of macrophages and infectious agent besides other cells and body matrix such as lymphocytes, neutrophils, eosinophils, fibroblasts and collagen.

In case of tuberculosis granulomas are formed at the site of infection where *Mycobacterium tuberculosis* remains as a latent infection. Infection to the macrophages of lungs leads to secretion of several of chemokines which attracts lymphocytes and neutrophils. These cells are able to contain pathogen inside granuloma, thus preventing the spread of bacterium to other parts of body and further inflammation. In other words granulomas are hiding place of bacteria in the infected organs. Final outcome of these interactions and whether it will lead to disease condition or not depends on the strength of host immune response.

Host immune response blocks spread of infection and prevents disease condition but it is not able to completely remove *M. tb* from body. Its persistent infection in a person converts into diseased condition when there is suppression of immunity such as in case of AIIDS. As HIV infection compromises immunity, the person will become highly susceptible to active tuberculosis as latent infection turns into active form (Goletti D, *et al.*, 1996). Co-existence of both TB and HIV fuel each other worsening the patient's condition. Immunosuppression in HIV patients occur as a result of decrease in number of $CD4^+$ T cells and leads to progression of TB. One report suggests that the chances of getting TB increases from 4% to 49% when there is decrease in $CD4^+$ T cells from 200 cells/µl to 100 cells/µl (Jones BE *et al.*, 1993). On the other hand *Mycobacterium tuberculosis* infection facilitates replication of HIV. This is done by cytokines such as TNF-α and IL-6 secreted from *M. tb* infected macrophages (Havlir DV and Barnes PF 1999; Nakata K, *et al.*, 1997). These cytokines creates a microenvironment which are inductive to HIV replication (Goletti D, *et al.* 1996). Thus, both HIV and *M. tb* can shorten the lifespan of patients by working together.

4. Bacillus Calmette–Gue´rin (BCG) and its efficacy

Bacillus Calmette-Gue´rin (BCG) vaccine is prepared from attenuated strain of *Mycobacterium bovis*. This strain has become avirulent due to continuous passages in artificial medium for a long time but still remained antigenic, being used as vaccine to prevent tuberculosis. But its effectiveness is not 100% and does not last longer (Colditz GA *et al.*, 1994). At the maximum it can provide protection up to 15 years depending on many factors including geographical conditions. Directly Observed Treatment, Short Course (DOTS) is a world health organisation (WHO) recommended treatment for tuberculosis. It was launched in India in 1997 as a revised national tuberculosis control programme. Before launching the programme, it was tested from 1993-1996. The key components of this programme are as follows-

i. Political commitment to control TB;
ii. Case detection by sputum smear microscopy examination among symptomatic patients;
iii. Patients are given anti- TB drugs under the direct observation of the health care provider/community DOT provider;
iv. Regular, uninterrupted supply of anti-TB drugs; and
v. Systematic recording and reporting system that allows assessment of treatment results of each and every patient and of whole TB control programme.

Treatment of tuberculosis involves- isoniazid, rifampicin, ethambutol, pyrazinamide daily for two months, followed by four months of isoniazid and rifampicin given three times a week. Sometimes one or the other drugs are omitted during treatment depending on the patient's condition. Later in 2006; WHO launched stop TB programme as a multi-dimensional approach to fight this disease at international level and better management of treatment strategies.

5. Mesenchymal stem cells (MSCs) and its role in *M. tb* infection

Discovered by A. J. Friedenstein in 1968 (Friedenstein, AJ. *et al.*,1974) MSCs are a subset of non-haematopoietic pleuripotent cells found in adult bone marrow and are capable of differentiating into adipocytes, fibroblasts and even myoblasts (Ren G. *et al.*, 2010). The mesenchymal stem cell name to these cells was given by Caplan. They have very high capacity to proliferate *in vitro* and don't loose proliferation capacity for a long time (Sundin, M. *et al.*, 2006). After their discovery and growing understanding of their role in the modulation of host immune response, they have been thought to be an important tool for regenerative medicine and immunotherapy. Although there are no exclusive markers for MSCs, they are characterized by their ability to differentiate into different kinds of cells mentioned above and by the combined surface expressions of $CD29^{+}CD44^{+}Sca\text{-}1^{+}CD45^{-}CD11b^{-}CD11c^{-}Gr\text{-}1^{-}F4/80^{-}MHC\text{-}II^{-}MHC\text{-}I^{low}$ (Ren G. *et al.*, 2008 and 2010).

MSCs are immuno-suppressive in nature and they exert their effect only when they are stimulated. Unstimulated MSCs are not capable of performing this effect (Yufang Shi *et al.*, 2010). MSCs have been shown to prevent rejection of allogenic skin grafts (Xu G, *et al.* 2007), graft versus host diseases (K. Le Blanc and O. Ringden, 2006), and therefore are helpful in treating auto-immune disorders. They are able to alter function of T cells, B cells, dendritic cells (DCs) and natural killer (NK) cells (Ren G. *et al.*, 2010). This is done by cytokines secreted by MSCs and through direct cell-cell contact. MSCs produce number of cytokines, signalling molecules and growth factors which can suppress inflammatory response and may also lead to trophic effects (Caplan AI and Dennis JE. 2006; Lin H. *et al.*, 2011). Their regulatory effect on immune system, such as anti-proliferative (Bartholomew A, *et al.*, 2002; Di Nicola M *et al.*, 2002; Le Blank K *et al.*, 2003; Sudres M, *et al.*, 2006) and anti-inflammatory roles makes them an important candidate for therapy of many inflammatory diseases (Newman RE *et al.*, 2009).

Mesenchymal stem cells have ability to create a microenvironment which helps in engraftment. The expressions of major histocompatibility I (MHC I) molecules are less on these cells and they lack human leukocyte antigen (HLA) class II and costimulatory molecules such as CD40, CD80 and CD86 (Krampera, M. *et al.*, 2003). Low level expression of MSC I can still activate T cells but they become anergic as there is no secondary signals or co-stimulation (Javazon EH. *et al.*, 2004; Wong RS. 2011). Also low level expression of MHC I prevent these cells from being destroyed by natural killer cells (Moretta A. *et al.*, 2001). They generally do not express MHC II molecules on their surface (Le Blank K. *et al.*, 2003) but could be immunogenic in certain circumstances (Le Blank K. *et al.*, 2003; Stagg J. *et al.*, 2006). The above characteristics help them to be less immunogenic (Herrero C. and Perez-Simon, J. A. 2010) and also have ability of interaction with components of both innate and adaptive immune system. Suppression of T and B cell proliferation and their activation makes them useful for treatment of different infectious and non-infectious diseases such as tuberculosis, graft versus host disease and various auto-immune diseases (Sundin, M. *et al.*, 2006). These cells have ability to migrate specifically to the site of injury. This has been shown in many of diseases involving injury of tissues and cartilages.

5.1 Effector molecules of mesenchymal stem cells

The molecular players which perform immunosuppression are mainly nitric oxide (NO), indoleamine 2,3-dioxygenase (IDO) and prostaglandin E2 (PGE2) (Ren G. *et al.*, 2008). Three nitric oxide synthases catalyse the synthesis of NO, which by interacting with many receptors and enzymes plays critical role in immune-suppression. It affects the phenotype of T cells and impairs its proliferation and function affecting TCR mediated signalling (Hoffman, RA. *et al.*, 2002). MSCs has been shown to express many chemokine receptors such as CCR1, CCR4, CCR5 and CCR10, thus in response to many of the cytokines, they move to desired destination (Von Luttichau *et al.*, 2005).

5.2 Host immune response

Both innate and adaptive immunity plays role against *Mycobacterium tuberculosis* infection. Host immune response against *Mycobacterium tuberculosis* is Th1 rather than Th2 mediated as IFN-γ knock out mice fails to mount immune response against its infection (Schroder K *et al.*, 2004). Of note, IFN-γ plays suppressive role for Th2 cell differentiation. *M. tb* evades host protective immune responses by modulating various immune mechanisms that includes down regulations of Major Histocompatibility Complex (MHCs), co-stimulatory molecules, and up-regulating production of immune suppressive cytokines viz. TGF-β and IL-10, and prostaglandins. Each of these targets is extensively studied for therapeutic interventions. However, it has been mostly unsuccessful. It is now evident that MSCs confine harbouring bacteria and segregate host protective responses. Cell mediated immunity is required for protection from *M. tb*. But *M. tb* has evolved mechanisms to evade the host immune response and remains as persistent infection inside the granuloma.

5.3 Balance between immune response and disease outcome

After *M. tb* infection, macrophage and lymphocytes are mobilized to the site of infection, resulting in formation of granuloma. Thus cells of innate and adaptive immune system of body surround the pathogen. Recognition of pathogen associated molecular patterns leads to activation of T cells which secrete IFN-γ. Since *M. tb* is an intracellular pathogen, effector T cells plays crucial role in host immunity against this pathogen. To evade the host defence mechanism, pathogen recruits MSCs at the periphery of granuloma (Raghuvanshi S. *et al.*,

2010). Reports from various groups suggest that MSC interferes with antigen presenting cell functionality, block the differentiation of B cells. They also suppress natural killer cell and T cell responses. Both naïve and memory T cell responses were inhibited by MSCs. The suppression is due to cell cycle arrest at G0/G1 stage of T cells (Glennie S. *et al.*, 2005). They induce Th2 cells to produce interleukin-4 (IL-4) and also inhibit the production of interferon-γ thus creating an anti-inflammatory state. MSCs also arrest B cells at G0/G1 stage of their cell cycle besides suppressing their differentiation (Corcione, A. *et al.*, 2006; Tabera, S. *et al.*, 2008) and inhibit immunoglobulin production (Herrero, C. and Perez Simon J. A. 2010). MSCs also hinder functional differentiation of dendritic cells (Jiang XX., *et al.*, 2005; Ramasamy R., *et al.*, 2007). Besides above mentioned roles there is conflicting reports regarding immune-suppression effect of MSCs in murine models *in vivo* (Muriel Sudres *et al.*, 2006).

Pro-inflammatory cytokines induces MSCs to secrete several cytokines/ chemokines (IL-10, TGF-β, IDO and PGE2) and nitric oxide (NO). Together they perform immuno-suppression (Ren G. *at al.*, 2008) and also induce regulatory T cells which prevent killing of *M. tb* by cytotoxic T cells (Scott-Browne JP *et al.*, 2007). NO inhibits T cell proliferation, production of cytokines, and induce tolerance (Niedbala, W. *et al.*, 2006; Ren G. *et al.*, 2008). NO diffuses rapidly to the vicinity but its active concentration drops very fast as it is highly unstable (Ren G. *et al.*, 2008). It is effective only up to a distance of 100 micrometer (J.R. Lancaster Jr., 1997). To perform immunosuppressive activity, T cells must be held in close proximity to the MSCs. This is done by MSC surface molecules such as intercellular adhesion molecule-1 (ICAM1) and vascular cell adhesion molecule-1 (VCAM1), which are shown to interact with T cells and hold them close to the mesenchymal stem cells (Ren G. *et al.*, 2010 and 2011). Thus besides soluble factors secreted from MSCs, cell surface molecules on MSCs also play crucial role in immune suppression against *Mycobacterium tuberculosis* (Xu G, *et al.* 2007; Shi Y. *et al.*, 2010).

In mice after infection by *Mycobacterium tuberculosis*, MSCs exclusively infiltrate to infected organs such as lungs and spleen (Raghuvanshi S. *et al.*, 2010). They have not been found to the uninfected organs of the infected person. This report suggests that immune suppression by MSC is local and confines to the infection site only. Although MSCs recruited at the site of infection contains pathogen inside granulomas, it also prevents killing of *Mycobacterium tuberculosis* by suppressing the host immunity. These cells intercept immune cells from the pathogen by being there physically and helping to establish equilibrium between host and the pathogen (Figure 1). In other words, *M. tb* rely on MSCs to establish long lasting infection which should be intervened to achieve objective of treating tuberculosis.

6. Issues in therapy with stem cells

Therapy with stem cells have shown hope for treatment of those diseases which otherwise seems to be untreatable. But this approach also has its own risks. Utilization of MSCs for therapeutic use is like a double edged sword putting patient at the danger of cancer. The anti-proliferative effects of these cells are often associated with anti-apoptotic effect also, which may leads to tumour progression, metastasis and drug resistance. So even with vast therapeutic potential of stem cells in various non-infectious and infectious diseases, there

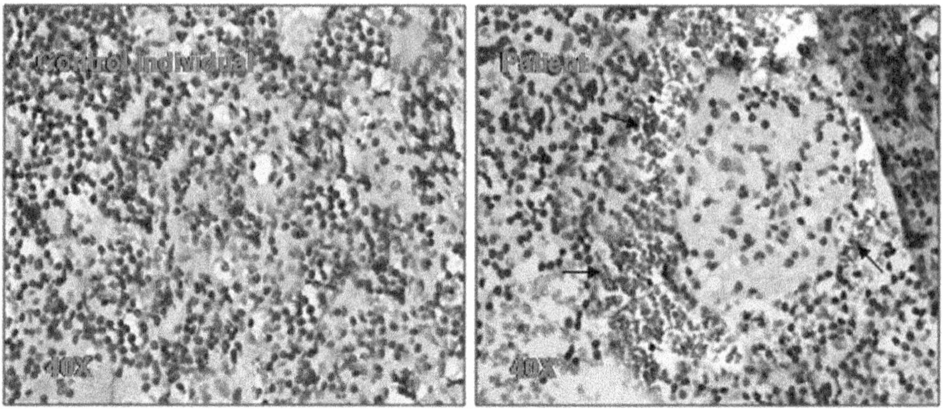

Fig. 1. Immunohistochemical staining for the presence of MSCs (arrows) in granuloma-containing lymph node of patients with tuberculosis. Adapted from Raghuvanshi S. *et al.*, PNAS, 2010.

are some issues which have to be addressed before its actual implementation. Some of them are as follows-

i. Reach of the administered stem cell to its desired destination such as injured tissue and infected/affected organ. Also the effect of endogenous population of the stem cells should be considered.
ii. Proper understanding of the host immune response against the administered stem cell.
iii. Dose of the transplanted stem cells. Also being animal product for administration into patients, long term safety issues has to be understood.
iv. Risk to the patient with secondary infections in case of immune suppression of the host by stem cells. Immuno-compromised condition of the patient may lead to infection of fungus, bacteria and viruses. This should be considered while going for stem cell infiltration and should be tested clinically (Sundin, M. *et al.*, 2006).
v. Although anti-tumor response of MSCs has been observed, they can also suppress anti-tumor immune response. MSCs can be potentially tumorogenic by direct transformation. So, use of MSCs for therapy of patients with high risk to cancer should be avoided.

Since allogenic MSCs are little immunogenic, the other choice should be administration of autologous MSCs. Clinical applications of autologous MSCs of bone marrow has been successfully shown in case of MDR tuberculosis (Erokhin VV., *et al.*, 2008). They have shown that systemic transplantation of the autologous MSCs stopped the bacterial discharge and lung tissue cavities were resolved in tuberculosis patients infected with resistant forms of *Mycobacterium tuberculosis*. Contrary to the role of MSCs in various diseases which have been discussed earlier, where transplantation of these cells is required for treatments of various diseases, report from our lab suggest them as a target for treatment of tuberculosis.

7. Conclusion and future perspectives

Use of stem cells for treatment of many diseases is the area of intensive research these days with many clinical trials undergoing. Mesenchymal stem cells are the main cell type being used due to their longevity and less ethical issues. Still there are many concerns as discussed including their immunogenicity. Suppression of immune system is the other major concern which poses serious threat of other infections to the patients. Studies from our lab using mouse model of tuberculosis suggest role of mesenchymal stem cells in this disease. Besides currently available strategies for treatment of tuberculosis, the probable new target such as MSCs holds promise in the current scenario of MDR and XDR tuberculosis. Targeting MSCs will also wouldn't lead to generation of any new resistance in pathogen as one does not need to target them directly rather manipulate the host immune response. In the coming future we may be able to use MSCs as an immuno-therapeutic target for the treatment of tuberculosis.

8. Acknowledgements

Authors would like to thank Wellcome-DBT India Alliance; Department of Biotechnology, Government of India and Council of Scientific and Industrial Research, Government of India for financial support.

9. References

Barry FP. and Murphy JM, Mesenchymal stem cells: clinical applications and biological characterization. Int J Biochem Cell Biol. 2004, 36 (4): 568-84.

Bartholomew A, Sturgeon C, Siatskas M, Ferrer K, McIntosh K, Patil S, Hardy W, Devine S, Ucker D, Deans R, Moseley A, Hoffman R, Mesenchymal stem cells suppress lymphocyte proliferation in vitro and prolong skin graft survival in vivo. Exp Hematol. 2002, 30 (1): 42-8.

Belyaev NN, Brown DE, Diaz AI, Rae A, Jarra W, Thompson J, Langhorne J, Potocnik AJ, Induction of an IL7-R(+)c-Kit(hi) myelolymphoid progenitor critically dependent on IFN-gamma signaling during acute malaria. Nat Immunol. 2010; 11(6): 477-85.

Bobis S, Jarocha D, Majka M; Mesenchymal stem cells: characteristics and clinical applications. Folia Histochem Cytobiol. 2006; 44(4): 215-30.

Caplan AI, and Dennis JE. Mesenchymal stem cells as trophic mediators. J Cell Biochem. 2006; 98(5): 1076-84.

Colditz GA, Brewer TF, Berkey CS (1994). "Efficacy of BCG Vaccine in the Prevention of Tuberculosis". J Am Med Assoc 271 (9): 698–702.

Corcione A, Benvenuto F, Ferretti E, Giunti D, Cappiello V, Cazzanti F, Risso M, Gualandi F, Mancardi GL, Pistoia V, Uccelli A., Human mesenchymal stem cells modulate B-cell functions. Blood, 2006, 1; 107 (1): 367-72.

Di Nicola M, Carlo-Stella C, Magni M, Milanesi M, Longoni PD, Matteucci P, Grisanti S, Gianni AM., Human bone marrow stromal cells suppress T-lymphocyte proliferation induced by cellular or nonspecific mitogenic stimuli, Blood. 2002; 99(10): 3838-43.

Erokhin VV, Vasil'eva IA, Konopliannikov AG, Chukanov VI, Tsyb AF, Bagdasarian TR, Danilenko AA, Lepekhina LA, Kal'sina SSh, Semenkova IV, Agaeva EV. Systemic transplantation of autologous mesenchymal stem cells of the bone marrow in the treatment of patients with multidrug-resistant pulmonary tuberculosis. Probl Tuberk Bolezn Legk. 2008; (10): 3-6.

Friedenstein AJ, Chailakhyan RK, Latsinik NV, Panasyuk AF, Keiliss-Borok IV. Stromal cells responsible for transferring the microenvironment of the hemopoietic tissues. Cloning in vitro and retransplantation in vivo, Transplantation. 1974; 17 (4): 331-40.

Glennie S, Soeiro I, Dyson PJ, Lam EW, Dazzi F, Bone marrow mesenchymal stem cells induce division arrest anergy of activated T cells, Blood. 2005; 105(7):2821-7.

Goletti D, Weissman D, Jackson RW, et al. Effect of *Mycobacterium tuberculosis* on HIV replication: role of immune activation. J Immunol. 1996; 157: 1271-1278.

Havlir DV, Barnes PF. Tuberculosis in patients with human immunodeficiency virus infection. N Engl J Med. 1999; 340: 367-373.

Herrero C, Pérez-Simón JA, Immunomodulatory effect of mesenchymal stem cells., Braz J Med Biol Res. 2010; 43(5): 425-30.

Hütter G, Nowak D, Mossner M, Ganepola S, Müssig A, Allers K, Schneider T, Hofmann J, Kücherer C, Blau O, Blau IW, Hofmann WK, Thiel E, Long-term control of HIV by CCR5 Delta32/Delta32 stem-cell transplantation. N Engl J Med. 2009; 360(7): 692-8.

Hoffman RA, Mahidhara RS, Wolf-Johnston AS, Lu L, Thomson AW, Simmons RL. Differential modulation of CD4 and CD8 T-cell proliferation by induction of nitric oxide synthesis in antigen presenting cells, Transplantation. 2002; 74(6): 836-45.

Holt N, Wang J, Kim K, Friedman G, Wang X, Taupin V, Crooks G. M., Kohn DB, Gregory PD, Holmes MC and Cannon PM. Human hematopoietic stem/ progenitor cells modified by zink-finger nucleases targeted to CCR5 control HIV-1 in vivo. Nature Biotechnol. 2010; 28 (8): 839-47.

Javazon EH, Beggs KJ, Flake AW. Mesenchymal stem cells: paradoxes of passaging. Exp Hematol. 2004; 32(5): 414-25.

Jiang XX, Zhang Y, Liu B, Zhang SX, Wu Y, Yu XD, Mao N., Human mesenchymal stem cells inhibit differentiation and function of monocyte-derived dendritic cells, Blood. 2005; 105(10): 4120-6.

Jones BE, Young SM, Antoniskis D, Davidson PT, Kramer F, Barnes PF, Relationship of the manifestations of tuberculosis to CD4 cell counts in patients with human immunodeficiency virus infection. Am Rev Respir Dis. 1993;148(5):1292-7.

Le Blanc K, Rasmusson I, Sundberg B, Götherström C, Hassan M, Uzunel M, Ringdén O. Treatment of severe acute graft-versus-host disease with third party haploidentical mesenchymal stem cells. Lancet. 2004; 363(9419):1439-41.

Le Blanc K and Ringdén O, Immunobiology of human mesenchymal stem cells and future use in hematopoietic stem cell transplantation, Biol Blood Marrow Transplant. 2005; 11(5): 321-34.

Le Blanc K and Ringden O., Mesenchymal stem cells: Properties and role in clinical bone marrow transplantation, Curr. Opin. Immunol. (2006), 18, pp. 586–591.

Le Blanc K, Tammik C, Rosendahl K, Zetterberg E, Ringdén O., HLA expression and immunologic properties of differentiated and undifferentiated mesenchymal stem cells, Exp Hematol. 2003; 31(10): 890-6.

Le Blanc K, Tammik L, Sundberg B, Haynesworth SE, Ringdén O., Mesenchymal stem cells inhibit and stimulate mixed lymphocyte cultures and mitogenic responses independently of the major histocompatibility complex., Scand J Immunol. 2003; 57(1): 11-20.

Kitchen SG, Bennett M, Galić Z, Kim J, Xu Q, Young A, Lieberman A, Joseph A, Goldstein H, Ng H, Yang O, Zack JA. Engineering antigen-specific T cells from genetically modified human hematopoietic stem cells in immunodeficient mice. PLoS One. 2009; 4(12)

Koç ON, Day J, Nieder M, Gerson SL, Lazarus HM, Krivit W. Allogeneic mesenchymal stem cell infusion for treatment of metachromatic leukodystrophy (MLD) and Hurler syndrome (MPS-IH), Bone Marrow Transplant. 2002; 30(4): 215-22.

Krampera M, Glennie S, Dyson J, Scott D, Laylor R, Simpson E, Dazzi F, Bone marrow mesenchymal stem cells inhibit the response of naive and memory antigen-specific T cells to their cognate peptide, Blood. 2003; 101(9): 3722-9.

Lancaster J.R. Jr., A tutorial on the diffusibility and reactivity of free nitric oxide. Nitric Oxide 1 (1997), pp. 18–30.

Lazebnik LB, Konopliannikov AG, Kniazev OV, Parfenov AI, Tsaregorodtseva TM, Ruchkina IN, Khomeriki SG, Rogozina VA, Konopliannikova OA. Use of allogeneic mesenchymal stem cells in the treatment of intestinal inflammatory diseases. Ter Arkh. 2010; 82(2): 38-43.

Lazebnik LB, Konopliannikov AG, Parfenov AI, Kniazev OV, Parfenov AI, Ruchkina IN, Khomeriki SG, Rogozina VA, Konopliannikova OA, Tsaregorodtseva TM. Application of allogeneic mesenchymal stem cells in complex patients treatment with ulcerative colitis. Eksp Klin Gastroenterol. 2009; (5): 4-12.

Lin H, Xu R, Zhang Z, Chen L, Shi M, Wang FS, Implications of the immunoregulatory functions of mesenchymal stem cells in the treatment of human liver diseases. Cell Mol Immunol. 2011, 8(1): 19-22.

Mei SH, Haitsma JJ, Dos Santos CC, Deng Y, Lai PF, Slutsky AS, Liles WC, Stewart DJ. Mesenchymal Stem Cells Reduce Inflammation while Enhancing Bacterial Clearance and Improving Survival in Sepsis. Am J Respir Crit Care Med. 2010 Oct 15; 182(8): 1047-57.

Melgar S and Shanahan F, Inflammatory bowel disease- from mechanisms to treatment strategies. Autoimmunity. 2010; 43(7): 463-77.

Moretta A, Bottino C, Vitale M, Pende D, Cantoni C, Mingari MC, Biassoni R, Moretta L. Activating receptors and coreceptors involved in human natural killer cell-mediated cytolysis. Annu Rev Immunol. 2001; 19: 197-223.

Nakata K, Rom WN, Honda Y, et al. *Mycobacterium tuberculosis* enhances human immunodeficiency virus-1 replication in the lung. Am J Respir Crit Care Med. 1997; 155: 996-1003.

Newman RE, Yoo D, LeRoux MA, Danilkovitch-Miagkova A. Treatment of inflammatory diseases with mesenchymal stem cells. Inflamm Allergy Drug Targets. 2009; 8(2):110-23.

Niedbala W., B. Cai and F.Y. Liew, Role of nitric oxide in the regulation of T cell functions, Ann. Rheum. *Dis.* 65 (Suppl 3) (2006), pp. iii37–iii40.

Ortiz LA, Gambelli F, McBride C, Gaupp D, Baddoo M, Kaminski N, Phinney DG. Mesenchymal stem cell engraftment in lung is enhanced in response to bleomycin exposure and ameliorates its fibrotic effects. Proc Natl Acad Sci U S A. 2003; 100(14): 8407-11.

Peter A. Otto, A. Agid, Suzan and Mushtaha, MDR-TB is in town; and might be tugging along XDR-TB. SSMJ Vol 2 Issue 3 (www.southernsudanmedicaljournal.com).

Raghuvanshi S, Sharma P, Singh S, Van Kaer L, Das G. Mycobacterium tuberculosis evades host immunity by recruiting mesenchymal stem cells. Proc Natl Acad Sci U S A. 2010, 107(50): 21653-8.

Ramasamy R, Fazekasova H, Lam EW, Soeiro I, Lombardi G, Dazzi F. Mesenchymal stem cells inhibit dendritic cell differentiation and function by preventing entry into the cell cycle, Transplantation. 2007; 83(1): 71-6.

Ren G, Zhang L, Zhao X, Xu G, Zhang Y, Roberts AI, Zhao RC, Shi Y. Mesenchymal stem cell-mediated immunosuppression occurs via concerted action of chemokines and nitric oxide. Cell Stem Cell. 2008, 7; 2(2): 141-50.

Ren G, Zhao X, Zhang L, Zhang J, L'Huillier A, Ling W, Roberts AI, Le AD, Shi S, Shao C, Shi Y. Inflammatory cytokine-induced intercellular adhesion molecule-1 and vascular cell adhesion molecule-1 in mesenchymal stem cells are critical for immunosuppression. J Immunol. 2010; 184(5): 2321-8.

Saei, A. A. and Ahmadian, S. Stem cell engineering might be protective against severe malaria Bioscience Hypotheses Volume 2, Issue 1, 2009, Pages 48-49.

Schroder K, Hertzog PJ, Ravasi T, Hume DA. Interferon-gamma: an overview of signals, mechanisms and functions". J. Leukoc. Biol. 2004, 75(2): 163–89.

Scott-Browne JP, Shafiani S, Tucker-Heard G, Ishida-Tsubota K, Fontenot JD, Rudensky AY, Bevan MJ, Urdahl KB. Expansion and function of Foxp3-expressing T regulatory cells during tuberculosis. J Exp Med. 2007;204(9): 2159-69.

Shi Y, Hu G, Su J, Li W, Chen Q, Shou P, Xu C, Chen X, Huang Y, Zhu Z, Huang X, Han X, Xie N, Ren G. Mesenchymal stem cells: a new strategy for immunosuppression and tissue repair. Cell Res. 2010; 20(5): 510-8.

Siegmund B and Zeitz M, Innate and adaptive immunity in inflammatory bowel disease. World J Gastroenterol. 2011; 17(27): 3178-83.

Stagg J, Pommey S, Eliopoulos N, Galipeau J, Interferon-gamma-stimulated marrow stromal cells: a new type of nonhematopoietic antigen-presenting cell, Blood. 2006; 107(6): 2570-7.

Steven G Deeks and Joseph M McCune, Can HIV be cured with stem cell therapy? Nature Biotechnology, 2010, 28, 807–810.

Sundin M, Orvell C, Rasmusson I, Sundberg B, Ringdén O, Le Blanc K, Mesenchymal stem cells are susceptible to human herpesviruses, but viral DNA cannot be detected in the healthy seropositive individual, Bone Marrow Transplant. 2006; 37(11): 1051-9.

Sudres M, Norol F, Trenado A, Grégoire S, Charlotte F, Levacher B, Lataillade JJ, Bourin P, Holy X, Vernant JP, Klatzmann D, Cohen JL. Bone marrow mesenchymal stem cells suppress lymphocyte proliferation in vitro but fail to prevent graft-versus-host disease in mice. J Immunol. 2006; 176(12): 7761-7.

Tabera S, Pérez-Simón JA, Díez-Campelo M, Sánchez-Abarca LI, Blanco B, López A, Benito A, Ocio E, Sánchez-Guijo FM, Cañizo C, San Miguel JF, The effect of mesenchymal stem cells on the viability, proliferation and differentiation of B-lymphocytes, Haematologica. 2008; 93(9):1301-9.

Teng YD, Lavik EB, Qu X, Park KI, Ourednik J, Zurakowski D, Langer R, Snyder EY; Functional recovery following traumatic spinal cord injury mediated by a unique polymer scaffold seeded with neural stem cells; Proc Natl Acad Sci U S A. 2002; 99(5): 3024-9.

Tse WT, Pendleton JD, Beyer WM, Egalka MC, Guinan EC., Suppression of allogeneic T-cell proliferation by human marrow stromal cells: implications in transplantation, Transplantation. 2003, 75(3): 389-97.

Xu G, Zhang L, Ren G, Yuan Z, Zhang Y, Zhao RC, Shi Y. Immunosuppressive properties of cloned bone marrow mesenchymal stem cells. Cell Res. 2007; 17(3): 240-8.

Von Lüttichau I, Notohamiprodjo M, Wechselberger A, Peters C, Henger A, Seliger C, Djafarzadeh R, Huss R, Nelson PJ. Human adult CD34- progenitor cells functionally express the chemokine receptors CCR1, CCR4, CCR7, CXCR5, and CCR10 but not CXCR4, Stem Cells Dev. 2005; 14(3): 329-36.

Wong RS, Mesenchymal stem cells: angels or demons? J Biomed Biotechnol. 2011; 2011: 459510.

10

The Importance of Haem vs Non-Haem Iron in the Survival and Pathogenesis of *Brucella abortus*

Marta A. Almirón[1], Nidia E. Lucero[2] and Norberto A. Sanjuan[3]
[1]*Universidad Nacional de San Martín/Instituto de Investigaciones Biotecnológicas*
[2]*Instituto Nacional de Enfermedades Infecciosas-ANLIS "Dr. C. G. Malbrán", Departamento de Bacteriología,*
[3]*Universidad de Buenos Aires/ Facultad de Medicina/ Departamento de Microbiología*
Argentina

1. Introduction

The genus *Brucella* belongs to the alpha-group of proteobacteria, along with plant pathogens as *Agrobacterium* and symbionts as *Rhizobium* and *Bradyrhizobium*. Several *Brucella* species, highly related at the genetic level, have been identified as the etiological agents of brucellosis. Each one has shown a preferred host although they can infect other animals. Animal brucellosis is usually endemic in developing countries and its main impact is economic. Human brucellosis is difficult to diagnose because symptoms are extremely variable. Few live vaccines are available for animals only, not for humans. The main problems with this pathogen are the lack of virulence factors commonly identified in other bacteria and the ability to establish a niche inside eukaryotic cells, where they replicate and survive evading the immune response and the action of other antibacterial molecules.

In general, the pathogenic mechanisms used by bacteria have been related to iron because this essential cellular nutrient is scarce and not easily available for bacteria either in body fluids or inside eukaryotic cells. Thus, the iron deficient environment that bacteria encounter during infection induces genes which products are needed to support effective survival and thus they became part of virulence factors. Most of them are related to the acquisition of ionic iron or iron-containing molecules (Schaible & Kaufmann, 2004).

In the case of *Brucella*, much effort has been put into the study of this organism under iron limitation. The first reports about the nutritional preferences showed an absolute requirement for iron (Gerhardt, 1958). Further studies, mainly on *Brucella abortus* (the causative agent of brucellosis in cattle) have shown that *Brucella* produce two catecholic compounds, 2,3-dyhidroxybenzoic acid (2,3-DHBA) and brucebactin, as siderophores under iron limitation (Gonzalez Carrero et al., 2002; Lopez-Goñi et al., 1992). However, experimental evidence on mutants unable to synthesize those molecules failed to demonstrate that their production is critical for bacterial replication inside macrophages (Bellaire et al., 1999; Jain et al., 2011). In addition, a mutant in the main iron-response regulator gene, with deficient synthesis of siderophores and increased intracellular haem content, showed a better replication pattern inside professional phagocytes than wild type (Martinez et al., 2006). On the other hand, a *B.*

abortus mutant that can not ensemble iron into protoporphyrin IX to produce its own haem was unable to survive inside professional phagocytes (Almiron et al., 2001). Another *B. abortus* mutant that can not internalize haem from the medium showed significant attenuation in cultured murine macrophages (Paulley et al., 2007). None of these two mutants could establish a wild-type pattern of infection in the mice model. Therefore, taking into consideration all these results, it seems that under iron limitation, as one of the stress conditions that probably *Brucella* face during infection, the acquisition or biosynthesis of haem renders more benefits to survive than the acquisition of iron. In agreement with this, we found that a mutation in the main iron-reservoir protein of *B. abortus* did not affect its replication inside professional phagocytes (Almiron & Ugalde, 2010).

For a long time, a link has been established between the preference of *Brucella* to use erythritol as a carbon and energy source and the pathogenesis of this organism, based on experimental data (Smith et al., 1962). This molecule is present at high concentrations in placental trophoblast, the preferred niche for *Brucella*. One of the plausible explanations to this link is the bacterial necessity for iron to catabolized erythritol. Without interfering with this theory, it is apparent that placenta is a membranous-vascular organ that receives nutrients from the mother´s blood providing in this way a high content of haem. Additionally, haem is known to be the main iron source inside eukaryotic cells.

2. Involvement of iron in the replication of *B. abortus*

B. abortus, like most pathogenic bacteria, presents an absolute requirement for the micronutrient iron to support growth (Gerardt, 1958). Bacteria utilize iron as a cofactor or as a prosthetic group for essential enzymes that participates in many biological processes, such as metabolism, respiration, oxygen transport, and gene regulation. Iron is one of the most abundant elements in nature but its bioavailability is reduced under physiological conditions. The oxidised Fe^{3+} ferric form is predominant in the environment under aerobic atmospheres with very low solubility at neutral pH (10^{-18} M), and even lower (10^{-36}M) in solution due to its tendency to hydrolyze and form polymers (Andrews et al., 2003). In animals, iron is bound to proteins in order to keep the metal soluble and to avoid toxic reactions due to its redox potential. Intracellularly, iron is chelated by a porphyrin ring giving rise to haem. However, the chelated metal iron can undergo reversible oxidative changes and thus haem is mainly associated to proteins. In this way, free iron is practically unavailable for bacteria in the host.

B. abortus is able to acquire iron in different ways. Directly, through the synthesis and secretion of two catecholic siderophores, 2,3-DHBA and the more complex compound derived from this known as brucebactin. Both of them are synthesized by the enzymes encoded in the *dhbCEBA* operon in response to iron limitation (Gonzalez Carrero et al., 2002; Lopez-Goñi et al., 1992). The indirect way is by the incorporation of haemin as an iron source (Almirón et al., 2001; Paulley et al., 2007).

B. abortus stores iron mainly in a bacterioferritin. This molecule represents a ferritin that contains haem. In *Brucella*, the bacterioferritin is a homopolymer that accumulates approximately 70% of the intracellular iron (Almirón & Ugalde, 2010). Another protein considered as a miniferritin, Dps, is expressed in *Brucella* and could be contributing with iron storage in this pathogen during the stationary phase of growth (Almiron et al., 1992;

Lamontagne et al., 2009). According to the phenotype of a *B. abortus bfr* mutant it was suggested that this microorganism senses the Bfr-bound iron available for metabolism, by an unknown mechanism, and thus regulates iron homeostasis independently of the external iron concentration (Almiron & Ugalde, 2010).

2.1 Extracellular survival

The acquisition of iron from the environment is a process tightly regulated by bacteria in order to keep iron homeostasis. An excess of free intracellular iron can be devastating for bacterial survival. The iron-uptake system by siderophores, low-molecular chelators with high-affinity towards ferric iron, means the production of the compounds plus the proteins needed for transportation and reception of ferric-siderophores complexes. The transport is usually mediated by the energy-transducing TonB-ExbB-ExbD system in Gram-negative bacteria (Andrews et al., 2003).

In this regard, the TonB system, an ABC transporter, and a putative GTPase were shown to be involved in iron acquisition of *B. melitensis*. The *exbB*, *dstC* and *dugA* genes are needed for the assimilation of DHBA and /or ferric citrate (Danese et al., 2004). Is it probably that they have the same effect in *B. abortus*.

2.1.1 The complex regulation of siderophore biosynthesis

The *B. abortus dhbCEBA* operon is repressed during growth under iron-sufficient conditions while it is highly induced under iron limitation (Lopez-Goñi et al., 1992). The transcriptional regulators acting on the promoter region of the *dhbCEBA* operon are Irr and DhbR. The iron-response regulator, Irr, is a member of the Fur family, and DhbR of the AraC family. Both proteins have demonstrated to interact with the DNA *in vitro* by the electrophoretic mobility shift assay (Anderson et al., 2008; Martinez et al., 2006). The *B. abortus irr* gene is constitutively transcribed regardless of the external iron concentration, but no protein could be detected under iron-sufficient conditions (Martinez et al., 2005). The transcription of *dhbR* is iron repressible and seems to be under the transcriptional control of Irr. A putative binding site for Irr was found between the -35 and -10 regions related to the transcriptional start of the *dhbR* gene (Anderson et al., 2008). The induction of *dhbC* transcription by Irr and DhbR has been correlated with the reduced production of siderophores in the culture media of the *irr* and *dhbR* mutants, respectively, and in comparison with the wild type. In both studies, the transcription was analyzed by constructing *dhbC*-lacZ fusions. To study the Irr regulation, the fusion was carried out to the *B. abortus* chromosome causing a mutation in the gene that enabled the strain to produce siderophores. In this case, a two-fold induction was observed in the wild type in comparison with the *irr* mutant (Martinez et al., 2006). In the other work, the authors assayed the β-galactosidase activity of a plasmid-borne lacZ fusion expressed in different genetic backgrounds. Interestingly, they found equivalent reduction in the enzyme activity expressed either in *B. abortus dhbR* or in *B. abortus dhbC* mutants. In this way, the authors corroborated that DhbR needs siderophores as a coinducer to repress transcription. This mode of action was described for other AraC-like regulators (Anderson et al., 2008). If DhbR acts in this way, the cause of the remaining levels of the enzyme activity detected in the *B. abortus irr dhbC* mutant under iron limitation should be investigated.

Neither Irr nor DhbR are involved in the transcriptional repression of the *dhbCEBA* operon. In order to have an accurate control of iron metabolism, the Irr protein is unstable under iron-sufficient conditions. The *Brucella* genome encodes two *irr* paralogues as other members of the alpha-proteobacteria group (Martinez et al., 2005). It has not been studied yet if the *B. abortus irr* ortologue is expressed and plays a role in iron-dependent regulation.

Other regulators that could be involved in iron homeostasis have been described by genomic sequence analysis, like RirA (Johnston et al., 2007; Rodionov et al., 2006). But, the lack of experimental results limits our understanding of this subject in *Brucella*.

Beyond this, the fact that more than two regulators modulate the transcription of the genes involved in the biosynthesis of both siderophores is an indication of the importance of the non-haem iron acquisition in the survival of *Brucella* under iron limitation. The idea that siderophores contribute to the virulence of several pathogens -such as *Escherichia coli* and *Vibrio cholerae*- is based on the capacity they give to the bacteria to acquire an essential nutrient under iron limitation. However, this role has not been well defined in *Brucella* yet, as we will discuss below.

2.1.2 Could erythritol be related to siderophore production due to its osmotic property?

The attenuation of a *B. abortus dhbC* mutant in pregnant cattle settled the bases for the relationship between iron acquisition and erythritol catabolism (Bellaire et al., 2003a). Bellaire and colleagues found that the production of siderophores was stimulated by the presence of erythritol in the media, and this effect was also observed at transcriptional level. The wild-type *B. abortus* harboring a plasmid-borne *dhbC-lacZ* fusion showed an increment in the β-galactosidase levels when grown in the presence of erythritol than that observed when this polyalcohol was not added. In order to explain this observation, they hypothesized that wild-type *B. abortus* experience an increased demand for iron in order to catabolize erythritol, since one of the enzymes involved in this metabolic pathway needs iron as a cofactor.

Interestingly, we found that if instead of the minimal media MG (usually employed to test siderophore production in *B. abortus* strains) we used the minimal media MM, no siderophores detection was possible after bacterial growth although iron was not present. The composition of this defined media is: $(NH_4)_2SO_4$ 2 g, KH_2PO_4 7 g, glucose 4 g, casaminoacids 10 g, $MnCl_2$ 100 μg, $MgSO_4$ 100 mg, biotin 2 μg, nicotinic acid 0.4 mg, piridoxal 0.4 mg, thiamin 0.4 mg and pantoteic acid 0.4 mg per liter; pH 7. A comparative look at the composition of both media led us to find a remarkable difference related to NaCl and glycerol, present in 7.5 g/l (128mM) and 37.5 g/l respectively in MG media. Thus, we decided to supplement MM with NaCl and glycerol and test for catechole production.

The results presented in Table 1 indicate that the *B. abortus* siderophore production was induced by increasing amounts of NaCl or glycerol. Moreover, both osmolytes act in a synergistic mode when added together to the MM media. An increment in siderophore production was also obtained when manitol was added to MM, suggesting that the phenotype was not restricted to ionic osmolytes. To test if this induction was exerted at transcriptional level, the β-galactosidase of the *B. abortus* chromosomal *dhbC-lacZ* fusion was

Medium	MM	MM	MM	MM	MM	MG
NaCl (g/l)	-	5	10	-	10	-
Glicerol (g/l)	-	-	-	37,5	37,5	-
[SD]/OD_{600}	1.9	13.0	34.4	21.3	122.6	51.4

Table 1. Effects of NaCl and glycerol on *B. abortus* siderophore production. *B. abortus* siderophore secretion expressed as nmol/ml related to cell density from the wild-type 2308 strain grown in MG or MM media supplemented with NaCl and glycerol at the indicated concentrations. Data are from one experiment made in duplicates and representative of more than four independent experiments.

measured in MM media supplemented with different amounts of NaCl. The results, as shown in Table 2, demonstrate that osmolality plays a role in *dhbC* transcription and consequently in siderophore secretion.

mM NaCl in MM	0	50	100	200
β-galactosidase (Miller units)	21.8	23.2	93.3	439.1

Table 2. Effects of NaCl on the *B. abortus dhbC* transcription. β-Galactosidase activity from *B. abortus dhbC-lacZ* grown in MM supplemented with NaCl at the indicated concentrations. Data are representative of at least three independent experiments.

Even though *Bacillus subtilis* is a Gram-positive bacterium, it produces a similar catechol molecule, 2,3-dihydroxybenzoate, that is finally modified to render the siderophore bacillibactin with stronger chelation capacity than the precursor. The enzymes that participate in their biosynthetic pathway are encoded in the *dhbACEBF* operon. It was reported that high salinity causes iron limitation in *B. subtilis* and triggers the derepression of iron-controlled genes present in the operon mentioned before (Hoffmann et al., 2002). Iron limitation as well as high salinity led to the accumulation of comparable amounts of siderophores in the bacterial culture. This phenotype as well as the growth deficiency observed under high salinity could be reduced by an excess of iron. In this microorganism, the ferric uptake regulator Fur is repressing the genes when sufficient iron is present (Hoffmann et al., 2002). In this relation, it should be noted that erythritol is an osmolyte and curiously, it has been shown that the growth of the *B. abortus dhbC* mutant in iron-limited media supplemented with erythritol is enhanced by the addition of iron (Bellaire et al., 2003a).

Similarly, a *B. abortus entF* mutant presented a growth deficiency under iron limitation in comparison with wild type, which was reverted by the addition of iron (Jain et al., 2011). The product of *entF* is involved in the production of brucebactin (Gonzalez Carrero et al., 2002). It was shown that the *B. abortus entF* mutant was not able to increase the number of viable cells when incubated under iron limitation. Interestingly, the mutant culture had not lost viability before a period of 192 h of incubation as an indication that the internal-iron content was enough to support metabolism in the experimental conditions used. Instead, a decrease in the number of viable cells was observed when the medium was supplemented with erythritol, but this phenotype was reverted by the addition of iron salts. These data indicate, besides the role that the product of *entF* could have in the erythritol metabolism as suggested, the relationship between siderophore production and erythritol. Is it possible that *Brucella* needs to acquire iron in order to survive under osmotic pressure?

No data about the growth phenotype of iron-depleted cells in media containing erythritol has been reported. This information may be important if it is considered that the host imposes iron limitation as a defense mechanism against microbial infection (Schaible & Kaufmann, 2004). Under this circumstance, it is likely to find iron-depleted bacteria from host's samples. A similar situation could be considered if the bacterial samples came from environment. Taking into account that *Brucella* modulates iron-dependent gene regulation according to their iron content and independently of the external iron concentration, it should be appropriate to test the survival efficiency of iron-depleted *brucella* in media that contain erythritol, such as the modified Brucella selective medium that has been developed to be used for diagnostic purposes (Her et al., 2010).

2.1.3 Fur regulation

Bfr is a homopolymeric hemoprotein that functions as the main iron-reservoir of *Brucella*. As other members of the alpha-proteobacteria group, the *Brucella* iron-dependent regulation responds to the internal iron concentration (Almirón & Ugalde, 2010). Hence, a mutation in the *B. abortus bfr* induces siderophore biosynthesis and secretion earlier than in the wild-type strain under iron limitation (Almirón & Ugalde, 2010). It has been described that the promoter region of the *dhbCEBA* operon is subjected to the regulation of Irr and DhbR proteins under iron limitation. Both were able to bind the promoter region *in vitro*. The same region has also two putative Fur boxes. Fur is the main iron-dependent regulator in many bacteria. It usually represses genes when bound to iron. Therefore, if iron is not available there should be a derepression of fur-regulated genes. In order to understand whether Fur participates in the *dhbCEBA* regulation we constructed mutants by inserting a kanamicin-resistant cassette in the amplified *fur* gene and then, by carring this mutation to the chromosome of the wild-type *B. abortus* 2308 and the isogenic *bfr* or *dhbC-lacZ* mutants by homologous recombination as described previously (Martinez, 2004). As shown in Figure 1, we determined the β-galactosidase activity of the chromosomal *dhbC*-lacZ fusion in the background of the parental and *fur* mutant strains. We included the *bfr dhbC* mutant strain for comparative purpose (Almirón & Ugalde, 2010).

The experiments were done when cells were grown in MG or iron-supplemented MG. Although the absence of Fur did not produce the same effect on the *dhbC* transcription, the small induction observed among cultures at $OD_{600} \leq 1$ led us to look more precisely at siderophore production in the wild-type, *bfr* and *fur* isogenic mutants.

It is interesting to note that when the cells have the possibility to acquire external iron by means of siderophores, the results can be different. While the wild type did not sense internal iron limitation during the first hours of incubation in MG, the consequence of Fur absence is equivalent to the internal-iron deficiency produced by the mutation in *bfr*, in terms of siderophore secretion (Figure 2A). In contrast, in the presence of external iron the *bfr* mutant represses the biosynthesis as wild type, while *fur* did not (Figure 2B). To determine if the repression observed in *bfr* mutant was due to Fur, a *B. abortus bfr fur* double mutant was constructed. The results suggest that Fur is regulating siderophore production

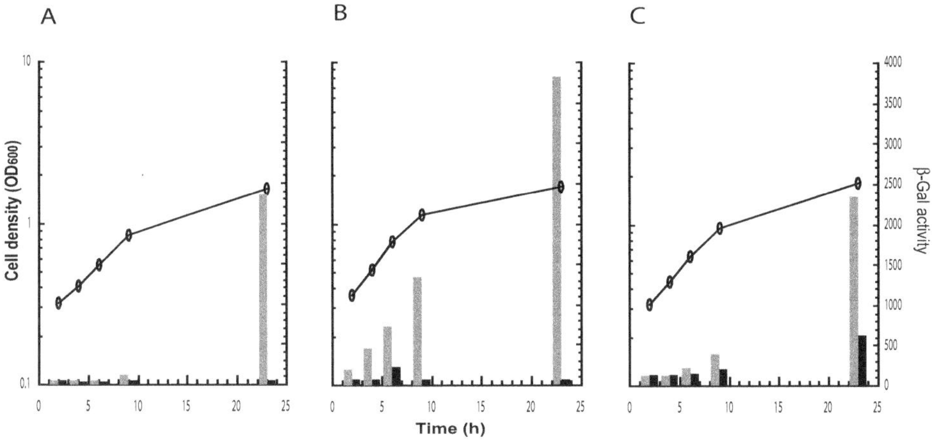

Fig. 1. Effect of iron concentration on *dhbCEBA* transcription. β-Galactosidase activity (Miller units) was determined from *B. abortus* 2308 derivatives growing in MG (gray bars) or in MG supplemented with 50 μM iron citrate (black bars). (**A**) *B. abortus* 2308 *dhbC,* (**B**) 2308 *bfr dhbC,* and (**C**) 2308 *fur dhbC.* Growth curves in MG were determined by measurment of OD_{600} (lines). Data are average of duplicates, standard deviation were less than 5%.

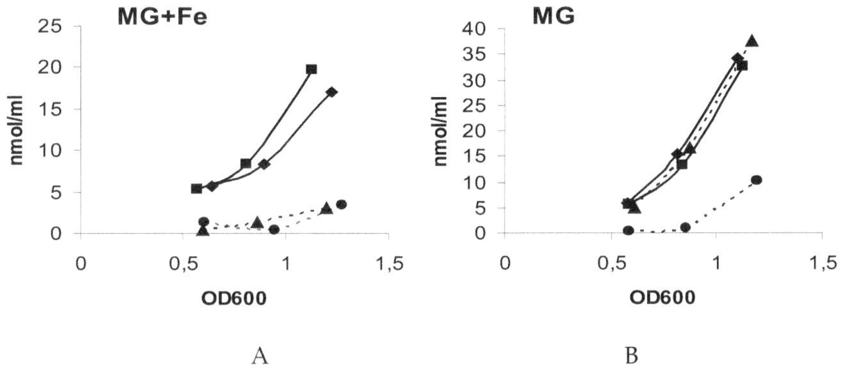

Fig. 2. *B. abortus* siderophore secretion in response to external iron concentration. Concentration of siderophores related to cell density from *B. abortus* 2308 (..●..), 2308 *fur* (-■-), 2308 *fur bfr* (-♦-), and 2308 *bfr* (..▲..).Values of catechol concentration (determined by the Arnow assay) are expressed from duplicates at three different time points during incubation. Results are representative of three independent experiments.

in *Brucella abortus* under iron sufficient conditions. Further studies are needed to determine the promoter region that interacts with Fur-Fe complexes.

There is a previous report showing that a *fur* mutant was producing less β-galactosidase activities than the wild type in MG. No differences were observed in the presence of iron. It should be noted that the data were obtained from a plasmid-borned *dhbC-lacZ* fusion expressed either in the wild-type *B. abortus* or in the isogenic *fur* mutant (Roop, et al., 2004).

Because the extracellular iron concentration does not represent the *Brucella* iron content, the experimental conditions used to test the *dhbC*-lacZ fusion, sometimes in a plasmid and others in the chromosome causing a mutation in the *dhbC* gene, do not result trivial, especially with Fur that needs intracellular free-iron to bind DNA near the promoter region of a gene. Thus, it should be important to determine the transcriptional level of the *dhbCEBA* operon relative to the internal iron content in *Brucella* strains in order to get comparable results and to better understand iron homeostasis in this pathogen.

2.1.4 Production of outer-membrane vesicles under iron limitation

The dogma that bacteria induce virulence factors under iron limitation and the possibility to find them concentrated in outer-membrane vesicles, as described for other pathogens, led us to isolate *B. abortus* membrane vesicles from cells grown in iron rich (2xYT) and iron-depleted (2xYT treated with 150 μM DIP) media at 37 °C for 1 week in a CO_2 incubator. Cells were collected in saline solution and heated at 60 °C for 30 minutes. Cells were discarded by centrifugation at 13,000 x g. Supernatants were centrifuged at 18,500 rpm for 30 min in the 70Ti Beckman-rotor. A second centrifugation of the supernatant was done at 43,500 rpm for 3 h in the same rotor for further purification. The pellet was suspended in PBS and tested under transmission-electron microscopy for the presence of pure vesicles. Samples of equal volume were subjected to electrophoresis in polyacrylamide gels and stained with Coomassie blue for protein detection. Proteins were detected only from cultures grown with iron limitation.

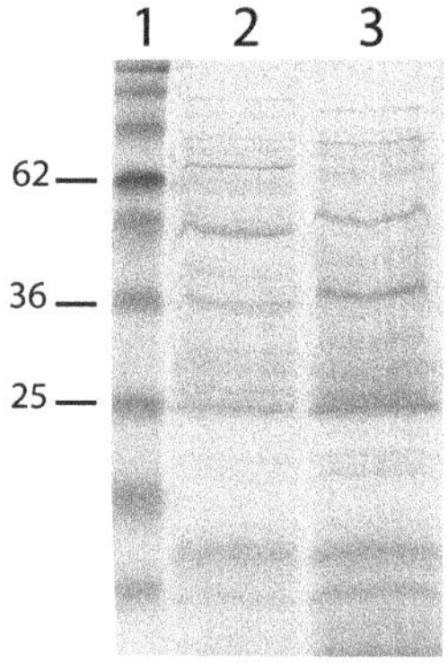

Fig. 3. Outer-membrane vesicles from *B. abortus* in response to iron limitation. 15% SDS-PAGE analysis of proteins obtained from outer-membrane vesicles preparations of *B. abortus* grown under iron limitation at 5 (line 2) and 15 days (line 3). Molecular mass standards (line1); kilodaltons are indicated on the left.

As shown in Figure 3, similar patterns were observed from cultures incubated between 5 and 15 days under the conditions mentioned before. Interestingly, it was also observed in samples prepared from *B. abortus irr* and *bfr* mutants.

The peptides obtained from the 36 KDa (adaivaxepeaveyv and ntvaednaxggiv) and the 25 KDa bands (enxgyv and adaivaqpateid) identified after trypsin digestion followed by HPLC-MS, led us to identify the porin Omp2b and OmpW as the major proteins expressed in *brucella* vesicles produced under iron limitation.

The bacterial liberation to the culture media of outer-membrane vesicles represents a phenomenon that has been described for many bacteria including *Brucella* (Gamazo et al., 1987; 1989). The origin of these bacterial structures and their function are still under investigation. So far, there is no genetic evidence supporting the idea that bacteria can regulate its production. In terms of function, it has been hypothesized that they can contribute to bacterial virulence by evading the immunological host-defense mechanisms and by redirecting or preserving the virulence factors accumulated in their lumen. In this regard, further studies are needed to understand whether the presence of these proteins in the *brucella* vesicles has a meaning in the virulence of this pathogen.

2.2 Intracellular growth

The growth- deficient phenotype of the B. *abortus bfr* observed under iron limitation *in vitro* was not reproduced when cells were growing intracellularly (Almiron & Ugalde, 2010). Nonetheless, we investigated whether siderophores were assisting *B. abortus bfr* for intracellular replication. The gentamicin protection assay was done in HeLa cells with the parental strain and the isogenic *bfr* and *bfr dhbC* mutants. Similar results were obtained for all strains (Figure 4) indicating that siderophores are not involved in *B. abortus bfr* intracellular survival.

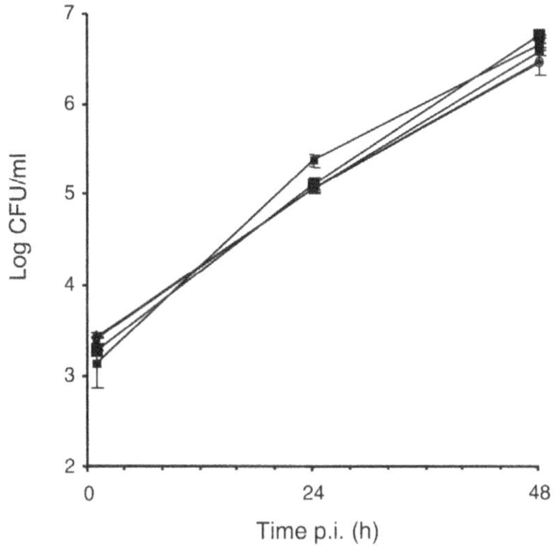

Fig. 4. Intracellular survival of *B. abortus* strains in HeLa cells. Monolayers of HeLa (10^5 cells/well) were infected with wild-type 2308 (■), 2308 *bfr* (•), 2308*dhbC* (Δ) and 2308 *bfr dhbC* (▲). At different times p.i. cells were lysed to determine the number of viable intracellular bacteria (CFU/ml). Data are expressed as means and standard deviations from one experiment performed in triplicate. They are representative of three independent experiments.

B. abortus mutants unable to produce 2,3-DHBA and brucebactin (*B. abortus dhbC* and *entF*) presented a wild-type behavior when infecting murine macrophages (Bellaire et al., 1999; Jain et al., 2011).

The role of *exbB, dstC* and *dugA* in the intracellular replication of *Brucella* were tested in bovine macrophages and in HeLa cells. None of these mutants showed attenuation in comparison to the wild type (Danese et al., 2004). These results are in agreement with those obtained with mutants that do not produce 2,3-DHBA.

A proteomic analysis of intracellular *B. abortus* recovered at different times after infection of murine macrophages revealed that proteins related to iron and haem transport were reduced during the first hours post-infection (p.i.) and interestingly, were induced after 20 or 44 h p.i (Lamontagne et al., 2009). These results suggest that once in the endoplasmic reticulum-related vacuole *Brucella* could get access to iron-sources facilitating the intracellular replication. In general, when *Brucella* infects a professional phagocytic cell-line, there is about one log reduction in the intracellular number of colony-forming units after 12 h p.i. Thus, it can not be discarded that the iron source encountered by *Brucella* latter in times have bacterial origin. The ferritins Bfr and Dps were reported to remain uninduced after 3 h of infection.

2.3 In animals

B. abortus dhbC was as virulent as wild type in the murine model using Balb/C mice, though this strain showed attenuation in pregnant cattle (Bellaire et al., 1999; 2003b). The author attributed the difference to the presence of erythritol in the bovine placental trophoblast which is absent in mice.

The *B. melitensis exbB, dstC* and *dugA* mutants were also tested for virulence in Balb/C mice. According to the bacterial counts obtained from mouse spleens at 1 and 4 weeks p.i., no difference was observed between wild type and mutants (Danese et al., 2004).

According to these data, the iron acquisition systems do not seem to be involved in *Brucella* pathogenicity when tested in a mouse model. The significance in the natural host requires further experimentation.

3. Involvement of haem in the replication of *B. abortus*

Whilst pathogenic bacteria possess different mechanisms for extracellular haem incorporation, their own biosynthesis is considered to be the main haem source.

The haem biosynthetic pathway in alpha-proteobacteria is similar to that in animal and yeast mitochondria. It starts with the action of the ALA synthase and finishes with the ferrochelatase. The last step, corresponding to the incorporation of a ferrous iron into protoporphyring IX, can be affected by the availability of intracellular iron, a condition usually faced by bacteria during infection. The oxidative characteristic of the chelated iron allows haem to participate as a cofactor in oxidative reactions. This type of reactions plays an important role in electron transfer for metabolism or energy generation (O'Brian & Thony-Meyer, 2002) and can also be employed in signal transduction systems. It has been described that haem participates in the sensing of diatomic gases and in the transcriptional and post-transcriptional regulation of several genes (Genco & Dixon, 2001).

Bacteria can produce cell lysis to gain access to the intracellular haem by secreting cellular proteases or haemolysins, or via complement. Also, bacteria can get extracellular haem through haemophores that will compete with haem-containing molecules for the haem group. Once haem is accessible, it is transported across the outer membrane via a TonB-dependent process. Because haem is hydrophobic and tends to aggregate at physiological pH it needs a recognition molecule at the bacteria surface and carrier proteins to be translocated to the cytoplasm. Then, haem can be used as an iron source after the action of haemoxigenases or incorporated to proteins (Lee et al, 1995; Wandersman & Delepelaire, 2004).

The synthesis of haem in *B. abortus* was reported to be altered by mutations in the *hemH* as an indication that *Brucella* is able to synthesize its own haem (Almirón et al, 2001). The protophorphyrin accumulation together with the decreased number of β-galactosidase units obtained from a plasmid-borne *hemB-lacZ* fusion expressed in the *irr* mutant under iron limitation, in contrast to the wild type, suggest that Irr down-regulates the haem biosynthesis. This kind of Irr regulation at the level of *hemB* has been described in *Bradyrhizobium japonicum* and in *Rhizobium leguminosarum* (Hamza et al., 1998; Wexler et al., 2003). Thus, it can be concluded that *B. abortus* has a haem biosynthetic pathway regulated by Irr.

Additionally, *B. abortus* can acquire haem from the environment for metabolic use (Almirón et al, 2001). The BhuA was shown to be involved in the internalization of haem during the stationary phase of *B. abortus* growth, under iron limitation. This outer-membrane protein is an homologue of Ton-B dependent haem transporters already characterized for other Gram-negative bacteria such as *Shigella dysenteriae, Yersinia pestis,* and *Bradyrhizobium japonicum* (Paulley et al., 2007).

The genome of *Brucella* possesses sequences coding for putative haemolysins. However no expression of such DNA has been described yet.

3.1 Extracellular survival

The auxothrophy of the *B. abortus hemH* mutant was restored only by the addition of haemin indicating the presence of some mechanisms in *Brucella* that allow the internalization and utilization of exogenous hemin as described for other bacteria (Almiron et al., 2001). Iron salts or hemoproteins did not revert the auxothorophy.

As predicted, a *B. abortus bhuA* mutant cannot use haem as an iron source. When this mutant and the parental strain were cultured in the low iron medium MG, no differences were observed during the logarithmic and the stationary phases of growth. However, the death phase of the mutant culture started earlier than the wild type. Since the addition of external iron salts prevented the loss of viability, the authors have suggested that BhuA plays a role in stationary-phase iron acquisition in *B. abortus*. It is hard not to relate iron with haem. In that sense, another data interpretation might suggest that iron allowed the cells to resume haem biosynthesis or instead, no more haem was used as an iron source thus, preserving this molecule. Is it haem or iron what *Brucella* needs to survive extracellularly under iron limitation or stationary phase? The growth capability of *B. abortus hemH* was not restored by the addition of iron salts, even under iron-sufficient conditions. This indicates that haem is essential for *B. abortus* to live as a free microorganism.

The transcription of *bhuA* is under the positive regulation of Irr in *B. abortus* (Anderson et al., 2011). Although this regulation was observed during the stationary phase, it should be considered that iron limitation occurs in *Brucella* when the internal iron content reaches a threshold, independently of the external iron concentration. This situation could be achieved by cells after several hours of incubation under iron-limited conditions. That is the stationary phase.

Interestingly, a mutation in the *B. abortus irr* has rendered an increase in haem content due to a derepression of the haem biosynthesis (Martinez et al., 2005; 2006). This phenotype assists *brucella* to survive under the oxidative stress produced by exposition to hydrogen peroxide. On the other hand, another mutation in the *B. abortus irr* prevented iron acquisition through siderophores, as previously reported, and haem internalization via the haem transporter BhuA (Anderson et al, 2011). Consequently, if a *Brucella irr* mutant is grown for several hours under iron limitation, it is expected that this mutant will not survive even if haem is added to the media. The iron depletion imposed does not support its own haem biosynthesis and the mutant is unable to internalize haem. But, if iron is added to the media, the *irr* mutant can resume the haem biosynthesis and survive. This hypothesis has been supported by the experimental data reported by Anderson. These data indicate that, besides the supply of iron that haem carries, haem itself is essential for *in vitro Brucella* growth.

3.2 Intracellular survival

Irr desregulation in *B. abortus* caused by a mutation in *irr* enables the microorganism with a better performance inside eukaryotic cells (Martinez et al., 2006). Thus, while wild type experienced a decrease in the number of intracellular bacteria during the first 24 h p.i. in HeLa or J774 cell lines, the *irr* mutant showed an increment in the bacterial count. Even though the invasion was not affected for the mutation, it is evident that it led *Brucella* to be better equipped than wild type for the survival strategy under iron limitation. Catalase as other haem-containing molecules can be considered as part of that equipment since the *irr* mutant showed higher intracellular haem content, catalase activity and resistance to hydrogen peroxide than the wild type. Paradoxically, the iron-acquisition system through siderophores was deficient in this mutant. This data is in agreement with those that indicate that siderophores are not involved in the intracellular replication of *Brucella*.

The *hemH* mutant was assayed for *in vitro* survival inside HeLa cells and J774 murine macrophages. This mutant was completely attenuated in both cell lines in comparison with the wild type. It was impaired in both invasion capability and intracellular survival. The mechanism that failed in this mutant remains unknown. Considering that haem is present in different kinds of molecules, it is possible to speculate that, with an outer-membrane haemoprotein deficiency, it could be involved in cell invasion. Once inside the cell, it is more likely that a synergistic effect from different haemoproteins leads to the unsuccessful survival.

Furthermore, the *B. abortus bhuA* mutant was attenuated in cultured murine macrophages compared to wild type (Paulley et al., 2007).

3.3 In animals

When Balb/C mice were infected with the *Brucella hemH* mutant it was interesting to note that as early as 2 weeks p.i. neither spleen nor liver colonization were observed in comparison with the wild type or the *hem*H mutant complemented with the wild-type *hemH*. In spite of this, the histological examination of the spleens revealed the same granulomatous reaction in mice infected with all three strains at 2 and 4 weeks p.i. Hyperplasia occurred to a lesser degree in mice inoculated with the *hemH* mutant.

Interestingly, mutations in *B. abortus* genes that affect the haem acquisition system, like *bhuA* or *irr*, were shown to be attenuated in C57BL6 mice at 4 weeks p.i. (Anderson et al., 2011; Paulley et al., 2007). When a different *B. abortus irr* mutant was previously tested in Balb/C mice, at 7 and 21 days after inoculation, neither the increment in catalase activity and haem content, nor the decline in siderophores biosynthesis affected the wild type virulence (Martinez et al., 2006). Although a different mice strain was used, the attenuation in the *brucella* virulence observed after 4 weeks p.i. could be an indication that *Brucella* suffers from iron limitation after one month of infection. Most importantly, it can be a clear indication that cells have access to haem but not to free iron at this stage in the infected animal.

4. Conclusion

It is as much impossible to dissociate free iron from haem as it is difficult to know whether bacteria incorporate haem in response to a real demand for this molecule or it just represents an iron source. Nonetheless, if we analyze the data presented here, there is a line of evidence that suggests the preferred value of haem over non-haem iron in the survival of *B. abortus* during its life cycle as a free organism or as an intracellular pathogen.

First of all, the transcriptional regulation as the protein stability of the major iron responsive regulator in *Brucella abortus* depends on haem. The *irr* gene is transcribed independently of the external iron concentration but it is autoregulated under low iron conditions. The Irr protein is able to bind haem in vitro and this situation probably contributes to the formation of dimers. Intracellularly, Irr is degraded when bacteria do not sense iron limitation. In this condition, bacteria are provided with both non-haem iron and haem.

In general, as it has been proved, the inability to acquire iron through siderophores does not alter the intracellular replication and the capacity to infect mice. On the contrary, the inability to synthesize its own haem or to acquire this molecule from the media affects both the *B. abortus* intracellular replication and the possibility to establish a normal infection in the mouse model.

5. Perspectives

Future research in haem biosynthesis under conditions that result more representative of those faced by *brucellae* during infection might help to increase our knowledge about the survival and pathogenesis of *B. abortus*.

6. Acknowledgment

This work was supported by grants from the Agencia Nacional de Promoción Científica y Tecnológica de la República Argentina PICT 6580 and PICT 651; and by Grant PIP 5463 obtained from the Consejo Nacional de Investigaciones Científicas y Técnicas de la Argentina (CONICET).

7. References

Almiron M, Link AJ, Furlong D, Kolter R (1992) A novel DNA-binding protein with regulatory and protective roles in starved *Escherichia coli*. *Genes Dev*, Vol.6, No.12B, pp. 2646-2654, ISSN 0890-9369

Almiron, M., Martinez, M., Sanjuan, N. & Ugalde, R.A. (2001) Ferrochelatase is present in *Brucella abortus* and is critical for its intracellular survival and virulence. *Infect Immun*, Vol. 69, No.10, pp. 6225-6230, ISSN 0019-9567

Almiron, M.A. & Ugalde, R.A. (2010) Iron homeostasis in *Brucella abortus*: the role of bacterioferritin. *J Microbiol* , Vol.48, No.5, pp. 668-673, ISSN 1976-3794

Anderson ES, Paulley JT, Roop RM, 2nd (2008) The AraC-like transcriptional regulator DhbR is required for maximum expression of the 2,3-dihydroxybenzoic acid biosynthesis genes in *Brucella abortus* 2308 in response to iron deprivation. *J Bacteriol* , Vol.190, No.5, pp.1838-1842, ISSN 1098-5530

Anderson, E.S., Paulley, J.T., Martinson, D.A., Gaines, J.M., Steele, K.H., et al. (2011) The iron responsive regulator Irr is required for wild-type expression of the gene encoding the heme transporter BhuA in *Brucella abortus* 2308. *J Bacteriol.*, Vol.193, No19, pp.5359-5364, ISSN 1098-5530

Anderson JD, Smith H (1965) The Metabolism of Erythritol by *Brucella Abortus*. *J Gen Microbiol*, Vol. 38, pp.109-124, ISSN 0022-1287

Andrews SC, Robinson AK, Rodriguez-Quinones F (2003) Bacterial iron homeostasis. *FEMS Microbiol Rev*, Vol. 27, No.2-3, pp. 215-237, ISSN 0168-6445

Bellaire BH, Elzer PH, Baldwin CL, Roop RM, 2nd (1999) The siderophore 2,3-dihydroxybenzoic acid is not required for virulence of *Brucella abortus* in BALB/c mice. *Infect Immun*, Vol.67, No.5, pp. 2615-2618, ISSN 0019-9567

Bellaire BH, Elzer PH, Baldwin CL, Roop RM, 2nd (2003) Production of the siderophore 2,3-dihydroxybenzoic acid is required for wild-type growth of *Brucella abortus* in the presence of erythritol under low-iron conditions in vitro. *Infect Immun*, Vol.71, No.5, pp. 2927-2832, ISSN 0019-9567

Bellaire BH, Elzer PH, Hagius S, Walker J, Baldwin CL, et al. (2003) Genetic organization and iron-responsive regulation of the *Brucella abortus* 2,3-dihydroxybenzoic acid biosynthesis operon, a cluster of genes required for wild-type virulence in pregnant cattle. *Infect Immun*, Vol.71, No. 4, pp. 1794-1803, ISSN 0019-9567

Burkhardt S, Jimenez de Bagues MP, Liautard JP, Kohler S (2005) Analysis of the behavior of *eryC* mutants of *Brucella suis* attenuated in macrophages. *Infect Immun*, Vol.73, No.10, pp. 6782-6790, ISSN 0019-9567

Danese I, Haine V, Delrue RM, Tibor A, Lestrate P, et al. (2004) The Ton system, an ABC transporter, and a universally conserved GTPase are involved in iron utilization by *Brucella melitensis* 16M. *Infect Immun*, Vol. 72, No.10, pp. 5783-5790, ISSN 0019-9567

Gamazo C, Moriyon I (1987) Release of outer membrane fragments by exponentially growing Brucella melitensis cells. *Infect Immun*, Vo.55, No.3, pp. 609-615, ISSN 0019-9567

Gamazo C, Winter AJ, Moriyon I, Riezu-Boj JI, Blasco JM, et al. (1989) Comparative analyses of proteins extracted by hot saline or released spontaneously into outer membrane blebs from field strains of *Brucella ovis* and *Brucella melitensis*. *Infect Immun*, Vol.57, No.5, pp. 1419-1426, ISSN 0019-9567

Garcia-Lobo JM, Sangari Garcia FJ (2004) Erythritol Metabolism and Virulence in *Brucella*. In: Lopez-Goni I, Moriyon I, editors. *Brucella*: Molecular and Cellular Biology. Norfolk: horizon bioscience. pp. 231-242.

Gerhardt P (1958) The nutrition of *brucellae*. *Bacteriol Rev*, Vol. 22, No.2, pp:81-98, ISSN 0005-3678

Genco CA, Dixon DW (2001) Emerging strategies in microbial haem capture. *Mol Microbiol* Vol.39, No.1, pp. 1-11, ISSN 0950-382X

Gonzalez Carrero MI, Sangari FJ, Aguero J, Garcia Lobo JM (2002) *Brucella abortus* strain 2308 produces brucebactin, a highly efficient catecholic siderophore. *Microbiology*, Vol.148, No.Pt2, pp. 353-360, ISSN 1350-0872

Hamza I, Chauhan S, Hassett R, O'Brian MR (1998) The bacterial irr protein is required for coordination of heme biosynthesis with iron availability. *J Biol Chem*, Vol.273. No.34, pp.21669-21674, ISSN 0021-9258

Her M, Cho DH, Kang SI, Cho YS, Hwang IY, et al. (2010) The development of a selective medium for the *Brucella abortus* strains and its comparison with the currently recommended and used medium. Diagn Microbiol *Infect Dis*, Vol. 67, No.1, pp. 15-21, ISSN 1879-0070

Hoffmann T, Schutz A, Brosius M, Volker A, Volker U, et al. (2002) High-salinity-induced iron limitation in *Bacillus subtilis*. *J Bacteriol*, Vol. 184, No.3, pp. 718-727, ISSN 0021-9193

Jain N, Rodriguez AC, Kimsawatde G, Seleem MN, Boyle SM, et al. (2011) Effect of entF deletion on iron acquisition and erythritol metabolism by *Brucella abortus* 2308. *FEMS Microbiol Lett* , Vol.316, No.1, pp. 1-6, ISSN 1574-6968

Johnston AW, Todd JD, Curson AR, Lei S, Nikolaidou-Katsaridou N, et al. (2007) Living without Fur: the subtlety and complexity of iron-responsive gene regulation in the symbiotic bacterium *Rhizobium* and other alpha-proteobacteria. *Biometals*, Vol. 20, No.3-4, pp. 501-511, ISSN 0966-0844

Lamontagne J, Forest A, Marazzo E, Denis F, Butler H, et al. (2009) Intracellular adaptation of *Brucella abortus*. *J Proteome Res*, Vol. 8, No.3,pp.1594-1609, ISSN 1535-3893

Lee BC (1995) Quelling the red menace: haem capture by bacteria. *Mol Microbiol*, Vol.18, No.3, pp. 383-390, ISSN 0950-382X

Lopez-Goni I, Moriyon I, Neilands JB (1992) Identification of 2,3-dihydroxybenzoic acid as a *Brucella abortus* siderophore. *Infect Immun* , Vol.60, No.11, pp. 4496-4503, ISSN 0019-9567

Martinez M, Ugalde RA, Almiron M (2005) Dimeric *Brucella abortus* Irr protein controls its own expression and binds haem. *Microbiology* Vol.151, No.Pt10, pp.3427-3433, ISSN 1350-0872

Martinez M, Ugalde RA, Almiron M (2006) Irr regulates brucebactin and 2,3-dihydroxybenzoic acid biosynthesis, and is implicated in the oxidative stress resistance and intracellular survival of *Brucella abort*us. *Microbiology*, Vol.152, No.Pt9, pp. 2591-2598, ISSN 1350-0872

O'Brian MR, Thony-Meyer L (2002) Biochemistry, regulation and genomics of haem biosynthesis in prokaryotes. *Adv Microb Physiol* , Vol.46, pp. 257-318, ISSN 0065-2911

Parent MA, Bellaire BH, Murphy EA, Roop RM, 2nd, Elzer PH, et al. (2002) *Brucella abortus* siderophore 2,3-dihydroxybenzoic acid (DHBA) facilitates intracellular survival of the bacteria. *Microb Pathog*, Vol.32, No.5, pp. 239-248, ISSN 0882-4010

Paulley JT, Anderson ES, Roop RM, 2nd (2007) *Brucella abortus* requires the heme transporter BhuA for maintenance of chronic infection in BALB/c mice. *Infect Immun*, Vol. 75, No.11, pp. 5248-5254, ISSN 0019-9567

Rodionov DA, Gelfand MS, Todd JD, Curson AR, Johnston AW (2006) Computational reconstruction of iron- and manganese-responsive transcriptional networks in alpha-proteobacteria. *PLoS Comput Biol* 2: e163.

Roop RM, Bellaire BH, Anderson E, Paulley JT (2004) Iron Metabolism in *Brucella*. In: Lopez-Goni I, Moriyon I, editors. *Brucella*: Molecular and Cellular Biology. Norfolk: Horizon Bioscience.

Schaible UE, Kaufmann SH (2004) Iron and microbial infection. *Nat Rev Microbiol*, Vol.2, No.12, pp. 946-953, ISSN 1740-1526

Smith H, Williams AE, Pearce JH, Keppie J, Harris-Smith PW, et al. (1962) Foetal erythritol: a cause of the localization of *Brucella abortus* in bovine contagious abortion. *Nature*, Vol. 193, pp.47-49, ISSN 0028-0836

Wandersman C, Delepelaire P (2004) Bacterial iron sources: from siderophores to hemophores. *Annu Rev Microbiol* , Vol.58, pp.611-647, ISSN 0066-4227

Wexler M, Todd JD, Kolade O, Bellini D, Hemmings AM, et al. (2003) Fur is not the global regulator of iron uptake genes in *Rhizobium leguminosarum*. *Microbiology*, Vol. 149, No. Pt5, pp. 1357-1365, ISSN 1350-0872

Permissions

The contributors of this book come from diverse backgrounds, making this book a truly international effort. This book will bring forth new frontiers with its revolutionizing research information and detailed analysis of the nascent developments around the world.

We would like to thank Dr. Priti Kumar Roy, for lending her expertise to make the book truly unique. She has played a crucial role in the development of this book. Without her invaluable contribution this book wouldn't have been possible. She has made vital efforts to compile up to date information on the varied aspects of this subject to make this book a valuable addition to the collection of many professionals and students.

This book was conceptualized with the vision of imparting up-to-date information and advanced data in this field. To ensure the same, a matchless editorial board was set up. Every individual on the board went through rigorous rounds of assessment to prove their worth. After which they invested a large part of their time researching and compiling the most relevant data for our readers. Conferences and sessions were held from time to time between the editorial board and the contributing authors to present the data in the most comprehensible form. The editorial team has worked tirelessly to provide valuable and valid information to help people across the globe.

Every chapter published in this book has been scrutinized by our experts. Their significance has been extensively debated. The topics covered herein carry significant findings which will fuel the growth of the discipline. They may even be implemented as practical applications or may be referred to as a beginning point for another development. Chapters in this book were first published by InTech; hereby published with permission under the Creative Commons Attribution License or equivalent.

The editorial board has been involved in producing this book since its inception. They have spent rigorous hours researching and exploring the diverse topics which have resulted in the successful publishing of this book. They have passed on their knowledge of decades through this book. To expedite this challenging task, the publisher supported the team at every step. A small team of assistant editors was also appointed to further simplify the editing procedure and attain best results for the readers.

Our editorial team has been hand-picked from every corner of the world. Their multi-ethnicity adds dynamic inputs to the discussions which result in innovative outcomes. These outcomes are then further discussed with the researchers and contributors who give their valuable feedback and opinion regarding the same. The feedback is then collaborated with the researches and they are edited in a comprehensive manner to aid the understanding of the subject.

Apart from the editorial board, the designing team has also invested a significant amount of their time in understanding the subject and creating the most relevant covers. They scrutinized every image to scout for the most suitable representation of the subject and create an appropriate cover for the book.

The publishing team has been involved in this book since its early stages. They were actively engaged in every process, be it collecting the data, connecting with the contributors or procuring relevant information. The team has been an ardent support to the editorial, designing and production team. Their endless efforts to recruit the best for this project, has resulted in the accomplishment of this book. They are a veteran in the field of academics and their pool of knowledge is as vast as their experience in printing. Their expertise and guidance has proved useful at every step. Their uncompromising quality standards have made this book an exceptional effort. Their encouragement from time to time has been an inspiration for everyone.

The publisher and the editorial board hope that this book will prove to be a valuable piece of knowledge for researchers, students, practitioners and scholars across the globe.

List of Contributors

Yoshiko Atsukawa, Sayoko Kawakami and Yukihisa Miyazawa
Department of Central Clinical Laboratory, Teikyo University Hospital, Tokyo, Japan

Ryuichi Fujisaki and Hajime Nishiya
Department of Internal Medicine, Teikyo University School of Medicine, Tokyo, Japan

Yasuo Ono
Department of Microbiology, Teikyo University School of Medicine, Tokyo, Japan

Ümit Kartoğlu
World Health Organization, Switzerland

Argiris Symeonidis
Hematology Division, University of Patras Medical School, Patras, Greece

Markos Marangos
Division of Infectious Diseases, Dept of Internal Medicine, University of Patras Medical School, Patras, Greece

Agnieszka Gniadek
Department of Medical and Environmental Nursing, Faculty of Health Sciences, Jagiellonian University Medical College, Kraków, Poland

Tetsuya Tanaka and Kozo Fujisaki
Laboratory of Emerging Infectious Diseases, Department of Frontier Veterinary Science, Faculty of Agriculture, Kagoshima University, Korimoto, Kagoshima, Japan

Xuenan Xuan
National Research Center for Protozoan Diseases, Obihiro University of Agriculture and Veterinary Medicine, Obihiro, Hokkaido, Japan

Kei-ichi Shimazaki
Laboratory of Dairy Food Science, Research Faculty Agriculture, Hokkaido University, Sapporo, Hokkaido, Japan

Ryan C. Ratts
Dartmouth Medical School, USA

John R. Murphy
Boston University School of Medicine, USA

Ardi Liaunardy Jopeace, Chris B. Howard, Ben L. Murton and Tom P. Monie
Department of Biochemistry, University of Cambridge

Alexander D. Edwards
School of Pharmacy, University of Reading, United Kingdom

Shanow Uthman and Flaviano Giorgini
Department of Genetics, University of Leicester, Leicester, UK

Shihui Liu
Laboratory of Bacterial Diseases, NIAID, NIH, Bethesda, MD, USA

Michael J. R. Stark
Wellcome Trust Centre for Gene Regulation & Expression, University of Dundee, Scotland

Michael Costanzo
The Donnelly Centre, University of Toronto, Toronto, Ontario, Canada

Raffael Schaffrath
Department of Genetics, University of Leicester, Leicester, UK
Institut für Biologie, Mikrobiologie, Universität Kassel, Kassel, Germany

Ramesh Chandra Rai, Debapriya Bhattacharya and Gobardhan Das
Immunology Group, International Centre for Genetic Engineering and Biotechnology, New Delhi, India

Marta A. Almirón
Universidad Nacional de San Martín/Instituto de Investigaciones Biotecnológicas, Argentina

Nidia E. Lucero
Instituto Nacional de Enfermedades Infecciosas-ANLIS "Dr. C. G. Malbrán", Departamento de Bacteriología, Argentina

Norberto A. Sanjuan
Universidad de Buenos Aires/ Facultad de Medicina/ Departamento de Microbiología, Argentina

Printed in the USA
CPSIA information can be obtained
at www.ICGtesting.com
JSHW011414221024
72173JS00004B/545

9 781632 422071